Tuberculosis Host-Pathogen Interactions

Jeffrey D. Cirillo • Ying Kong
Editors

Tuberculosis Host-Pathogen Interactions

Springer

Editors
Jeffrey D. Cirillo
Department of Microbial Pathogenesis
and Immunology
Texas A&M University College of Medicine
Bryan, TX, USA

Ying Kong
The University of Tennessee Health Science
Center
Memphis, TN, USA

ISBN 978-3-030-25380-6 ISBN 978-3-030-25381-3 (eBook)
https://doi.org/10.1007/978-3-030-25381-3

This Springer imprint is published by the registered company Springer Nature Switzerland AG
The registered company address is: Gewerbestrasse 11, 6330 Cham, Switzerland

Preface

Tuberculosis was one of the earliest organisms associated with disease in humans, along with leprosy or Hansen's disease, and anthrax. Koch demonstrated that a specific disease, tuberculosis, could be caused by *Mycobacterium tuberculosis* using guinea pigs in the 1880s. The resulting host-bacteria system was used to develop Koch's postulates, one of the foundations of infectious diseases research, illustrating the importance of understanding both sides of the disease process for infections, the host and pathogen. Prior to the late 1980s, the study of the pathogen that causes tuberculosis was very limited due to the inability to genetically manipulate the organism, but a little over 100 years after Koch's discovery, molecular genetics became possible in *M. tuberculosis*, opening a vast array of new studies on these bacteria along with endless possibilities to create novel interventions. Many of the chapters in this book come out of having new abilities to manipulate tuberculosis host-pathogen interactions beyond those previously possible.

Our aim is to present some of these more recent findings and novel technologies that have come out of research in host-pathogen interactions. In this book, we aim to provide insight into many aspects of tuberculosis host-pathogen interactions, though we would not even attempt to be comprehensive, since the breadth of knowledge and the pace of advancement in the field are great. Attempting to be comprehensive in the tuberculosis field is no longer possible, mostly because that would require many volumes of reviews, rather than a single volume. We requested authors to provide their thoughts on topics within host-pathogen interactions from their own perspective and believe that the resulting chapters give insight into the breadth of the field currently. We cover many individual components of the bacteria that are involved in host-pathogen interactions as well as aspects of the host and comorbidities in disease. In some cases, it is obvious there remains a great deal more to do and examination of much biology in mycobacteria remains to be explored. Latent infections, in particular, represent a problematic issue that is difficult to model and gain insight into the actual situation in humans. This problem is partially due to the difficulty of tracking and study of very few bacteria directly in humans. New technologies on the horizon in imaging may help to contribute to our understanding of the bacteria without having to isolate them, and the state of the art in this area is presented.

The combination of the ability to track very few bacteria during infections as well as monitor the host response during all aspects of disease could ultimately provide a more comprehensive picture of tuberculosis host-pathogen interactions. The understanding of mesenchymal, myeloid, and T cells during all stages of disease, including latency, combined with understanding epigenetic changes could provide much of the necessary information regarding how different hosts respond to tuberculosis that is sorely needed. We present information on these cells and would suggest that the ability to evaluate these populations of cells and their ability to respond in patients may be key to the development of intervention strategies that may be used to improve vaccine and therapeutic technologies.

Overall, the information provided in these chapters is only a taste of the tuberculosis field, and we would suggest interested readers look to a number of additional resources that are available such as the extensively informative source of B. R. Bloom (*Tuberculosis: Pathogenesis, Protection, and Control*, 653 p., ASM Press, 1994), the important general molecular overview of Hatfull and Jacobs (*Molecular Genetics of Mycobacteria*, 363 p., ASM Press, 2000), the genetics methods compendium of Jacobs et al. (Genetic Systems of Mycobacteria in *Methods in Enzymology Vol. 204 Bacterial Genetic Systems*, J.H. Miller (Ed.), 537–555 p., Academic Press, 1991), the valuable overview by Grosset and Chaisson (*Handbook of Tuberculosis*, 221 p., Springer, 2017), and the key overview by Shinnick (*Tuberculosis*, 307 p., Springer, 1996), just to name a few of the available resources. We provide a supplement and update to these prior publications with a focus on how each area impacts interactions of *M. tuberculosis* with its human host.

Areas that are covered include surface molecules, lipids, and cell wall, with how they play a role in direct modulation of the host and how tuberculosis can affect the host and the role of these modulatory effects on HIV. Specific cell types play an important role in tuberculosis, such as stem cells, myeloid cells, and T cells, all of which have been examined in overviews that are included. Latent infections can persist for the life of a host, reactivating at any time, and aspects of the bacterial interactions are covered in multiple chapters to emphasize their importance and the complexity of the issues involved. We are also on the cusp of new key discoveries through exploration of new research directions, including the use of imaging technologies and examination of the role of epigenetic relationships in disease processes that are explored in two other chapters. Thus, although not at all comprehensive, this overview summarizes several key areas of tuberculosis host-pathogen interactions with the goal of stimulating additional enthusiasm in readers that will translate into further advances that will contribute in the fight against this devastating disease.

We thank all of the authors for their patience and tireless effort as we completed this project. Everyone included did their part quickly and without complaint, despite all of our busy schedules, making the project very enjoyable and easier than expected. We look forward to working with everyone well into the future in our own efforts to make more rapid progress in the tuberculosis field.

Bryan, TX, USA Jeffrey D. Cirillo

Contents

Cell Wall Biosynthesis and Latency During Tuberculosis Infections

Michio Kurosu

Abstract *Mycobacterium tuberculosis* (Mtb) uses a wide range of mechanisms to survive the host immune system. Mtb can persist in host tissues for months to decades without replicating, however, non-replicating (or dormant) Mtb has the ability to resume growth at any time. Persons with latent TB infection do not have typical TB symptoms, and dormant forms of Mtb are not considered transmissible. Several factors (e.g. HIV infection, cancers, and immunosuppressive drug therapy) alter the course of latent TB and are thought to have the potential to cause reactivation, leading to active TB. Treatment regimens for latent TB infection require long durations in order to prevent relapse. It is difficult to eradicate latent forms of the relatively drug resistant Mtb in short periods of time with the currently available TB therapies. Thus, it is very important to develop new drugs for the treatment of latent or persistent forms of Mtb that reduce treatment time required for TB patients. Mycobacterial cell walls consist of complex mixtures of polysaccharides and mycolic acids, and they play an important role in escaping from the host immune systems and in surviving within granulomas that form in response to the bacteria. This chapter reviews the potential drug targets that exist in cell wall biosynthesis for non-replicating (or dormant) Mtb based on bioinformatics, genomic and proteomic analyses and *in vitro* data with replicating and non-replicating bacilli.

Keywords Cell wall biosynthesis · Non-replicating *Mycobacterium tuberculosis* · Dormant bacilli · Latent tuberculosis infections · Granuloma · Anti-TB drugs · Mycolic acid biosynthesis inhibitors · Bacterial phosphotransferase inhibitors · Arabinogalactan biosynthesis inhibitors · Peptidoglycan biosynthesis inhibitors

M. Kurosu (✉)
Department of Pharmaceutical Sciences, College of Pharmacy, University of Tennessee Health Science Center, Memphis, TN, USA
e-mail: mkurosu@uthsc.edu

J. D. Cirillo, Y. Kong (eds.), *Tuberculosis Host-Pathogen Interactions*,
https://doi.org/10.1007/978-3-030-25381-3_1

Introduction

The non-replicating (or dormant state) of *Mycobacterium tuberculosis* (Mtb) is characterized by non-dividing or slowly replicating bacilli with a low metabolic state as well as resistance to standard anti-tuberculosis (anti-TB) agents [1]. The majority of Mtb infections are thought to occur in alveolar macrophages [2, 3]. Chemotactic cytokines produced by alveolar macrophages stimulate inflammatory cells (e.g. neutrophils, monocyte derived macrophages, NK cells, and T-cells) that further promote inflammation and tissue remodelling, establishing granulomas [4]. Granulomas are a cluster of immune cells including infected and uninfected macrophages, differentiated macrophages, epithelioid cells, and giant cells. Granuloma formation is a well-known pathological characteristic of TB [5]. In most healthy individuals, Mtb infection causes few problems in health and display no symptoms due to control of infection by the innate immune response. Mtb infected alveolar macrophages frequently escape from the early immune response [6]. In a small number of cases (~10% of infected people), the infection spreads via macrophages and dendritic cells to the draining lymph nodes and other organs, leading to clinically significant disease [7].

Mtb is a facultative intracellular bacterium. Entry of Mtb into alveolar macrophages is facilitated by several mechanisms, including specific receptor-mediated and signal transduction pathways. During the last decade, mycobacterial genetic analyses of *ex-vivo* and *in vivo* gene expression has allowed elucidation of a number of components that contribute to survival and replication within macrophages [8–12]. Because it is commonly believed that the dormant form of Mtb is non-replicating bacteria within granulomas, cell wall biosynthesis is often not considered a favourable drug target to treat dormant TB. However, recent studies have demonstrated that several cell wall biosynthesis enzymes are essential to maintain viability of dormant Mtb in granulomas and macrophages [13–16]. We summarize in this chapter many of the unique metabolic pathways associated with cell wall biosynthesis and the potential drug targets that are effective against non-replicating (or dormant) Mtb.

Mycobacterial Cell Wall

The complexity of mycobacterial cell wall is relatively unusual as compared to other Gram-positive and -negative bacteria (Fig. 1). The core structure of the mycobacterial cell wall is commonly termed mycoly-arabinogalactan-peptidoglycan complex. The biosynthesis of peptidoglycan (PG) of *E. coli* has been discussed extensively in reviews by van Heijenoort [17]. Most of the genes involved in peptidoglycan biosynthesis in *E. coli* are known, and orthologues have been identified in Gram-positive genomes. However, some of the genes responsible for the unique features found in mycobacterial peptidoglycan remain unknown. Detailed analyses

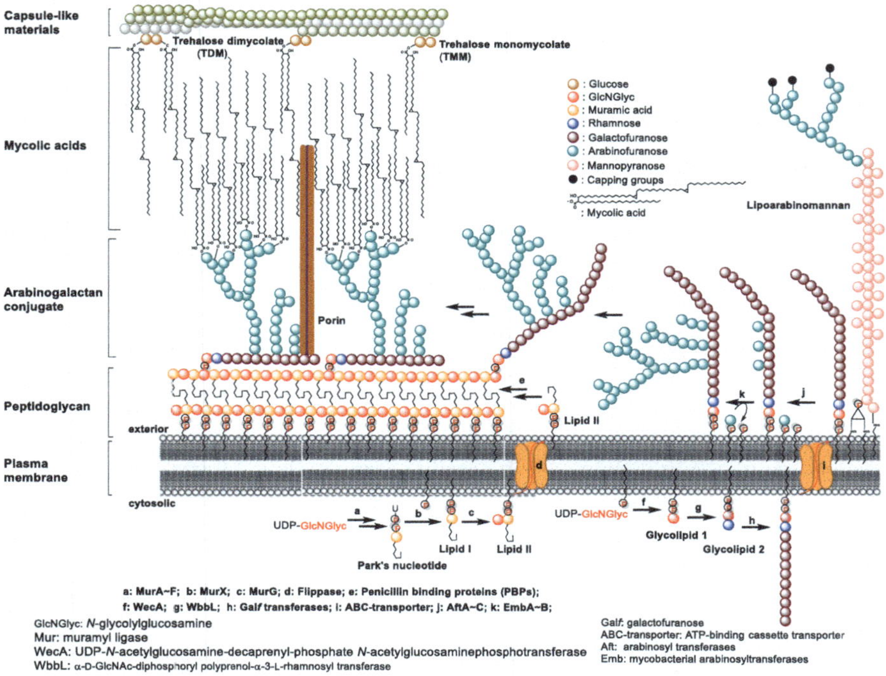

Fig. 1 *Mycobacterium tuberculosis* cell wall and cell wall biosynthesis pathways

of the components of mycobacterial PG revealed that it contains a variety of modified molecules including *N*-glycolyl (NGlyc) in addition to *N*-acetyl (NAc) groups on muramic acid (Mur), amidation of the carboxylic acids, and additional glycine or serine residues [18, 19]. Although the precise functions of these modified molecules have not yet been elucidated, it is speculated that the additional coordinated groups participate in electrostatic interactions contributing to reinforcement of the PG layer [20].

Lipid II, a precursor of PG, is synthesized in the cytosol initially and then in the inner portion of the plasma membrane from UDP-GlcNGlyc (and UDP-GlcNAc) by Mur enzymes (MurA~F, MurX, and MurG). Lipid II is required to flip-flop so that it can localize to the outer plasma membrane where penicillin-binding proteins (*e.g.* PBPa and PBPb) polymerize lipid II to form PG. Approximately 10–12% of the C6-hydroxy groups of muramic acid form phosphodiester bonds with the L-α-rhamnopyranosyl-(1→3)-D-α-GlcNGlyc-(1→P) unit (Fig. 2), which serves as linker to conjugate arabinogalactan (AG) [16].

AG biosynthesis commences with WecA (polyprenyl phosphate-GlcNGlyc-1-phosphate transferase)-catalysed synthesis of glycolipid-1 (D-GlcNGlyc-P-P-C_{50} and D-GlcNAc-P-P-C_{50}) with UDP-GlcNGlyc (and UDP-GlcNAc) and decaprenylphosphate (C_{50}-P) (Fig. 3). Glycolipid-1 is anchored into the intracellular plasma membrane where WbbL (a rhamnosyltransferase) transfers L-Rha*p* to the

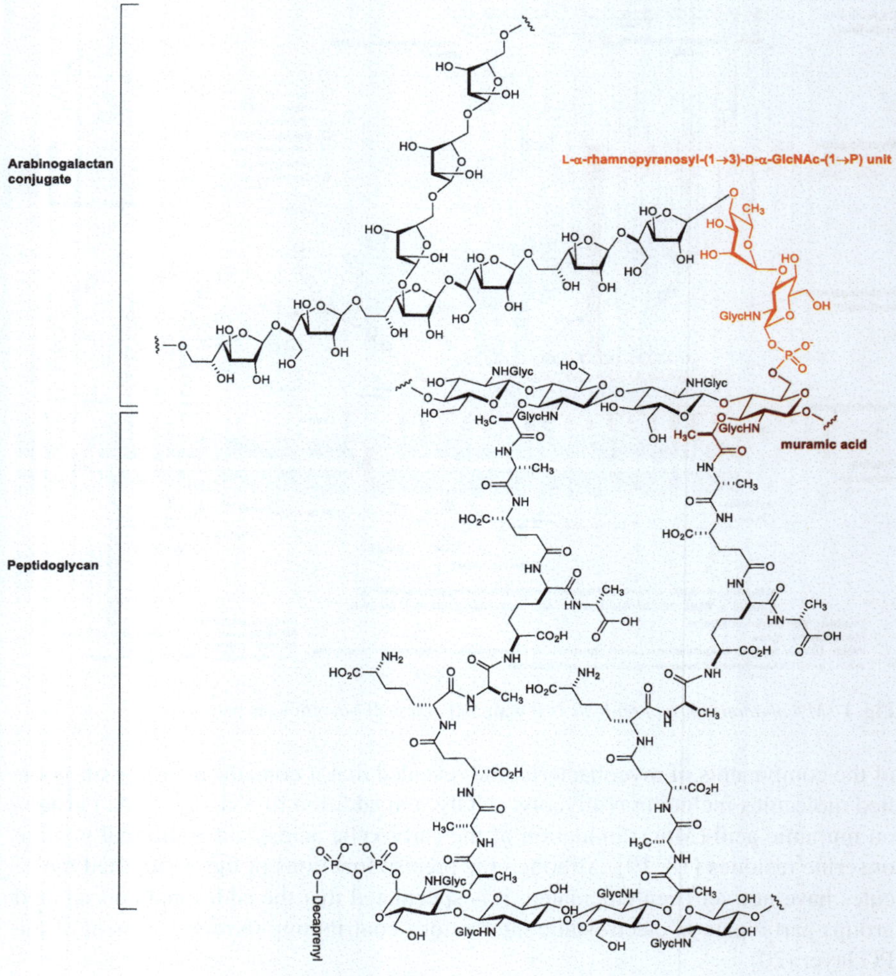

Fig. 2 Stereochemistries of the carbohydrate and peptide portions of mycobacterial cell wall, L-α-rhamnopyranosyl-(1→3)-D-α-GlcNAc-(1→P) unit is highlighted

GlcNGlyc with dTDP-rhamnose, furnishing glycolipid-2 (L-Rha*p*-(α1→3)-D-GlcNGlyc-P-P-C_{50}).

Two galactofuranosyltransferases (Gal*f*Ts) are responsible for completion of galactan biosynthesis. The first and second transfers of Gal*f* residues are catalysed by GalT1 (a GT-A superfamily) using UDP-Gal*f*, forming glycolipid-4 (D-Gal*f*-(α1→4)-D-Gal*f*-(α1→4)-L-Rha-(α1→3)-D-GlcNGlyc-P-P-C_{50}). Glycosylations of ~30 Gal*f* residues with alternating β(1→5) and β(1→6) linkages are catalysed by GalT2, which possesses dual enzymatic functions of UDP-Gal*f*: β-D-(1→5) GalT and UDP-Gal*f*: β-D-(1→6) GalT activities. These decaprenyl-diphosphate linked-polysaccharides, D-Gal*f*-(α1→5)-[D-Gal*f*-(α1→6)-D-Gal*f*-(α1→5)]$_n$-D-

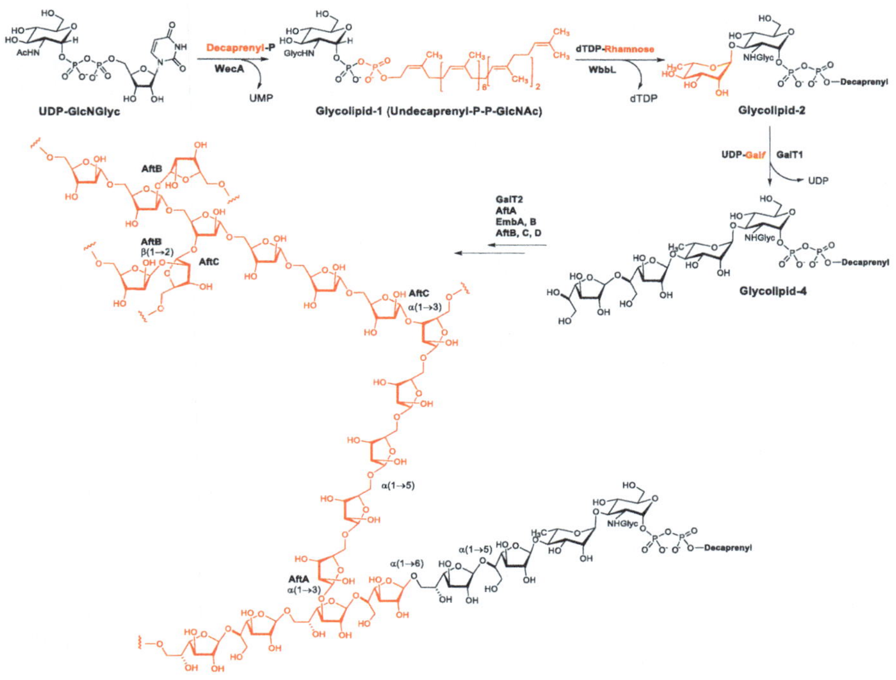

Fig. 3 Biosyntehsis of arabinogalactan

Gal*f*-(α1→4)-D-Gal*f*-(α1→4)-L-Rha-(α1→3)-D-GlcNAc-P-P-C_{50} are transported across the cytoplasmic membrane by the ABC (ATP-binding cassette)-transporter [21]. The translocated galactans are further modified with the arabinofuranoses by arabinosyltransferases with decaprenylphosphoryl-D-arabinofuranose, forming the AG conjugate. Several mycobacterial arabinosyltransferases such as EmbA, EmbB, AftA, AftB, AftC, and AftD have been characterized and implicated to be involved in arabinosylations of the galactan moiety. A number of distinct types of 22 arabinofuranose (Ara*f*) residues with alternating α(1→5), α(1→3), and β(1→2) linkages have been characterized in AG in *Mycobacterium spp.* [22].

Mycolic acids (MAs) are a hallmark of the cell wall of *Mycobacterium spp.* [23] They exist as esters of trehalose and/or glycerol and of the terminal penta-arabinofuranosyl moiety of AG. The former MA-esters are not linked with the cell wall components via covalent bond, but comprise the cell wall via electrostatic interaction. MAs play a critical role in localization of Mtb in the lung tissue and formation of granulomas. A large number of long-chained fatty acids have been characterized from different bacteria. The total carbon chain of C_{66}–C_{90} of MAs have been determined in fatty acid analyses of Mtb. MAs display a large diversity of chemical structures (Fig. 4). The general structures of MAs are referred to as α-branched β-hydroxy long-chain fatty acids. The α-branched moiety is composed of the C_{22}–C_{26} fatty acids. The main carbon chain where the long-alkyl group is

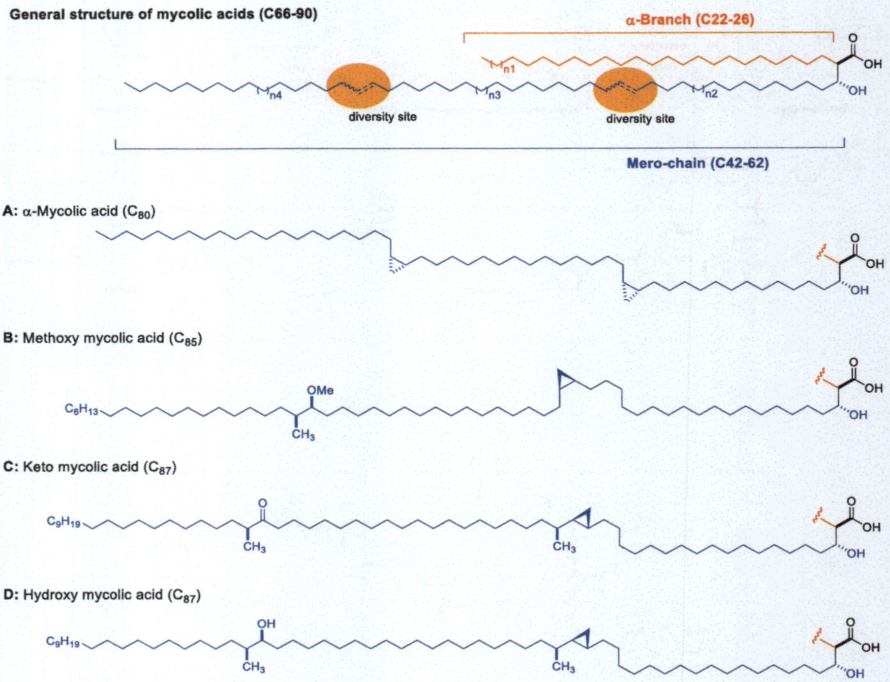

Fig. 4 Structure of mycolic acids

attached at the C3 (or β)-position is designated mero-mycolic chain composed of ω-42 to -62 fatty acids. The degree of unsaturation (*cis* or *trans* geometry or cyclopropyl) of the mero-mycolic chain is generally one or two. In some Mtb strains, a longer mero-mycolic chain and higher degree of unsaturation have been identified. Additional functional modifications observed are the carbonyl (ketone), hydroxy, methoxy, epoxy, methyl, and ester groups in the mero-mycolic chain [24]. The biosynthesis of MAs is achieved by fatty acid synthases FAS-I, FAS-II, Fab, and several modification enzymes. Unlike the enzymes in FAS-I, the enzymes of FAS-II and FabH and are not found in humans. Fatty acid biosynthesis has been reviewed in a number of scientific articles and books (Fig. 5) [23, 25]. In Mtb, β-ketoacyl-(acyl-carrier-protein) synthase III (designated MtFabH) compensates the gap in the mycobacterial fatty acid biosynthesis via FAS-I and FAS-II pathways. FAS-I produces C_{16}–C_{18} and C_{24}–C_{26} acyl CoAs. FAS-II elongates C_{12}–C_{16} fatty acids to furnish C_{18}–C_{30} acyl carrier proteins (ACPs) for the synthesis of meromycolic acid. MtFabH carries out the initial coupling (Claisen-type) reaction of fatty acid biosynthesis with malonyl-ACP and acetyl-CoA, producing short-chain fatty acid primers [24]. The generated β-ketoacyl-ACPs are reduced by NADPH-dependent β-ketoacyl-ACP reductase (MabA). The resulting β-hydroxy ACPs are dehydrated by dehydrases (HadAB, HadBC, or HadABC complexes) and saturations of the double bond(s) are accomplished by NADH-dependent trans-2-enoyl-ACP reductase

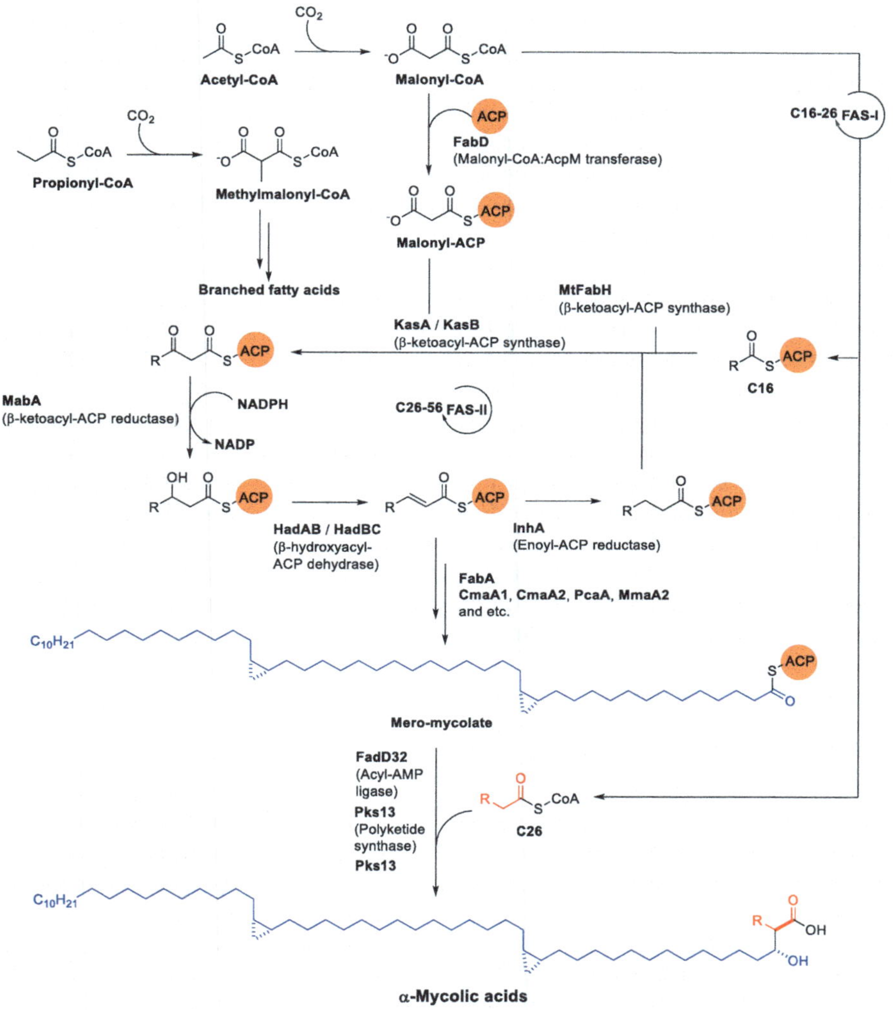

Fig. 5 Mycolic acid biosynthesis

(InhA), leading to saturated acyl-ACPs [26]. The other carbon-chain elongations are performed by β-ketoacyl-ACP synthases (KasA and KasB). KasA elongates C16-CoA to monounsaturated fatty acids with the average length of ~C40. In the presence of KasA, KasB produces a longer chain with multiunsaturated hydrocarbons with the average length of ~C54. These β-ketoacyl-ACP synthases are essential for the synthesis of mero-mycolic acids. Biochemical analyses of the Mtb ΔkasB mutant strain revealed that it synthesizes mycolic acids with shorter carbon-chain lengths. In addition, the loss of acid-fastness and ketomycolic acids and a reduction of trans-cyclopropanated mycolic acids and methoxymycolic acids were observed.

The exact mechanisms of unsaturation and formation of trans/cis-isomerizations are still in the hypothesis stage. Isomerization of the *trans*-double bond to the corresponding *cis*-geometric isomer is catalysed by dehydrase/isomerase (FabA of FAS-II) in *E. coli*. The enzymes that have the functions of dehydrase or isomerization activity have been found in other bacteria. Similarly, Mtb may express isomerases that have *trans/cis*-isomerization activity in the FAS-II cycle. Cyclopropanations are catalysed by *S*-adenosyl-methionine (SAM)-mediated methyltransferases. Four methyltransferases (CmaA1, CmaA2, PcaA, and MmaA2) are identified in Mtb that are responsible for cyclopropanations of mero-mycolic acids [24, 27].

Lipoarabinomannans are important glycoconjugates that are integrated into the mycobacterial cell wall. The glycolipid lipoarabinomannan (LAM) consists of three primary structural domains including a glycosylphosphatidyl moiety, which anchors LAM to the cell wall, D-mannan core, and D-arabinan (Fig. 1). The terminal D-arabinan creates a large number of LAM structures. The cell wall components (PG, AG, and MA) discussed above provide the chemical space for insertion of materials such as LAM, lipomannan, phthiocerol-containing lipids, trehalose mycolates, phosphatidylinositol mannosides, and their related molecules [28]. LAM plays an important role in mediating host-bacterial interactions and is involved in modulation of the immune response. These mechanisms include inhibition of macrophage microbicidal activity via a diminished IFN-γ response and neutralization of reactive oxygen free radicals produced by macrophages [29].

Granuloma Formation

The enzymes involved in mycolic acid-arabinogalactan conjugates are essential for survival of Mtb in the host macrophages. Many *in vitro* studies have supported entry of Mtb into alveolar macrophages; an array of different surface receptor molecules and cholesterol of macrophages are involved in phagocytotic entry of Mtb. The infected macrophages trigger innate immune signalling pathways, leading to the production of various chemokines and cytokines. These signalling proteins recruit other macrophages, dendritic cells, and lymphocytes to the infection sites (Fig. 6) [30]. They organise the granuloma, which is defined as a focal accumulation of activated macrophages and epithelioid cells, often with giant cells, and lymphocytes. The granulomas of TB tend to become necrotic, causing chronic inflammatory reactions. In the early stages of granuloma formation, TNF-α produced by macrophages infected with Mtb and type I T-helper (TH1 T) cells play a critical role in maintaining the granuloma structure. Mycobacterial granulomas are believed to be a host defence mechanism used to wall-off Mtb infected cells. However, Mtb can survive within macrophages and enter into a dormant from, thus, the granuloma also serves as a protective structure to prevent killing by the host immune system. When the host immune system is weakened, dormant Mtb in latent tuberculosis infection undergoes a change to growing, leading to the reactivation state. Understanding the pathology of TB lung granulomas is critical for discovery of new TB drugs effective against dormant Mtb [5, 31].

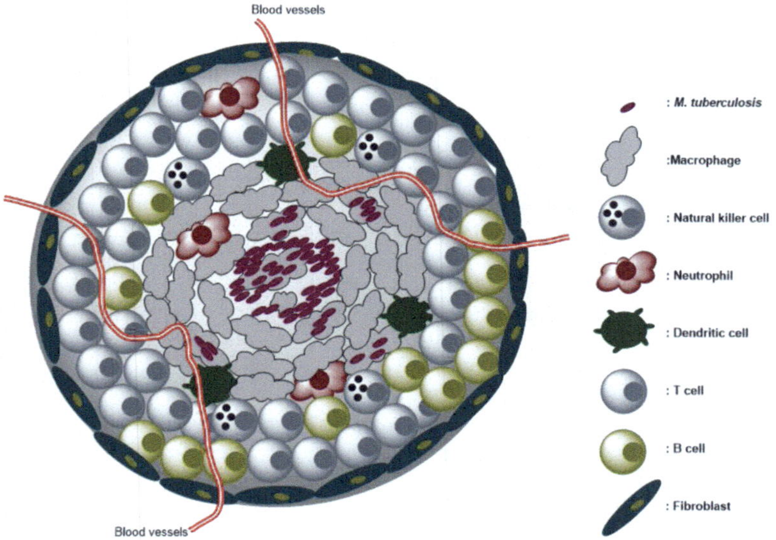

Fig. 6 Architecture of a *Mycobacterium tuberculosis* granuloma

Cell Wall Remodelling

Because of the limited understanding of mycobacterial physiology during dormancy, TB drug development towards discovery of drugs effective against dormant Mtb is one of the most challenging subjects. To date, very few antibacterial agents have been identified that are effective against latent tuberculosis infections. In stationary phase cultures of *Staphylococcus aureus*, the cell wall structure is different from that in the exponential phase; the peptidoglycan (PG) mass for a stationary phase is significantly increased. Similarly, structural dynamics of PG during endospore formation (dormancy) and germination of spores of *Bacillus subtilis* have been reported. Like many other bacteria, Mtb varies the cross-linking of PG in its dormant states. During the exponential phase, (D,D) 4→3 transpeptide linkages (linkages between the 4th (D-alanine) amino acids the 3rd (*meso*-diaminopimelic acid) of PG are predominantly produced by penicillin binding proteins (D,D-transpeptidases) (Fig. 7). However, the nonclassical (L,D) 3→3 linkages predominate the transpeptide, networking the PG layer of non-replicating Mtb. The latter transformation is catalysed by β-lactam insensitive L,D-transpeptidase (Ldt_{Mt2}). An Mtb strain lacking Ldt_{Mt2} loses virulence and attenuates growth during the chronic phase of the disease [32].

The mycolic acid-arabinogalactan conjugate is one of the most important cell wall components, playing a critical role in survival of Mtb within macrophages. The *in vitro* experimental data reported by Wayne et al. suggest that low-oxygen triggers mycobacterial dormancy and adaptation to anaerobiosis is a feature of persistent

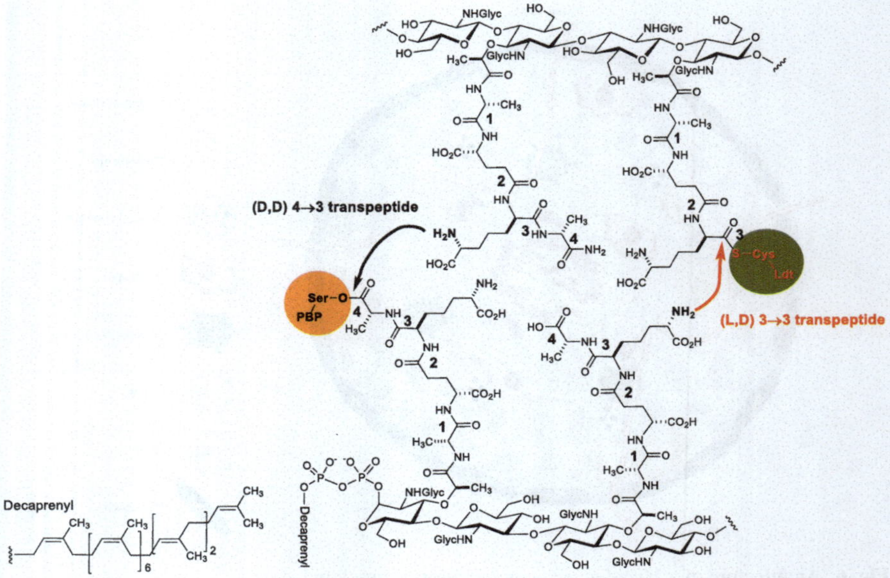

Fig. 7 Cross-linkages with classical (D,D) 4→3 transpeptide and nonclassical (L,D) 3→3 transpeptide bonds in peptidoglycan biosynthesis

tubercle bacilli. In addition, thickening of the cell wall outer layer in Mtb is observed when cultured bacteria establish the non-replicating state under anaerobic conditions. Scanning electron micrographic images coupled with specific staining of non-replicating Mtb revealed that an extracellular material composed of carbohydrate conjugates is over-produced. Non-replicating Mtb exhibit a distinctive phenotype characterized by increased extractable (free) mycolic acids and lipoglycans, along with increased arabinosylation. Despite over-expression of the genes associated with these cell wall biosynthesis pathways, substantial down-regulation of the genes involved in energy metabolism is observed in non-replicating Mtb [33].

Cell Wall Biosyntheses as Drug Targets Effective Against Non-replicating Bacilli

Among the first-line TB drugs, rifampicin, a DNA-dependent RNA polymerase inhibitor is known to be effective against non-replicating Mtb at a higher concentration than the minimal inhibitory concentration (MIC) against replicating bacilli. High-dose rifampicin is currently being evaluated in phase II clinical studies that aim to shorten treatment time for TB without causing adverse effects [34]. The hypothesis is that higher doses of rifampicin will increase its blood concentration and may also kill non-replicating Mtb within granulomas. In addition to DNA-dependent RNA polymerase, electron transport systems, menaquinone biosynthesis, F_oF_1 ATP synthase, protein kinases, DosS/DosR systems, the glyoxylate pathway, DNA gyrase, and protein biosynthesis have been studied to validate their essentiality during dormancy.

Maintaining the cell wall structure inside macrophages is one of the important factors that allows Mtb to persist in granulomas for a long time. However, until recently cell wall biosynthesis has not received much attention for development of inhibitors for treatment of dormant tuberculosis. This is most likely because dormant forms of Mtb are thought to persist without replication, leading to speculation that there is very little metabolism of cell wall components occurring during persistence. The observations that specific cell wall synthesis inhibitors kill non-replicating Mtb oppose this traditional view [13, 35]. Potential cell wall biosynthesis inhibitors that may be effective against non-replicating Mtb are discussed below.

Mycolic Acid Biosynthesis Inhibitors

Fatty acid analysis of Mtb reveals that free mycolic acid is increased in stationary phase and the non-replicating state. Gene expression DNA microarray and RNA microarray experiments support the concept that fatty acid synthesis and pyruvate metabolism pathways remain active under dormant conditions. A bicyclic nitroimidazole anti-TB drug, delemanid (formerly OPC-67683) has been reported to inhibit Mtb mycolic acid biosynthesis (Fig. 8) [36]. A member of the superfamily of

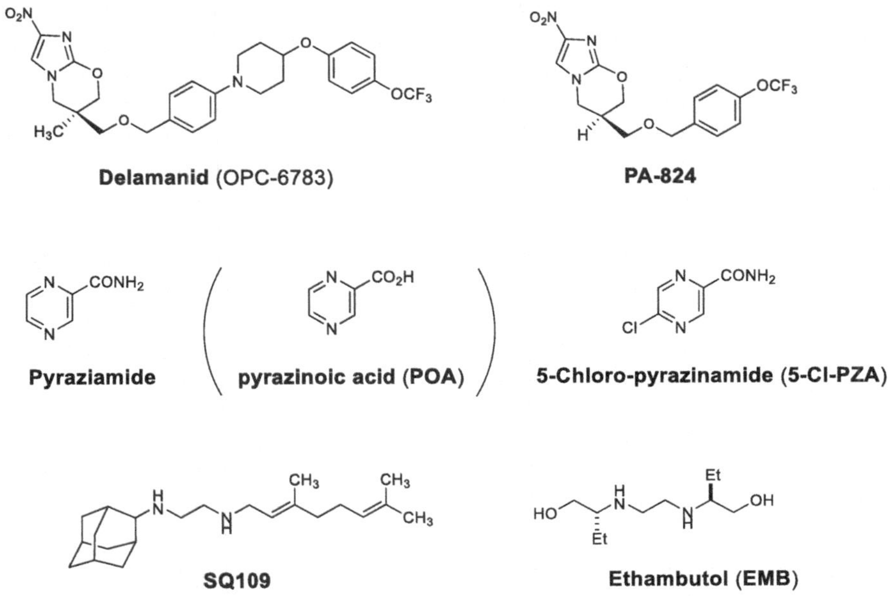

Fig. 8 Mycolic acid biosynthesis inhibitors. (Drugs effective against non-replicating Mtb are highlighted)

classical nitroreductases are flavin mononucleotide (FMN)-binding proteins that remain active under hypoxic conditions similar to tuberculosis dormancy. In general, nitroimidazole antibacterial agents require activation by reductase(s) to exert their antibacterial activities. Delemanid may be reduced by nitroreductase Rv3547 to generate the radical intermediate which, in turn, inhibits biosynthesis of mycolic acids. Studies with *Mycobacterium bovis* BCG demonstrated that delemanid inhibits production of methoxymycolic acid and ketomycolic acid (Figs. 4 and 5). Delemanid resistant Mtb strains display cross-resistance to the other nitroimidazole being developed for TB treatment, PA-824 [40]. Both compounds exhibit bactericidal activity against replicating and dormant bacilli at relatively low concentrations. The transcriptional response profile of Mtb to PA-824 indicates that it acts as a respiratory poison, releasing nitric oxide (NO). NO inhibits members of the electron transport chain, blocking ATP production. A detailed mode of action of delemanid is needed, but it is likely to share molecular targets with PA-824 [37].

Pyrazinamide (PZA), a first-line TB drug, is a prodrug that is thought to kill non-replicating Mtb [38]. A PZA analogue, 5-chloro-pyrazinamide (5-Cl-PZA) inhibits Mtb fatty acid synthase type I (FAS-I). The mode of action of 5-Cl-PZA is assumed to be identical to PZA. Pyrazinamidase/nicotinamidase (PncA) hydrolyses 5-Cl-PZA to produce the active form, pyrazinoic acid (POA) [39]. In C_{16} fatty acid biosynthesis inhibition assays with bacterial whole cells, pH-dependent activity of PZA and its analogues is observed. Under acidic conditions accumulation of POA may disrupt membrane potential and interfere with the electron transport, which is essential for both replicating and non-replicating Mtb ATP production [40, 42].

A 1,2-ethylenediamine analogue, SQ109 is a phase clinical TB drug that exhibits activity against MDR- and XDR-Mtb strains. The mode of action for SQ109 is different from ethambutol (EMB); SQ109 is effective against a number of EMB-resistant strains, and the transcriptional response to SQ109 is different from that of EMB. Analysis of the Mtb mutants that are resistant to molecules closely related to SQ109 suggested that MmpL3, the putative transporter of trehalose monomycolates (TMM) is one of the likely drug targets of SQ109. By contrast, the mode of action for EMB has been extensively studied; it disrupts arabinogalactan biosynthesis by inhibiting arabinosyl transferases (EmbA, EmbB, and EmbC). Interestingly, SQ109 effectively kills intracellular Mtb and dormant forms of Mtb *in vitro*; however, EMB does not affect viability of non-replicating Mtb. In addition to a unique mode of action of SQ109 against Mtb, SQ109 has the ability to disrupt the transmembrane electrochemical proton gradient [41]. Electron transport inhibitory activity may be the primary target for other bacteria and certain fungi that do not synthesize mycolic acids.

Bacterial Phosphotransferase Inhibitors

Two-types of phosphotransferases have been studied for the development of new TB drugs. The mycobacterial translocase I (MurX) and WecA utilize decaprenyl phosphate as the acceptor substrate, but use different UDP-2-deoxy-2-*N*-acetyl-D-hexosamine donor substrates. The MurX-type transferase is highly specific for

UDP-*N*-acetylmuramate-pentapeptide; whereas, WecA is selective for UDP-*N*-acetylglucosamine (UDP-GlcNAc). Translocase I (MraY or MurX) is essential in the growth of many bacteria listed in the NIAID Category A, B, and C Priority Pathogens. However, WecA-type phosphotransferase is not essential in the growth of many bacteria, including Gram-negatives, but is essential in growth of Mtb and viability in the hypoxic dormant state [42]. WecA is a polyprenylphosphate *N*-acetylhexosamine-1-phosphate transferase that catalyzes transformation from UDP-GlcNAc to decaprenyl-GlcNAc-pyrophosphate (decaprenyl-P-P-GlcNAc) in Mtb [43]. As illustrated in Fig. 1, WecA is the first membrane-associated step that anchors the phospho-GlcNAc moiety of UDP-GlcNAc to decaprenyl phosphate (C_{50}-P), leading to the formation of mycolyl-arabinogalactan conjugate. On the other hand, MurX catalyzes transformation from UDP-*N*-glycorylmuramyl-pentapeptide (Park's nucleotide) to decaprenyl-diphosphoryl-*N*-glycorylmuramyl-pentapeptide (lipid I, Fig. 9). MurX inhibitors are effective in killing only replicating Mtb under aerobic conditions. On the other hand, WecA inhibitors kill both replicating and non-replicating Mtb at low concentrations *in vitro* [44]. It is important to

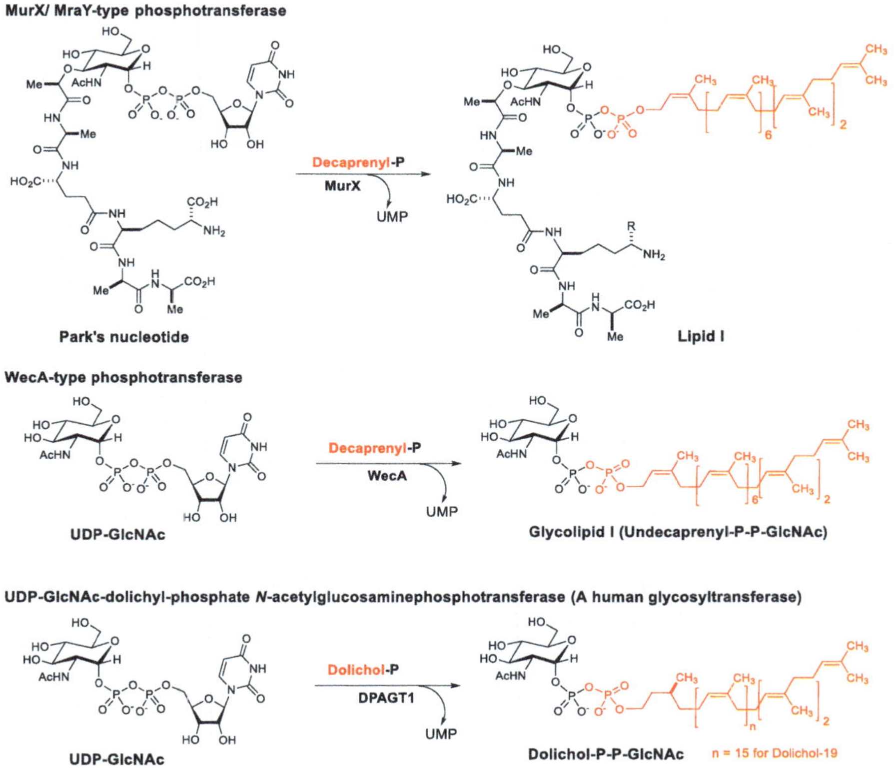

Fig. 9 Mycobacterial phosphotransferases (MurX and WecA) and a human glycosyltransferase (DPAGT1)

note that a *murX* gene homologue does not exist in humans; however, WecA inhibitors have the potential to interfere with an existing human homologue, dolichyl-phosphate GlcNAc-1-phosphotransferase 1 (DPAGT1, Fig. 9). DPAGT1 is responsible for the first step of the protein *N*-glycosylation process in humans [45]. Historically, several groups of nucleoside antibiotics have extensively been studied for the development of new antibacterial agents by targeting translocase I. The major source of MraY inhibitors is divided into four classes: capuramycins, tunicamycins, ribosaminouridines, and uridylpeptides. WecA enzyme inhibitory activity of nucleoside-based antibiotics has not received much attention until recently [46]. Tunicamycin is a laboratory tool that displays a wide range of biological activities associated with phosphotransferase inhibition. For example, tunicamycin has been studied in the anticancer field (ER stress, protein misfolding, ATP-binding cassette subfamily G member 2 (ABCG2), and apoptosis).

Interestingly, tunicamycin shows >10 times stronger inhibitory activity against WecA (IC_{50} 0.120 μg/mL) than that of MraY or MurX. A promising preclinical TB drug, CPZEN-45 was reported to inhibit both MurX and WecA activity *in vitro* [47]. However, efficacy of CPZEN-45 against non-replicating Mtb has not been thoroughly characterized. Capuramycin is a strong MurX inhibitor that kills only replicating Mtb. In contrast, 2'*O*-methyl capuramycin does not exhibit MurX inhibitory activity, but displays strong WecA inhibitory activity. Thus, methylation at the C2'-hydroxy group of capuramycin alters the molecular target. 2'*O*-Methyl capuramycin exhibits bactericidal activity against non-replicating Mtb with the same range of MIC values for replicating Mtb (Fig. 10). In screening against WecA, it

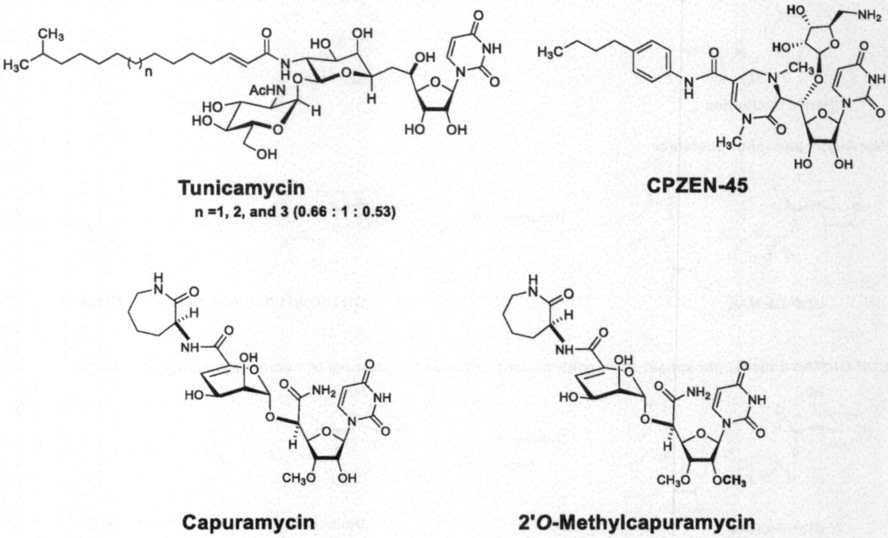

Fig. 10 Bacterial phosphotransferase inhibitors. (Drugs effective against non-replicating Mtb are highlighted)

was revealed that several MraY inhibitor nucleoside antibiotics also possess WecA inhibitory activity [48]. Thus, reinvestigation of MraY/MurX inhibitors could likely identify WecA inhibitors that have the ability to kill both replicating and non-replicating Mtb.

Arabinogalactan Biosynthesis Inhibitors

Arabinogalactan (AG) is the major cell wall polysaccharide that serves to connect peptidoglycan (PG) with the mycolic acid layer. A variety of distinctive glycosyltransferases are involved in its assembly. The L-rhamnosyl residues are a characteristic of AG that does not exist in humans. Importantly, there is no salvage pathway (degradative pathway for biosynthesis of nucleotides) for the formation of the L-rhamnosyl donor, dTDP-β-L-rhamnose in Mtb [48, 49]. Thus, the enzymes (RmlA, RmlB, RmlC, and RmlD) associated with the pathway of dTDP-β-L-rhamnose from α-D-glucose-1-phospahte are attractive drug targets. Biosynthesized glycolipid 2 (L-Rha-(α1→3)-D-GlcNAc-P-P-C_{50}) is functionalized by bifunctinal galactofuranosyltransferases, GalfT1 Gal*f*T2 and arbinosyltransferases to complete AG synthesis (Fig. 2). A large number of inhibitor molecules have been designed and synthesized by targeting these glycosyltransferases. They are moderate enzyme inhibitors, and very few molecules displayed strong growth inhibitory activity against Mtb *in vitro* [50]. Unfortunately, none of the *de novo* inhibitors of galactofuranosyltransferases or arbinosyltransferases have been investigated for dormant forms of Mtb.

Ethambutol (EMB, Fig. 8) interferes with the biosynthesis of AG and lipoarabinomannan (LAM). Among the characterized arabinosyltransferases (*e.g.* EmbA, EmbB, AftA, AftB, AftC, and AftD), EmbA and EmbB are required for the biosynthesis of AG, and EmbA is essential for growth of Mtb [51]. EMB is known to target EmbC, which is responsible for biosynthesis of lipoarabinomannan (LAM) that is essential for the viability of Mtb [5, 52]. LAM is thought to combat the host immune response to TB, and is an important component of the cell wall to maintain viability within macrophages. Suppression of host immunity is associated with a diminished interferon (INF)-γ response and enhancement of lipopolysaccharide (LPS)-stimulated release of tumour necrosis factor (TNF)-α, which triggers inflammatory reactions [5]. An additional function of LAM is thought to be neutralizing toxic oxygen radicals produced by macrophages [53]. EMB alone is not an effective drug against dormant or latent Mtb *in vitro* or *in vivo*. Gene expression profiles for LAM biosynthetic genes indicate that the expression levels for *ubiA* (encodes decaprenylphosphate 5-phosphoribosyltransferase synthase), *embC* (encodes arabinosyltransferase), and *pmmA* (encordes phosphomannose mutase) are significantly reduced in the non-replicating state *in vitro* [13]. These data suggest that the majority of enzymes associated with LAM biosynthesis are reduced in expression for non-replicating Mtb as compared to exponentially replicating bacilli, and thus, are not useful drug targets for latent TB infections.

The dehydrogenase/reductase (SDR) superfamily involves oxidation/reduction with NADH or FADH as a co-factor. Several epimerases, such as UDP-glucose 4-epimerase and decaprenyl-phosphoribose-2′-epimerase (DprE1), are key enzymes in AG biosynthesis [54]. Although expression levels of oxidoreductases involved in AG are not known, several epimerases have the potential to be effective targets for non-replicating Mtb, since many oxidoreductases (*e.g.* respiratory enzymes) are viable drug targets for both replicating and non-replicating Mtb [55].

Peptidoglycan Biosynthesis Inhibitors

The D,D (4→3) transpeptide linkages are targeted by β-lactam antibiotics (Fig. 7). Mtb shows resistance against β-lactam antibiotics by producing the β-lactamase, BlaC. It was discovered that Mtb produces nonclassical L,D (3→3) transpeptidase type 1 and 2 (Ldt_{Mt1} and Ldt_{Mt2}) [5, 32]. An Mtb strain lacking Ldt_{Mt2} loses virulence and is more susceptible to β-lactam antibiotics. During the exponential phase, the degree of L,D (3→3) linkages in Mtb is as high as 80%, whereas, in *E. coli*, a large portion of PG consists D,D 4→3 linkages [5]. The accumulated data support that Ldt_{Mt1} is upregulated during dormancy of Mtb. It was demonstrated that a combination of meropenem, a carbapenem and clavulanate, a β-lactamase inhibitor, effectively inhibits growth of Mtb and also kills non-replicating Mtb in the Wayne model (Fig. 11) [56–58]. Meropenem is not a drug of choice for *in vivo* studies due to its short half-life under physiological conditions. Thus, identification of β-lactams that are metabolically stable and sufficiently tolerated for treatment of TB is a challenge.

Conclusion

Dormant *M. tuberculosis* (Mtb) exhibits resistance to the majority of the FDA-approved TB drugs at what are considered therapeutic concentrations. Among the marketed TB drugs, only rifampicin, a RNA polymerase inhibitor, appears to have promise for efficacy against dormant Mtb. High doses of rifampicin monotherapy or multi-drug therapies using high doses of rifampicin, have the potential to shorten

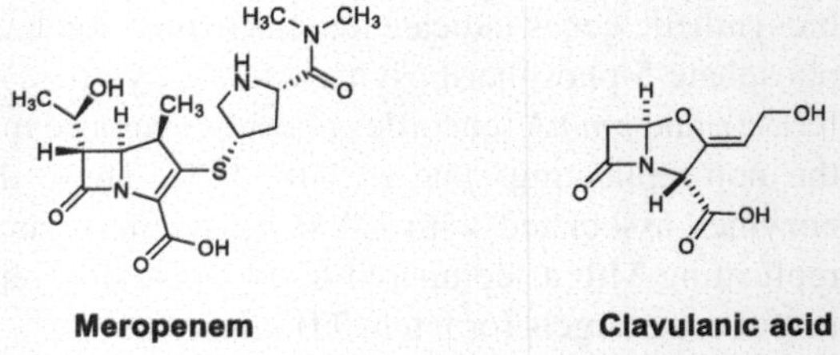

Fig. 11 An Mtb L,D-transpeptidase inhibitor

treatment for TB. However, MDR- and XDR-Mtb infections remain a public health crisis and a health security threat that may not be solved by re-engineering and repositioning older anti-TB drugs. Sustaining the viability of the dormant form in macrophages (or granulomas) requires remodelling of the Mtb cell wall. Thickening of the mycobacterial cell wall upon hypoxia *in vitro* was demonstrated more than 30 years ago. Thus, the importance of cell wall biosynthesis during dormancy has been discussed in a number of publications. However, most TB drugs that target cell wall biosynthesis are not effective against dormant Mtb. Interestingly, INH monotherapy for a period of 6–12 months is currently recommended for latent TB infection. The side effects associated with the long regimen and emergence of MDR-Mtb strains have led to poor adherence to INH therapy. These facts may discourage scientists from developing new cell wall biosynthesis inhibitors for latent tuberculosis infection.

Bioinformatics, genomic, and proteomic approaches reveal genes and their products that are essential to sustain the Mtb dormant state. Out of 3977 genes classified in Mtb (~600 of unknown function), 742 genes are associated with cell wall processes and lipid metabolism. Structural changes in the extracellular materials (e.g. lipoarabinomannan (LAM), lipomannan (LM), free mycolic acids) have been observed when Mtb enters the non-replicating state. Among the genes associated with glycolipid and lipoglycan macromolecules, only select genes are up-regulated in the non-replicating state. In addition, no selective lipoglycan biosynthesis inhibitor is available to perform proof-of-pharmacological concept studies that establish new molecular targets for development of TB drugs effective against latent TB infections. These facts make drug discovery targeting LAM and LM very challenging.

Many key enzymes are involved in Mtb mycolic acid biosynthesis. As discussed above, mycolic acids are an important cell wall component that plays a key role in survival of Mtb within granulomas. The biosynthesis of mycolic acids is accomplished by type I (Fas-I) and type II (Fas-II) enzymes, including FabH, KasA/KasB, MabA, HadABC, and InhA, and the modification enzymes (SAM-dependent methyltransferases (MTases)). The other key enzymes include: Malonyl-CoA:ACP transferase (FabD), transporters (MmpL3), acyl-AMP ligase (FadD32), and polyketide synthase (Pks13, terminates fatty acid synthesis). Among these enzymes, a few have been validated as potential targets that may be effective against non-replicating Mtb. Over the decades, a large number of fatty acid biosynthesis inhibitors have been isolated from natural sources, and small inhibitor molecules have been designed and synthesised. Although they display strong inhibitory activity against the selective targets, due primarily to the very hydrophobic characteristics of the protein surfaces and their inhibitor molecules, PK/PD properties of the majority of bacterial fatty acid biosynthesis inhibitors do not appear to be desirable. Out of 15 TB drugs being used clinically, six drugs interfere with mycolic acid biosynthesis. Although the effectiveness of delemanid against non-replicating Mtb is a very attractive biochemical discovery, it is approximately 25 times less active against non-replicating Mtb than replicating bacilli *in vitro*. Delemanid, INH, and pyrazinamide analogues are prodrugs that require activation by bacterial enzyme(s). If activation processes are diminished by lower expression levels of activation enzymes due to dormancy or drug resistance because of mutations in the activation enzyme coding region, prodrugs would exhibit less or no activity against non-replicating bacilli. Thus, efforts to identify a new class of mycolic acid biosynthesis inhibitors that do not require prodrug activation would be valuable.

Effectiveness of WecA (polyprenyl phosphate-GlcNAc-1-phosphate transferase) inhibitors on dormant Mtb has been reported. A selective WecA inhibitor displays a narrow-spectrum of antibacterial activity (against some Gram-positive bacteria and *Mycobacterium spp.*). WecA catalyzes the first committed step in mycolic acid-arabinogalactan conjugate biosynthesis. Thus, inhibition of WecA may influence the biosynthesis of the entire outer cell wall. To date, all bacterial phosphotransferase inhibitors are nucleoside antibiotics or analogues of them. Several studies suggest that a nucleoside antibiotic requires uptake through a membrane transporter, and thus, efficacy of these molecules may depend on bacterial transport mechanisms. In this regard, WecA inhibitors that do not require transport are preferable for use as bactericidal molecules against non-replicating Mtb.

Activity of peptidoglycan biosynthesis is down-regulated in the stationary phase and non-replicating state of Mtb. Nonclassical L,D (3→3) transpeptidases (Ldt_{Mt1} and Ldt_{Mt2}) are attractive drug targets to reinvestigate β-lactams effective against latent TB infections. Due to the large library of β-lactam antibiotics available to screen, more pharmacologically beneficial L,D (3→3) transpeptidase inhibitors are likely to be discovered.

In summary, the cell wall synthesis inhibitor molecules summarized in this chapter have been demonstrated their efficacy against non-replicating Mtb *in vitro*. Some of molecules target specific to mycobacterial cell wall biosynthesis that are beneficial for developing antibacterial agents focus against *Mycobacterium spp*. Bacterial cell walls need to be reconstructed during the adaptation processes to environmental stresses. The dormant forms of Mtb require maintenance of functional integrity of their cell walls to escape from endogenous macrophage attack. Thus, certain cell wall synthesis enzymes responsible for maintaining Mtb dormancy inside macrophages are attractive drug targets; the development of their inhibitor molecules having drug-like property will result in a shorting of duration of current tuberculosis treatment.

References

1. Wayne LG, Hayes LG. An in vitro model for sequential study of shiftdown of Mycobacterium tuberculosis through two stages of nonreplicating persistence. Infect Immun. 1996;64:2062–9.
2. Hume DA, Ross IL, Himes SR, Sasmono RT, Wells CA, Ravasi T. The mononuclear phagocyte system revisited. J Leukoc Biol. 2002;72:621–7.
3. Guirado E, Schlesinger LS, Kaplan G. Macrophages in tuberculosis: friend or foe. Semin Immunopathol. 2013;35:563–83. https://doi.org/10.1007/s00281-013-0388-2.
4. Cooper AM, Flynn JL. The protective immune response to Mycobacterium tuberculosis. Curr Opin Immunol. 1995;7:512–6.

5. Ramakrishnan L. Revisiting the role of the granuloma in tuberculosis. Nat Rev Immunol. 2012;12:352–67. https://doi.org/10.1038/nri3211.
6. Chen K, Kolls JK. T cell-mediated host immune defenses in the lung. Annu Rev Immunol. 2013;31:605–33. https://doi.org/10.1146/annurev-immunol-032712-100019.
7. Polena H, Boudou F, Tilleul S, Dubois-Colas N, Lecointe C, Rakotosamimanana N, et al. Mycobacterium tuberculosis exploits the formation of new blood vessels for its dissemination. Sci Rep. 2016;6:33162. https://doi.org/10.1038/srep33162.
8. Ragno S, Estrada-Garcia I, Butler R, Colston JM. Regulation of macrophage gene expression by Mycobacterium tuberculosis: down-regulation of mitochondrial cytochrome c oxidase. Infect Immun. 1998;66:3952–8.
9. Ragno S, Romano M, Howell S, Pappin DJ, Jenner PJ, Colston MJ. Changes in gene expression in macrophages infected with Mycobacterium tuberculosis: a combined transcriptomic and proteomic approach. Immunology. 2001;104:99–108.
10. Rengarajan J, Bloom BR, Rubin EJ. Genome-wide requirements for Mycobacterium tuberculosis adaptation and survival in macrophages. PNAS. 2005;102:8327–32. https://doi.org/10.1073/pnas.0503272102.
11. Smith I. Mycobacterium tuberculosis pathogenesis and molecular determinants of virulence. Clin Microbiol Rev. 2003;16:463–96. https://doi.org/10.1128/CMR.16.3.463-496.2003.
12. Hampshirea T, Sonejic S, Baconb J, Jamesb BW, Hindsa J, Lainga K, et al. Stationary phase gene expression of Mycobacterium tuberculosis following a progressive nutrient depletion: a model or persistent organisms? Tuberculosis (Edinb). 2004;84:228–38. https://doi.org/10.1016/j.tube.2003.12.010.
13. Bacon J, Alderwick LJ, Allnutt JA, Gabasova E, Watson R, Hatch KA, et al. Non-replicating Mycobacterium tuberculosis elicits a reduced infectivity profile with corresponding modifications to the cell wall and extracellular matrix. PLoS One. 2014;9:e87329. https://doi.org/10.1371/journal.pone.0087329.
14. Abrahams KA, Besra GS. Mycobacterial cell wall biosynthesis: a multifaceted antibiotic target. Parasitology. 2018;145:116–33. https://doi.org/10.1017/S0031182016002377.
15. Gengenbacher M, Kaufmann SHE. Mycobacterium tuberculosis: success through dormancy. FEMS Microbiol Rev. 2012;36:514–32. https://doi.org/10.1111/j.1574-6976.2012.00331.x.
16. Alderwick LJ, Harrison J, Lloyd GS, Birch HL. The mycobacterial cell wall-peptidoglycan and arabinogalactan. Cold Spring Harb Perspect Med. 2015;5:a021113. https://doi.org/10.1101/cshperspect.a021113.
17. van Heijenoort J. In: Ghuysen JM, Hakenbeck R, editors. Bacterial cell wall in biosynthesis of bacterial peptidoglycan. Amsterdam: Elsevier Science; 1994. p. 39–54. ISBN: 9780080860879.
18. Mahapatra S, Scherman H, Brennan PJ, Crick DC. N-Glycolylation of the nucleotide precursors of peptidoglycan biosynthesis of Mycobacterium spp. is altered by drug treatment. J Bacteriol. 2005;187:2341–7. https://doi.org/10.1128/JB.187.7.2341-2347.2005.
19. Raymond JB, Mahapatra S, Crick DC, Pavelka MS Jr. Identification of the namH gene, encoding the hydroxylase responsible for the N-glycosylation of the mycobacterial peptidoglycan. J Biol Chem. 2005;280:326–33. https://doi.org/10.1074/jbc.M411006200.
20. Jackson M, McNeil MR, Brennan PJ. Progress in targeting cell envelope biogenesis in Mycobacterium tuberculosis. Future Microbiol. 2013;8:855–75. https://doi.org/10.2217/fmb.13.52.
21. Bi Y, Mann E, Whitfield C, Zimmer J. Architecture of a channel-forming O-antigen polysaccharide ABC transporter. Nature. 2018;553:361–5. https://doi.org/10.1038/nature25190.
22. Zhang J, Angala SK, Pramanik PK, Li K, Crick DC, Liav A, Jozwiak A, Swiezewska E, Jackson M, Chatterjee D. Characterization of a distinct arabinofuranosyltransferase in Mycobacterium smegmatis. J Am Chem Soc. 2007;129:9650–62. https://doi.org/10.1021/ja070330k.
23. Marrakchi H, Lanéelle M-A, Daffe M. Mycolic acids: structures, biosynthesis, and beyond. Chem Biol. 2014;21:67–85. https://doi.org/10.1016/j.chembiol.2013.11.011.
24. Takayama K, Wang C, Besra GS. Pathway to synthesis and processing of Mycolic acids in Mycobacterium tuberculosis. Clin Microbiol Rev. 2005;18:81–101. https://doi.org/10.1128/CMR.18.1.81-101.2005.

25. North JE, Jackson M, Lee RE. New approaches to target the mycolic acid biosynthesis pathway for the development of tuberculosis therapeutics. Curr Pharm Des. 2014;20:4357–78.
26. Cantaloube S, Veyron-Churlet R, Haddache N, Daffé M, Zerbib D. The Mycobacterium tuberculosis FAS-II dehydratases and methyltransferases define the specificity of the mycolic acid elongation complexes. PLoS One. 2011;6:e29564. https://doi.org/10.1371/journal.pone.0029564.
27. Barkan D, Rao V, Sukenick DG, Glickman MS. Redundant function of cmaA2 and mmaA2 in Mycobacterium tuberculosis cis cyclopropanation of oxygenated mycolates. J Bacteriol. 2010;192:3661–8. https://doi.org/10.1128/JB.00312-10.
28. Kaur D, Berg S, Dinadayala P, Gicquel B, Chatterjee D, et al. Biosynthesis of mycobacterial lipoarabinomannan: role of a branching mannosyltransferase. PNAS. 2006;103:13664–9. https://doi.org/10.1073/pnas.0603049103.
29. Mishra AK, Krumbach K, Rittmann D, Appelmelk B, Pathak V, Pathak AK, et al. Lipoarabinomannan biosynthesis in Corynebacterineae: the interplay of two α(1→2)-mannopyranosyltransferases MptC and MptD in mannan branching. Mol Microbiol. 2011;80:1241–59. https://doi.org/10.1111/j.1365-2958.2011.07640.x.
30. Orme IM, Basaraba RJ. The formation of the granuloma in tuberculosis infection. Semin Immunol. 2014;16:601–9. https://doi.org/10.1016/j.smim.2014.09.009.
31. Ehlers S, Schaible UE. The granuloma in tuberculosis: dynamics of a host-pathogen collusion. Front Immunol. 2013;3:2–9. https://doi.org/10.3389/fimmu.2012.00411.
32. Erdemli SB, Gupta R, Bishai WR, Lamichhane G, Amzel ML, Bianchet MA. Targeting the cell wall of Mycobacterium tuberculosis: structure and mechanism of L,D-transpeptidase 2. Structure. 2012;20:2103–15. https://doi.org/10.1016/j.str.2012.09.016.
33. Dubnau E, Fontán P, Manganelli P, Soares-Appel S, Smith I. Mycobacterium tuberculosis genes induced during infection of human macrophages. Infect Immun. 2002;70:2787–95. https://doi.org/10.1128/IAI.70.6.2787–2795.2002.
34. Milstein M, Lecca L, Peloquin C, Mitchison D, Seung K, Pagano M, et al. Evaluation of high-dose rifampin in patients with new, smear-positive tuberculosis (HIRIF): study protocol for a randomized controlled trial. BMC Infect Dis. 2016;16:453–60. https://doi.org/10.1186/s12879-016-1790-x.
35. Starck J, Källenius G, Marklund B-I, Andersson DI, Åkerlund T. Comparative proteome analysis of Mycobacterium tuberculosis grown under aerobic and anaerobic conditions. Microbiology. 2004;150:3821–9. https://doi.org/10.1099/mic.0.27284-0.
36. Chen X, Hashizume H, Tomishige T, Nakamura I, Matsuba M, Fujiwara M, et al. Delamanid kills dormant mycobacteria in vitro and in a Guinea pig model of tuberculosis. Antimicrob Agents Chemother. 2017;61:e02402–16. https://doi.org/10.1128/AAC.02402-16.
37. Manjunatha U, Boshoff HIM, Barry CE III. The mechanism of action of PA-824. Commun Integr Biol. 2009;2:215–8.
38. Zhang Y, Wade MY, Scorpio A, Zhang H, Sun Z. Mode of action of pyrazinamide: disruption of Mycobacterium tuberculosis membrane transport and energetics by pyrazinoic acid. J Antimicrob Chemother. 2003;52:790–5. https://doi.org/10.1093/jac/dkg446.
39. Sayahi H, Pugliese KM, Zimhony O, Jacobs WR Jr, Shekhtman A, Welch JT. Analogs of the antituberculous agent pyrazinamide are competitive inhibitors of NADPH binding to M. tuberculosis fatty acid synthase I. Chem Biodivers. 2012;9:2582–96. https://doi.org/10.1002/cbdv.201200291.
40. Zhang Y, Shi W, Zhang W, Mitchison D. Mechanisms of pyrazinamide action and resistance. Microbiol Spectr. 2013;4:1–12. https://doi.org/10.1128/microbiolspec.MGM2-0023-2013.
41. Sacksteder KA, Protopopova M, Barry CE 3rd, Andries K, Nacy CA. Discovery and development of SQ109: a new antitubercular drug with a novel mechanism of action. Future Microbiol. 2012;7:823–37. https://doi.org/10.2217/fmb.12.56.
42. Jin Y, Xin Y, Zhang W, Ma Y. Mycobacterium tuberculosis Rv1302 and Mycobacterium smegmatis MSMEG4947 have WecA function and MSMEG4947 is required for the growth of M. smegmatis. FEMS Microbiol Lett. 2010;310:54–61. https://doi.org/10.1111/j.1574-6968.2010.02045.x.

43. Mitachi K, Siricilla S, Yang D, Kong Y, Skorupinska-Tudek K, Swiezewska E, et al. Fluorescence-based assay for polyprenyl phosphate-GlcNAc-1-phosphate transferase (WecA) and identification of novel antimycobacterial WecA inhibitors. Anal Biochem. 2016;512:78–90. https://doi.org/10.1016/j.ab.2016.08.008.
44. Siricilla S, Mitachi K, Wan B, Franzblau SG, Kurosu M. Discovery of a capuramycin analog that kills nonreplicating Mycobacterium tuberculosis and its synergistic effects with translocase I inhibitors. J Antibiot. 2015;68:271–8. https://doi.org/10.1038/ja.2014.133.
45. Kurosu M. Inhibition of N-glycosylation towards novel anti-cancer chemotherapeutics. J Mol Pharm Org Process Res. 2018;6:141–3. https://doi.org/10.4172/2329-9053.1000141.
46. Mitachi K, Aleiwi BA, Schneider CM, Siricilla S, Kurosu M. Stereocontrolled total synthesis of muraymycin D1 having a dual mode of action against Mycobacterium tuberculosis. J Am Chem Soc. 2016;138:12975–80. https://doi.org/10.1021/jacs.6b07395.
47. Ishizaki Y, Hayashi C, Inoue K, Igarashi M, Takahashi Y, Pujari V, et al. Inhibition of the first step in synthesis of the mycobacterial cell wall core, catalyzed by the GlcNAc-1-phosphate transferase WecA, by the novel caprazamycin derivative CPZEN-45. J Biol Chem. 2013;288:30309–19. https://doi.org/10.1074/jbc.M113.492173.
48. Kolita B, Gogoi D, Dutta PP, Bordoloi M, Bezbaruah RL. Arabinosyl transferase inhibitor design against Mycobacterium tuberculosis using ligand based drug design approach. Bangladesh J Pharmacol. 2014;9:225–9. https://doi.org/10.3329/bjp.v9i2.18270.
49. Ma Y, Stern RJ, Scherman MS, Vissa VD, Yan W, Jones VC, et al. Drug targeting Mycobacterium tuberculosis cell wall synthesis: genetics of dTDP-rhamnose synthetic enzymes and development of a microtiter plate-based screen for inhibitors of conversion of dTDP-glucose to dTDP-rhamnose. Antimicrob Agents Chemother. 2001;45:1407–16. https://doi.org/10.1128/AAC.45.5.1407-1416.2001.
50. Favrot L, Ronning DR. Targeting the mycobacterial envelope for tuberculosis drug development. Expert Rev Anti-Infect Ther. 2012;10:1023–36. https://doi.org/10.1586/eri.12.91.
51. Amin AG, Goude R, Shi L, Zhang J, Chatterjee D, Parish T. EmbA is an essential arabinosyltransferase in Mycobacterium tuberculosis. Microbiology. 2008;154:240–8. https://doi.org/10.1099/mic.0.2007/012153-0.
52. Goude R, Amin AG, Chatterjee D, Parish T. The Arabinosyltransferase EmbC is inhibited by Ethambutol in Mycobacterium tuberculosis. Antimicrob Agents Chemother. 2009;53:4138–46.
53. Gilleron M, Bala L, Brando T, Vercellone A, Puzo G. Mycobacterium tuberculosis H37Rv parietal and cellular lipoarabinomannans. J Biol Chem. 2000;275:677–84. https://doi.org/10.1074/jbc.275.1.677.
54. Kolly GS, Mukherjee R, Kilacsková E, Abriata LA, Raccaud M, Blaško J, et al. GtrA protein Rv3789 is required for arabinosylation of arabinogalactan in Mycobacterium tuberculosis. J Bacteriol. 2015;197:3686–97. https://doi.org/10.1128/JB.00628-15.
55. Brecik M, Centárová I, Mukherjee R, Kolly GS, Huszár S, Bobovská S, et al. DprE1 is a vulnerable tuberculosis drug target due to its cell wall localization. ACS Chem Biol. 2015;10:1631–6. https://doi.org/10.1021/acschembio.5b00237.
56. Kumar K, Arora K, Lloyd JR, Lee Y III, Nair V, Fischer E, et al. Meropenem inhibits D,D-carboxypeptidase activity in Mycobacterium tuberculosis. Mol Microbiol. 2012;86:367–81. https://doi.org/10.1111/j.1365-2958.2012.08199.x.
57. Forsman DL, Giske CG, Bruchfeld J, Schön T, Juréen P, Ängeby K. Meropenem-clavulanate has high in vitro activity against multidrug-resistant Mycobacterium tuberculosis. Int J Mycobacteriol. 2015;4:80–1. https://doi.org/10.1016/j.ijmyco.2014.10.018.
58. Kim HS, Kim J, Im HN, Yoon JY, An DR, Yoon HJ, et al. Structural basis for the inhibition of Mycobacterium tuberculosis L,D-transpeptidase by meropenem, a drug effective against extensively drug-resistant strains. Acta Cryst. 2013;69:420–31. https://doi.org/10.1107/S0907444912048998.

The Silent Plague: Regulation of Latent Tuberculosis Infections

Parnia Behinaein and Jeffrey D. Cirillo

Abstract Nearly one-third of the world's population carries viable tubercle bacilli in their bodies but do not display disease. This represents the clinical definition of a latently infected patient who can reactivate and produce active disease at any time. Despite a great deal of investigation, it remains unclear exactly where or what state the bacteria responsible, *Mycobacterium tuberculosis*, are in during this latent phase of infection and how they enter and leave dormancy. Neither the exact signals nor the complete regulatory pathways involved are fully understood. This review is not meant to be a comprehensive overview of tuberculosis latency, but is meant to briefly raise some of the more critical and controversial issues in the literature related to latent infections, focusing primarily on bacterial gene expression and offering suggestions for directions of future research. We conclude that there are several signals involved in establishment of the persistent state during latent infections and reactivation from that state that remain to be elucidated. Interestingly, the clinical definition of latency is not likely to be due to bacteria in the same state in all patients. The complexity of these events offers opportunities to combat tuberculosis through manipulation of the bacterial persistent state and the interacting host immune response. Exploitation of bacterial persistence during latent infections as well as the signals that control these events may be critical to the ultimate goal of eradicating this ongoing plague of mankind.

Keywords Transcription · Signals · Pulmonary · Dissemination · Genetics · Networks · Reactivation · Respiratory · Molecular · *Mycobacterium*

P. Behinaein · J. D. Cirillo (✉)
Department of Microbial Pathogenesis and Immunology, Texas A&M University College of Medicine, Bryan, TX, USA
e-mail: jdcirillo@tamu.edu

J. D. Cirillo, Y. Kong (eds.), *Tuberculosis Host-Pathogen Interactions*,
https://doi.org/10.1007/978-3-030-25381-3_2

Introduction

Tuberculosis is normally a respiratory disease of the lungs, but can present itself in nearly any organ. Infection leads to a chronic cough, night sweats and often wasting of the body, with pathological lesions called tubercles observed in infected organs. There has been a great deal of effort focused on eradication of tuberculosis such that the World Health Organization has targeted elimination in over 30 countries [1]. Despite this effort tuberculosis remains the most frequent cause of death due to an infectious agent worldwide and infects nearly one-third of the world's population [2, 3]. The majority (~50–90%) of individuals infected with *Mycobacterium tuberculosis* are considered latent [4–8], which means that they do not display active clinical symptoms and 2–9 times more individuals acquire latent tuberculosis as compared to those actually diagnosed with active tuberculosis. During clinically defined latent infection people carry persistent bacteria as shown by a positive skin test with purified protein derivative (PPD), the result of a positive delayed type hypersensitivity reaction when bacterial antigens are injected beneath the skin or a positive IFN-γ release assay, a blood test that measures the T-cell response to specific *M. tuberculosis* antigens. It is often thought that during clinically latent infections the bacteria are in a non-replicating state, but this assumption may not be true. There may well be a number of different bacterial replication states present during the latent phase of infection in humans, varying from patient to patient and even within a single patient. We will discuss the current understanding of the proteins involved in regulating initiation of the bacterial state thought to be present during latent infections and novel strategies under development that can be used to diagnose latent infections, interfere with initiation of the bacterial state present during latency and prevent infections that arise from transmission from individuals that are latently infected and reactivate.

Establishing Latent Infections

Patients become infected via aerosols from infectious individuals and latency can then be established via two routes [6–9]. First, the person may be infected and never become actively ill, but keep the bacilli at bay continuously as long as 50 years, during which reactivation could occur at any time. Second, the individual could develop tuberculosis, be treated for infection and not fully eliminate the bacilli, but not develop active disease until many years later. These two mechanisms may occur in exactly the same manner from the bacterial perspective or could represent two completely different ways of setting up the same balance between dormant and replicating bacilli [10]. In the case of individuals that develop latency immediately after infection instead of active disease, they most likely have very few bacteria present initially and maintain that low number by either inhibiting further growth or killing the bacilli as rapidly as they replicate. Differentiating models where the bacteria continue to replicate from inhibition of growth is extremely difficult, since there are very few bacteria present and any method of monitoring their physiological state has an impact upon that state. Similarly, after treatment of active disease, very few bacteria are present and the immune response is already primed, allowing the low number of bacilli to be maintained afterward [11–14]. The relationship between replication and killing is not known for this condition either, making it extremely important to develop strategies to measure bacterial replication that are not influenced by the stressful conditions that may be present when bacterial growth is inhibited during infection. Since DNA mutation rates can increase or decrease under stressful conditions, solely measuring incorporation of mutations or single-nucleotide polymorphisms (SNPs) over time does not solve this problem. Quantitative measures of bacterial replication during infection represent a major challenge to fully understanding latent infections.

Problems Modeling Latent Infections

One of the reasons that our knowledge is limited is that there is not a system where latency can be studied accurately in the laboratory, there are only approximations and there is little evidence for how well they fit the situation in humans. There are other models, but those primarily used are the Wayne model [15], the Cornell model [16–18], nutrient limitation [19–21] and the chronic phase of infection in mice [22]. One common feature of each model is that the growth rate of the bacteria is either very slow or not measurable, emphasizing the concept that in latency they are not thought to be growing or at least not very rapidly. However, whether or not the bacteria are actually growing during latent infections in humans has not been proven in any animal model [8], including primates. There are some data suggesting replication can occur in the chronic phase in mice [12], but whether this model is similar to human latent infections is unclear. Possibly the bacteria are not growing because, although evidence of DNA in tissue from latently infected people is sometimes present, it is difficult to demonstrate the presence of actual bacteria [23, 24]. The Wayne model is a nutrient limitation model, since it involves using sealed tubes and growth of the bacteria to deplete oxygen present, causing the bacteria to enter into a non-replicating state [15]. Mouse models for latency, such as the Cornell and chronic phase of infection models, are likely different from the Wayne model, since nutrients are present, immune factors are involved and oxygen levels are different in different microenvironments within diseased lungs. In the Cornell model, mouse infection is allowed to progress, the number of bacteria present is decreased by use of antibiotics, and then the antibiotics are removed [16, 17]. Over time, the mice reactivate in a nearly random manner, though an immunosuppressive treatment can be used to cause a higher frequency of reactivation in a more synchronized fashion [25]. The Cornell model has less than 100 bacteria present and reactivation can be demonstrated by measurable numbers (>100 bacteria) being present in tissues when mice display illness; whereas, for the chronic phase of infection in mice there are usually $>10^6$ bacteria present with no apparent disease until the mice get old and succumb to disease [14, 18]. In both cases, it is not clear whether the bacteria are replicating and being killed at the same rate, or just not growing. Which model more closely represents human latent infections is unclear, but despite this issue of relevance, all genes that are described as playing a role in latency have been identified using one of these models. Interestingly, there are numerous *M. tuberculosis* genes that have the ability to transport host lipids into the bacteria and many of these are involved in persistence during infection [26–28] and transitioning from the replicating to non-replicating state by the bacteria [29]. Taking all of this into account, it is likely that both during persistence and latent infections, fatty acids are used as the primary carbon source [22], since lipids are readily available in macrophages and all other infected tissues.

Importance of Signals and Regulatory Proteins

Regardless of the specific manner in which clinical latency develops, regulatory proteins in the bacteria are responsible for the transition from actively replicating to a persisting state that is maintained during these infections [19, 30]. This means that there are specific signals that must be present either external to or within the bacilli that indicate that this state is necessary to survive and persist within the host [31–38]. There has been a great deal of research focused on understanding the regulatory factors involved in initiation of latency, but there remain many gaps in our knowledge. The DosR regulatory protein has been identified as a factor thought to be involved as well as the Rel_{Mtb} regulatory protein that controls the stringent response. There is likely a link between these pathways and there is some evidence for this link through SigE [33, 39], but how these different pathways are modulated and their resulting impact on persistence are not fully understood. Since both DosR and Rel_{Mtb} play a role in persistence of tuberculosis bacilli in the host, a better understanding of the pathways they control or that control them could offer new targets for therapeutic intervention and possibly also impact vaccines and diagnostics focused on latent infections.

Despite the clear importance of the genes involved, understanding the signals that may control latency can be confusing because the same fatty acid utilization pathways are regulated by different proteins including RamB [40], MprAB [33], SigG [41], SigE [42], PhoPR [32, 43–45] and possibly others [46]. The multiple pathways involved in regulating this switch suggest that, rather than fatty acid utilization being a specific switch to or from latency, this transition is metabolic and can be triggered by a number of different pathways that require fatty acids. Identified for its role in surviving hypoxic environments [47–51], DosR is one of the primary regulators thought to play a role in persistence during latent infections. The Clp system transcriptional regulator ClgR regulates DosR and components of the SigH/E regulons and is induced by hypoxia, but is also regulated by several other conditions or signals [30]. The presence of lipids as the only carbon source results in broad differential regulation of the DosR and WhiB3 regulons, suggesting that hypoxia alone is not an exact approximation of conditions during infection that lead to latency [52]. One of the signals that triggers the DosR regulon is cAMP, which is important in signaling the presence of different nutrient environments and host cell infection [53]. The Rel_{Mtb} protein, which controls the stringent response, a response that occurs in bacteria under nutrient limiting conditions [35, 54–58] is another important regulator thought to play a role in latency. These observations suggest that there are many signals involved in triggering pathways that are important for bacterial persistence during latency, including hypoxia and nutrient composition.

Development of strategies to interfere with the various persistent bacterial states will require identification of additional factors involved in induction of and reactivation from latency. Recent data suggest that there is a unique niche for *M. tuberculosis* outside of diseased tissue in the lungs, mesenchymal and hematopoietic stem cells [59–61]. Although these may not be the only cells where *M. tuberculosis* can be sequestered and persist after treatment, including epithelial cells or adipocytes, these data argue that *M. tuberculosis* responds to signals in mammalian cells to enable persistence within an intracellular environment. Signals that are present in an intracellular niche would include each of those already known to trigger pathways relevant to persistence (Fig. 1): pH changes, stress, fatty acids as a carbon source, hypoxia, reduced iron and reduced access to nutrients. Since multiple signals are present, it is likely that only a model that involves several of these signals at appropriate levels would closely resemble conditions relevant to human latent infections. Although there are latency models in development that utilize multiple signals [20, 62], the complexity of these models makes it difficult to ascertain whether each signal is at the most appropriate level to trigger and maintain natural dormancy. The apparent phenotypic differences between bacteria that are grown under the conditions used in these multiple signal models for latency suggest that there are a number of genes differentially expressed. Overall, these observations emphasize the importance of identifying factors involved in conditions that mimic the natural latent environment, combined with analysis of any overlap between the genes expressed under these new conditions and those previously identified. However, nearly comprehensive modulation of the conditions to optimize similarities observed between in vitro and in vivo models, as well as analysis of expression during human latent infections will be necessary if we are to ever fully mimic latency in humans using an in vitro latent growth condition.

The Importance of Hypoxia

Another major gap in our knowledge is whether or not latent bacilli are present within granulomas or are under hypoxic conditions. Metronidazole, an antibiotic that is thought to function strictly under anaerobic conditions [15], kills *M. tuberculosis* in hypoxic granulomas [51], supporting a role for hypoxia in disease. The confounding issue is that the impact of metronidazole on humans has only been

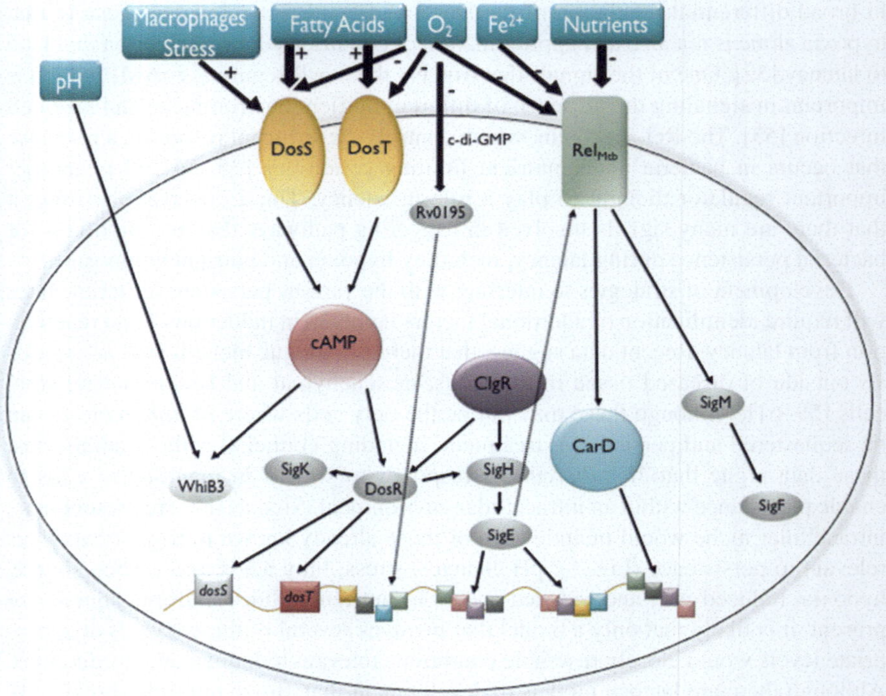

Fig. 1 A partial summary of regulators and regulatory pathways related to latent tuberculosis infections. Known signals that evidence exists for a role in the induction of establishment of bacterial persistence during latent infections and potentially could play a role in spontaneous reactivation are shown at the top of the figure and these trigger specific pathways downstream that have transcriptional and post-transcriptional effects on numerous genes in *Mycobacterium tuberculosis*. Arrows indicate directions of interactions between specific components involved in persistence. Dashed arrows indicate directions of known interactions that most likely have more than one component, but the specific components involved are not known. Curved line at bottom of cell indicates chromosomal DNA and genes thought to be regulated at the transcriptional level during persistence. Groups of boxes on DNA indicate multiple genes within regulons and specific genes are indicated within a single box along with their gene name. Plus and minus symbols next to arrows indicate whether the interaction is inductive or repressive, respectively. Not all interactions are shown for the sake of clarity and only key players discussed in this review are included. Rv0195 and DosR both regulate a large number of genes and have a similar phenotype, but none of the genes in their regulons are the same. The DosR regulon and Rel_{Mtb} regulon interact through SigE and interactions with other sigma factors are shown. Each sigma factor and WhiB3 regulates a large number of genes, but these regulons are not shown to prevent the depiction from being unnecessarily complex and better allow focus on key pathways

explored in active tuberculosis [63, 64]. The ability of metronidazole to prevent reactivation in latently infected patients would need to be examined to evaluate the role of hypoxic tissues in latency. Studies with human tissues suggest that neither granulomas nor any obvious pathology need to be present in tissues where the bacteria are present during latent infections in humans [23, 24]. When hypoxia is observed within *M. tuberculosis* infected tissues it is found inside necrotic granulomas. Thus, the absence of granulomas in sites where bacteria can be found in latently infected individuals is evidence against the possibility that clinical latency involves hypoxia or even that hypoxic granulomas play an important role in latency. Considering that much of the current data regarding latency arises from hypoxic conditions, these observations create a paradox that does not appear resolvable using available animal models. However, at least in terms of latency and reactivation, Cynomolgus macaques have proven to be a useful model that allows observation of entry into and exit from this clinical state [65–69]. In the Cynomolgus model increased inflammation, number of granulomas and extrapulmonary disease correlate with increased likelihood of reactivation [67]. Although the Cynomolgus studies used TNF neutralization to initiate reactivation, the correlation of reactivation with inflammation and granulomas suggests that an active host response is involved in development of active disease, which seems logical since pathology due to a host response and clinically observable disease occur together. These data emphasize the importance of better models for latency both in vitro and in animals to gain insight into the signals involved in latency and reactivation. These issues could be explored by examining modified Cornell models in other non-murine animals, but even when using models cheaper than macaques, these studies would be costly and require development of new technologies that will allow analysis of both the non-granulomatous tissue that appears to carry bacteria during latent infections and the granulomatous tissue that has been the focus of most studies on active disease.

Downstream Factors Involved

Recent studies have identified numerous downstream genes that are controlled by these regulators. Detailed characterization of their biological mechanisms of action represents a major bottleneck in the tuberculosis field, similar to research in every bacterial species, but magnified by the time it takes to conduct such studies in *M. tuberculosis* due to its slow growth and relatively complicated genetic manipulation [70, 71]. DosR regulates the sensor kinases DosS and DosT that are involved in survival under hypoxic conditions in the laboratory or in Kramnik mice, which have more hypoxic granulomas than C57BL/6 wild type mice [72]. Another regulator CarD is important globally and is controlled by Rel_{Mtb}, a protein involved in persistence and the response to nutrient limitation. However, both CarD and Rel_{Mtb} were evaluated during the chronic phase of mouse infection, a crude approximation of true latent infections due to the large number of bacteria present [73]. The key role of nutrient limitation is further emphasized by the involvement of DosR in control of iron acquisition, including mycobactin genes that are important in iron scavenging [50]. When nutrients are present and the bacteria are invading host tissues, DosR-regulated genes are repressed and genes for pathways involved in invasion, aerobic growth and metabolism are increased [74]. Both the signals that control these regulatory proteins and the predicted functions of downstream genes controlled by them suggest that hypoxia and iron limitation are two of the most important signals in establishing the persistent state(s) present during latent infections. The signals involved in reactivation may be similar, through a process of reversing these conditions, most likely by changes in the host that result in the bacteria being exposed to an environment that has additional nutrients and sufficient oxygen to trigger renewed growth.

There are numerous additional genes present in the *M. tuberculosis* genome that are thought to encode regulatory proteins and have either completely unknown functions or their functions are only poorly understood. One such protein, encoded by the Rv0195 gene, is controlled similarly to DosR, in that it is regulated by hypoxia and nutrient limitation [75]. Interestingly, although the Rv0195 protein regulates more than 180 genes, there is no overlap between the genes it regulates and the DosR regulon. These observations suggest that our understanding of hypoxia, whether or not it truly represents clinically relevant latent conditions, is only scratching the surface of what there is to discover. Clearly there are numerous potential signals that can play a role in initiation and exit from the persistent bacterial state that is present during latent infections (Fig. 1), but their interactions and whether some of them play a more or less important role, remain to be elucidated.

Latent Infections as a Therapeutic Target

Since a large portion of the world's population is latently infected [2], the ability to interfere with establishment or reactivation from latency would dramatically change the landscape of tuberculosis infections worldwide and save numerous lives. Blocking bacterial genes thought to play a role in persistence during latent infections does not have an impact on the early phases of infection when bacterial replication is occurring, but leads to a reduction in bacterial numbers once replication slows or stops. A defect only in later stages of infection in animals has been observed with bacteria that lack DosR [76], Rel_{Mtb} [56] and downstream genes that play roles during the chronic phase of infection, including the Mel2 genes [77]. These genes play roles in persistence of *M. tuberculosis* during the chronic phase of infection, but have no impact on growth during the early acute phase of infection where the bacteria replicate rapidly. Bacterial mutants in these genes display improved clearance from tissues during the chronic phase of infection, so they replicate normally initially and then are rapidly cleared after about 4 weeks post-infection [56, 76, 77]. Thus, if the functions of the proteins these genes encode can be interfered with, persisting bacteria would no longer be able to maintain persistence during the chronic phase of infection and clearance would occur. It should be possible to design inhibitors for proteins that play a role in persistence during latent infections. This type of inhibitor would be expected to improve clearance from tissues, similar to mutants in the genes that encode them, and, hopefully, result in a complete cure rather than latent infection. Use of this strategy would prevent latency and, thereby, reactivation, a critical problem throughout the world, but particularly important in countries where transmission rates are low.

Since the majority of human infections are latent, the ability to interfere with any aspect of latency could prove critical to eradication of tuberculosis [78]. Interestingly, during infections bacteria within the population are relatively resistant to antimicrobial therapy, as shown by the drug tolerance displayed by a sub-population of the bacteria present in sputum from patients [79]. Possibly the drug resistance observed is due to the non-replicating persistent state that the bacteria enter when in lipid rich sputum [80]. The fact that drug-resistant bacteria are likely present during latent infections makes it critical that alternative strategies to antimicrobial therapy are explored. There are three main steps in latent infections that could be targeted: establishment, throughout the infection or reactivation. The strategies for targeting different stages of latency may be different, but the more information there is regarding the details of the signals, receptors and pathways involved, the greater the chances are that strategies can be developed to interfere with them. Interfering with the signals involved in establishing persistence themselves is an attractive therapeutic strategy, resulting in a poorly persistent population of bacteria that would be more prone to clearance and antimicrobial therapy. Persistent bacteria can also be targeted, either by partially preventing the mechanisms that allow avoidance of clearance or directly blocking metabolic or catabolic pathways required for survival during latent infections.

One strategy that could be used to cause clearance during latency would be stimulation of the host response specifically targeted toward persistent bacilli. Caution is warranted with this approach, since it is possible that a host response to persistent bacteria could reactivate them in a similar manner to how the resuscitating promotion factors (Rpf) may function, partially digesting the cell wall [81, 82]. The Rpfs are five proteins that appear to be redundant in tuberculosis [83] and were originally identified from *Micrococcus* [84], but have the ability to resuscitate dormant bacteria that cannot normally be grown from sputum and other clinical material as well as culture [34, 81, 85–88]. Structural analyses ultimately found that Rpfs are very similar to lysozymes and have similar cell wall digesting ability [82, 89, 90]. Although the specificity of Rpfs as peptidoglycan hydrolases might suggest similar reactivation mechanisms are unlikely, mammalian peptidoglycan recognition proteins often have enzymatic activity that includes specific peptidoglycan hydrolase activities [91, 92]. The similarity of these activities leaves the potential for a host response to have similar effects to Rpfs, either through production of stimulatory cell wall components or a bacterial response to externally catalyzed cell wall remodeling. Reactivation of a small number of persistent bacteria when the host remains immune-competent may result in either improved recognition and clearance or active disease, making careful testing prior to attempting this approach critical. Presumably, the potential to reactivate could be an issue with any perturbation of persistent bacilli, making latency a valuable target, but with caveats that should be considered carefully. An appealing alternative is blocking reactivation itself, but there are few models for reactivation and those that exist are time consuming and expensive [25, 93–96]. The absence of inexpensive and rapid models to test inhibitors of reactivation are likely to make investigation of this type of therapeutic approach difficult without specifically targeted funding.

Importance of Biomarkers to Track Latency

Regardless of the method used to target latency, the ability to track latent infection will be important in assessing newly infected patients as well as those that are treated, to ensure each patient is managed appropriately. Biomarkers for the host response have the potential for use in tracking latent infection, but most often they do not differentiate previous infection from ongoing, due to immune memory. The ability to directly measure the presence of very low numbers of viable bacteria would prove useful to track latency, but the primary concern with this approach is that markers for the bacteria may be very different when they are actively growing as compared to persistent bacteria. Further examination of the biology of persistent bacilli is needed to identify the best targets for use to quantify latent bacteria. Although potentially appropriate targets, including BlaC [97–100], DosR [47, 76], DosR regulated genes [101], Rpf antigens [101] and ESAT-6 [101, 102] have already been identified, validation for use to quantify bacteria during latent infections in animal models and humans is needed. Not only does the marker need to be present, but it needs to be sensitive enough to detect very few bacteria, even those that are not very metabolically active. The quest for sensitive markers represents a major challenge. At present, reporter enzyme techniques to detect BlaC display some promise for having this level of sensitivity [103], but none have yet been developed to directly detect DosR, members of the DosR regulon or other proteins associated with LTBI, though indirect detection of DosR through detection of host responses to these antigens can potentially be used [101, 104]. Host biomarkers have been identified that appear to have the ability to differentiate latent from active infections at least in some individuals [105–107], but whether these biomarkers will be consistent in diverse populations needs to be investigated. However, in many cases host response-based methods are plagued by difficulty differentiating latent infections from past or currently active infections [104] as well as vaccinated individuals that have not been exposed to *M. tuberculosis* [108–112]. These observations suggest that continued identification of additional markers and development of technologies for their use to detect and quantify bacilli or the host response in latent and active infections are critical to improving management of latency.

Reactivation from Latency

Reactivation is when a latently infected individual begins to display symptoms, without being re-infected [6, 18, 113]. The bacilli are actively replicating after reactivation and will cause symptoms that are indistinguishable from the disease that occurs when someone is initially infected and develops active disease. An individual with latent tuberculosis has a 5–10% likelihood of reactivating at any time throughout their life until death. The frequency of reactivation increases dramatically to 5–10% per year with any immunocompromised state, including infection with HIV, which is considered a co-indicator of likely *M. tuberculosis* infection [114]. Any immunocompromised state or reduction in the ability to mount a robust immune response, such as during aging, has some likelihood for increasing the potential for reactivating infection and producing active disease. There is no obvious contact with active tuberculosis patients or travel to tuberculosis-endemic areas when reactivation occurs. The absence of any indicators of reactivation means that there no way to diagnose it until active disease is recognized in the same manner as other patients. Diagnosis of tuberculosis normally occurs after an extended chronic cough, night sweats and often wasting due to disease. Because of the extended time to diagnosis, transmission to a new host frequently occurs prior to recognition of reactivation and treatment. These facts make reactivation within a non-endemic population very difficult to predict and a constant critical source of new infections anywhere in the world. Since reactivation is the result of the presence of persistent bacilli in tissues of an infected individual, interfering with the transition of bacilli into the state they persist in during latent infections could prevent reactivation-related infections [11, 23].

Patients that are reactivating from latency represent a key group to identify, monitor and properly treat, since they provide an important source of new infections, particularly in countries where the frequency of active disease is low. The fact that bacterial numbers are very low during latency has made the search for immunological biomarkers that correlate with reactivation a major target of research in this area. Although a few host biomarkers can be found that at least partially correlate with latent infection, it remains unclear whether there are any that are consistent in all individuals that reactivate [115–119] and whether this inconsistency is due to differences in individual immune responses and/or immune memory. However, whether bacterial or host biomarkers are identified that allow recognition of patients that are reactivating, this type of early warning system would be extremely valuable. In healthy individuals reactivation is rare, but in HIV positive, immunocompromised or elderly, reactivation frequencies increase dramatically indicating that immunological deficiencies are linked to reactivation. Recognition of reactivating patients would allow treatment at a stage where fewer bacteria are present, helping ensure a positive treatment outcome. Furthermore, identification of these patients could allow treatment of the underlying issue in the host that is leading to reactivation. It is important to intervene at an early time point after reactivation to prevent transmission of *M. tuberculosis* to new patients and further spread, creating new active disease clusters.

Future Prospects

Recent studies have made great strides in our understanding of latent tuberculosis infections [49, 120], but they remain a critical problem with many unanswered questions. Are the bacteria actively replicating and being killed at the same rate, not replicating at all or in states in between? Could there be multiple types of latent infections where many of these are true? Do latent bacteria reside in a single niche or multiple niches? Could latent bacilli survive extracellularly, only within a cell or both? Is immune recognition of latent bacilli suppressed or does the immune system see the bacilli but is unable to sterilize infection? Exploring these questions could lead to novel intervention strategies and improve our ability to track latent infections to prevent active disease due to reactivation.

On the surface, the fact that isoniazid or rifampin prophylaxis can help prevent active tuberculosis might be taken as evidence that at least some bacteria present during latent infections are replicating. Examining the data more deeply we find that prophylaxis has primarily been studied in HIV positive patients where it has a 33–97% efficacy [121] or in the general at risk population to prevent infection where the efficacy is 31–69% [122–126]. In all cases, the risk of infection and reactivation correlates with efficacy as does the duration of treatment, where increased time allows a larger window where changes in bacterial replication in the host can occur. Since portions of these patient populations may have replicating bacteria due to reactivation, re-infection or new infection during prophylaxis, correlation of efficacy with time and patient risk factors would be expected and suggests that the efficacy may be very low in fully latent infections, leaving open the question of whether bacterial replication occurs at all in some cases. Furthermore, it is clear that the question of bacterial replication during latent infections is unanswered by a recent study that found no efficacy of prophylaxis subsequent to treatment, even though prophylaxis itself prevented tuberculosis during the course of therapy [127]. All of these observations suggest that there are likely multiple routes to latent infections and that many bacterial states can exist in patients that are classified as latently infected.

The fact that multiple routes could lead to latent infections makes it difficult to completely prevent latency, but greater insight into how, where and why latency occurs could allow better management. The fact that there are very low numbers of bacteria present during latent infections offers the potential that they may not be recognized well by the immune system and vaccination to stimulate a response could help eliminate them from tissues. The large number of latent infections worldwide makes developing strategies to combat this stage of infection critical to reducing tuberculosis worldwide, whether or not reactivation can be prevented. Our understanding of the complexity of signals involved in latency has expanded over time (Fig. 1), but each pathway involved represents a potential target for therapeutics or modulation of the signal to interfere with entry or exit from latency. Transmission after reactivation to new populations can be prevented if initiation of latent infections, persistence or reactivation can be interfered with and lead to clearance of infection. Since many of the signals thought to be involved in latency and reactivation are accessible extracellularly, they represent excellent targets for small molecules that could interfere with or modulate their pathways to result in better host-response mediated killing of the bacteria. Future studies will be focused on better understanding the specific niche(s) occupied by *M. tuberculosis* during latent infections as well as the levels of different signals involved. Only through an improved understanding of these signals and the environment where the bacteria are located will it be possible to utilize this relatively unique stage of disease, that the majority of patients are in and lasts the longest period of time, to combat tuberculosis and potentially eradicate one of the most successful bacterial pathogens of humans worldwide.

Acknowledgements We thank Raul Barletta for critical review of the manuscript.

Funding Information NIH, NIAID provided funding to Jeffrey D. Cirillo under grant number R01AI104960.

References

1. Ippoliti C. WHO targets elimination of TB in over 30 countries. Cent Eur J Public Health. 2014;22(3):158–63. WHO/ERS joint news release, July 3, 2014.
2. WHO. Global tuberculosis report 2013. Geneva: World Health Organization; 2013.
3. WHO. Global tuberculosis report 2016. Geneva: World Health Organization; 2016.
4. Bloom BR, Murray CJL. Tuberculosis: commentary on a reemergent killer. Science. 1992;257:1055–64.
5. Gedde-Dahl T. Tuberculous infection in the light of tuberculin matriculation. Am J Hyg. 1952;56:139–214.
6. Lillebaek T, Dirksen A, Baess I, Strunge B, Thomsen VO, Andersen AB. Molecular evidence of endogenous reactivation of *Mycobacterium tuberculosis* after 33 years of latent infection. J Infect Dis. 2002;185:401–4.
7. Parrish NM, Dick JD, Bishai WR. Mechanisms of latency in *Mycobacterium tuberculosis*. Trends Microbiol. 1998;6:107–12.
8. Vynnycky E, Fine PE. Lifetime risks, incubation period, and serial interval of tuberculosis. Am J Epidemiol. 2000;152:247–63.
9. Barry CE 3rd, Boshoff HI, Dartois V, Dick T, Ehrt S, Flynn J, Schnappinger D, Wilkinson RJ, Young D. The spectrum of latent tuberculosis: rethinking the biology and intervention strategies. Nat Rev Microbiol. 2009;7:845–55.
10. Manina G, Dhar N, McKinney JD. Stress and host immunity amplify *Mycobacterium tuberculosis* phenotypic heterogeneity and induce nongrowing metabolically active forms. Cell Host Microbe. 2015;17:32–46.
11. Gideon HP, Flynn JL. Latent tuberculosis: what the host "sees"? Immunol Res. 2011;50:202–12.
12. Gill WP, Harik NS, Whiddon MR, Liao RP, Mittler JE, Sherman DR. A replication clock for *Mycobacterium tuberculosis*. Nat Med. 2009;15:211–4.
13. Munoz-Elias EJ, Timm J, Botha T, Chan WT, Gomez JE, McKinney JD. Replication dynamics of *Mycobacterium tuberculosis* in chronically infected mice. Infect Immun. 2005;73:546–51.
14. Tufariello JM, Chan J, Flynn JL. Latent tuberculosis: mechanisms of host and bacillus that contribute to persistent infection. Lancet Infect Dis. 2003;3:578–90.
15. Wayne LG, Hayes LG. An in vitro model for sequential study of shiftdown of *Mycobacterium tuberculosis* through two stages of nonreplicating persistence. Infect Immun. 1996;64:2062–9.
16. McCune RM Jr, McDermott W, Tompsett R. The fate of *Mycobacterium tuberculosis* in mouse tissues as determined by the microbial enumeration technique. II. The conversion of tuberculous infection to the latent state by the administration of pyrazinamide and a companion drug. J Exp Med. 1956;104:763–802.
17. McCune RM Jr, Tompsett R. Fate of *Mycobacterium tuberculosis* in mouse tissues as determined by the microbial enumeration technique. I. The persistence of drug-susceptible tubercle bacilli in the tissues despite prolonged antimicrobial therapy. J Exp Med. 1956;104:737–62.

18. Scanga CA, Mohan VP, Joseph H, Yu K, Chan J, Flynn JL. Reactivation of latent tuberculosis: variations on the Cornell murine model. Infect Immun. 1999;67:4531–8.
19. Cunningham AF, Spreadbury CL. Mycobacterial stationary phase induced by low oxygen tension: cell wall thickening and localization of the 16-kilodalton alpha-crystallin homolog. J Bacteriol. 1998;180:801–8.
20. Gold B, Warrier T, Nathan C. A multi-stress model for high throughput screening against non-replicating *Mycobacterium tuberculosis*. Methods Mol Biol. 2015;1285:293–315.
21. Imboden P, Schoolnik GK. Construction and characterization of a partial *Mycobacterium tuberculosis* cDNA library of genes expressed at reduced oxygen tension. Gene. 1998;213:107–17.
22. McKinney JD, Zu Bentrup KH, Munoz-Elias EJ, Miczak A, Chen B, Chan W-T, Swenson D, Sacchettini JC, Jacobs WR Jr, Russell DG. Persistence of *Mycobacterium tuberculosis* in macrophages and mice requires the glyoxylate shunt enzyme isocitrate lyase. Nature. 2000;406:735–8.
23. Hernandez-Pando R, Jeyanathan M, Mengistu G, Aguilar D, Orozco H, Harboe M, Rook GA, Bjune G. Persistence of DNA from *Mycobacterium tuberculosis* in superficially normal lung tissue during latent infection. Lancet. 2000;356:2133–8.
24. Opie EL, Aronson JD. Tubercle bacilli in latent tuberculosis lesions and in lung tissue without tuberculous lesions. Arch Pathol Lab Med. 1927;4:1–21.
25. Scanga CA, Mohan VP, Yu K, Joseph H, Tanaka K, Chan J, Flynn JL. Depletion of CD4(+) T cells causes reactivation of murine persistent tuberculosis despite continued expression of interferon gamma and nitric oxide synthase 2. J Exp Med. 2000;192:347–58.
26. Forrellad MA, McNeil M, Santangelo Mde L, Blanco FC, Garcia E, Klepp LI, Huff J, Niederweis M, Jackson M, Bigi F. Role of the Mce1 transporter in the lipid homeostasis of Mycobacterium tuberculosis. Tuberculosis (Edinb). 2014;94:170–7.
27. Khan S, Islam A, Hassan MI, Ahmad F. Purification and structural characterization of Mce4A from *Mycobacterium tuberculosis*. Int J Biol Macromol. 2016;93:235–41.
28. Pandey AK, Sassetti CM. Mycobacterial persistence requires the utilization of host cholesterol. Proc Natl Acad Sci U S A. 2008;105:4376–80.
29. Daniel J, Sirakova T, Kolattukudy P. An acyl-CoA synthetase in *Mycobacterium tuberculosis* involved in triacylglycerol accumulation during dormancy. PLoS One. 2014;9:e114877.
30. McGillivray A, Golden NA, Kaushal D. The *Mycobacterium tuberculosis* Clp gene regulator is required for in vitro reactivation from hypoxia-induced dormancy. J Biol Chem. 2015;290:2351–67.
31. Banaiee N, Jacobs WR Jr, Ernst JD. Regulation of Mycobacterium tuberculosis whiB3 in the mouse lung and macrophages. Infect Immun. 2006;74:6449–57.
32. Gonzalo Asensio J, Maia C, Ferrer NL, Barilone N, Laval F, Soto CY, Winter N, Daffe M, Gicquel B, Martin C, Jackson M. The virulence-associated two-component PhoP-PhoR system controls the biosynthesis of polyketide-derived lipids in Mycobacterium tuberculosis. J Biol Chem. 2006;281:1313–6.
33. He H, Hovey R, Kane J, Singh V, Zahrt TC. Mprab is a stress-responsive two-component system that directly regulates expression of sigma factors SigB and SigE in Mycobacterium tuberculosis. J Bacteriol. 2006;188:2134–43.
34. Mukamolova GV, Turapov OA, Young DI, Kaprelyants AS, Kell DB, Young M. A family of autocrine growth factors in Mycobacterium tuberculosis. Mol Microbiol. 2002;46:623–35.
35. Primm TP, Andersen SJ, Mizrahi V, Avarbock D, Rubin H, Barry CE 3rd. The stringent response of Mycobacterium tuberculosis is required for long-term survival. J Bacteriol. 2000;182:4889–98.
36. Sherman DR, Voskuil M, Schnappinger D, Liao R, Harrell MI, Schoolnik GK. Regulation of the Mycobacterium tuberculosis hypoxic response gene encoding alpha -crystallin. Proc Natl Acad Sci U S A. 2001;98:7534–9.
37. Voskuil MI, Schnappinger D, Visconti KC, Harrell MI, Dolganov GM, Sherman DR, Schoolnik GK. Inhibition of respiration by nitric oxide induces a Mycobacterium tuberculosis dormancy program. J Exp Med. 2003;198:705–13.

38. Zahrt TC, Deretic V. Mycobacterium tuberculosis signal transduction system required for persistent infections. Proc Natl Acad Sci U S A. 2001;98:12706–11.
39. Sureka K, Ghosh B, Dasgupta A, Basu J, Kundu M, Bose I. Positive feedback and noise activate the stringent response regulator rel in mycobacteria. PLoS One. 2008;3:e1771.
40. Micklinghoff JC, Breitinger KJ, Schmidt M, Geffers R, Eikmanns BJ, Bange FC. Role of the transcriptional regulator RamB (Rv0465c) in the control of the glyoxylate cycle in Mycobacterium tuberculosis. J Bacteriol. 2009;191:7260–9.
41. Lee JH, Geiman DE, Bishai WR. Role of stress response sigma factor SigG in Mycobacterium tuberculosis. J Bacteriol. 2008;190:1128–33.
42. Manganelli R, Voskuil MI, Schoolnik GK, Smith I. The Mycobacterium tuberculosis ECF sigma factor sigmaE: role in global gene expression and survival in macrophages. Mol Microbiol. 2001;41:423–37.
43. Gonzalo-Asensio J, Mostowy S, Harders-Westerveen J, Huygen K, Hernandez-Pando R, Thole J, Behr M, Gicquel B, Martin C. PhoP: a missing piece in the intricate puzzle of Mycobacterium tuberculosis virulence. PLoS One. 2008;3:e3496.
44. Sinha A, Gupta S, Bhutani S, Pathak A, Sarkar D. PhoP-PhoP interaction at adjacent PhoP binding sites is influenced by protein phosphorylation. J Bacteriol. 2008;190:1317–28.
45. Walters SB, Dubnau E, Kolesnikova I, Laval F, Daffe M, Smith I. The Mycobacterium tuberculosis PhoPR two-component system regulates genes essential for virulence and complex lipid biosynthesis. Mol Microbiol. 2006;60:312–30.
46. Guo M, Feng H, Zhang J, Wang W, Wang Y, Li Y, Gao C, Chen H, Feng Y, He ZG. Dissecting transcription regulatory pathways through a new bacterial one-hybrid reporter system. Genome Res. 2009;19:1301–8.
47. Boon C, Dick T. How Mycobacterium tuberculosis goes to sleep: the dormancy survival regulator DosR a decade later. Future Microbiol. 2012;7:513–8.
48. Lenaerts AJ, Hoff D, Aly S, Ehlers S, Andries K, Cantarero L, Orme IM, Basaraba RJ. Location of persisting mycobacteria in the Guinea pig model of tuberculosis revealed by R207910. Antimicrob Agents Chemother. 2007;51:3338–45.
49. Rustad TR, Sherrid AM, Minch KJ, Sherman DR. Hypoxia: a window into Mycobacterium tuberculosis latency. Cell Microbiol. 2009;11:1151–9.
50. Schreuder LJ, Parish T. Mycobacterium tuberculosis DosR is required for activity of the PmbtB and PmbtI promoters under hypoxia. PLoS One. 2014;9:e107283.
51. Via LE, Lin PL, Ray SM, Carrillo J, Allen SS, Eum SY, Taylor K, Klein E, Manjunatha U, Gonzales J, Lee EG, Park SK, Raleigh JA, Cho SN, McMurray DN, Flynn JL, Barry CE 3rd. Tuberculous granulomas are hypoxic in Guinea pigs, rabbits, and nonhuman primates. Infect Immun. 2008;76:2333–40.
52. Rodriguez JG, Hernandez AC, Helguera-Repetto C, Aguilar Ayala D, Guadarrama-Medina R, Anzola JM, Bustos JR, Zambrano MM, Gonzalez YMJ, Garcia MJ, Del Portillo P. Global adaptation to a lipid environment triggers the dormancy-related phenotype of Mycobacterium tuberculosis. MBio. 2014;5:e01125–14.
53. Ranganathan S, Bai G, Lyubetskaya A, Knapp GS, Peterson MW, Gazdik M, Al CG, Galagan JE, McDonough KA. Characterization of a camp responsive transcription factor, Cmr (Rv1675c), in TB complex mycobacteria reveals overlap with the DosR (DevR) dormancy regulon. Nucleic Acids Res. 2016;44:134–51.
54. Avarbock A, Avarbock D, Teh JS, Buckstein M, Wang ZM, Rubin H. Functional regulation of the opposing (p)ppGpp synthetase/hydrolase activities of RelMtb from Mycobacterium tuberculosis. Biochemistry. 2005;44:9913–23.
55. Boutte CC, Crosson S. Bacterial lifestyle shapes stringent response activation. Trends Microbiol. 2013;21:174–80.
56. Dahl JL, Kraus CN, Boshoff HI, Doan B, Foley K, Avarbock D, Kaplan G, Mizrahi V, Rubin H, Barry CE 3rd. The role of RelMtb-mediated adaptation to stationary phase in long-term persistence of Mycobacterium tuberculosis in mice. Proc Natl Acad Sci U S A. 2003;100:10026–31.

57. Rifat D, Bishai WR, Karakousis PC. Phosphate depletion: a novel trigger for *Mycobacterium tuberculosis* persistence. J Infect Dis. 2009;200:1126–35.
58. Weiss LA, Stallings CL. Essential roles for *Mycobacterium tuberculosis* Rel beyond the production of (p)ppGpp. J Bacteriol. 2013;195:5629–38.
59. Das B, Kashino SS, Pulu I, Kalita D, Swami V, Yeger H, Felsher DW, Campos-Neto A. CD271(+) bone marrow mesenchymal stem cells may provide a niche for dormant *Mycobacterium tuberculosis*. Sci Transl Med. 2013;5:170ra13.
60. Garhyan J, Bhuyan S, Pulu I, Kalita D, Das B, Bhatnagar R. Preclinical and clinical evidence of *Mycobacterium tuberculosis* persistence in the hypoxic niche of bone marrow mesenchymal stem cells after therapy. Am J Pathol. 2015;185:1924–34.
61. Tornack J, Reece ST, Bauer WM, Vogelzang A, Bandermann S, Zedler U, Stingl G, Kaufmann SH, Melchers F. Human and mouse hematopoietic stem cells are a depot for dormant mycobacterium tuberculosis. PLoS One. 2017;12:e0169119.
62. Deb C, Lee CM, Dubey VS, Daniel J, Abomoelak B, Sirakova TD, Pawar S, Rogers L, Kolattukudy PE. A novel in vitro multiple-stress dormancy model for *Mycobacterium tuberculosis* generates a lipid-loaded, drug-tolerant, dormant pathogen. PLoS One. 2009;4:e6077.
63. Carroll MW, Jeon D, Mountz JM, Lee JD, Jeong YJ, Zia N, Lee M, Lee J, Via LE, Lee S, Eum SY, Lee SJ, Goldfeder LC, Cai Y, Jin B, Kim Y, Oh T, Chen RY, Dodd LE, Gu W, Dartois V, Park SK, Kim CT, Barry CE 3rd, Cho SN. Efficacy and safety of metronidazole for pulmonary multidrug-resistant tuberculosis. Antimicrob Agents Chemother. 2013;57:3903–9.
64. Desai CR, Heera S, Patel A, Babrekar AB, Mahashur AA, Kamat SR. Role of metronidazole in improving response and specific drug sensitivity in advanced pulmonary tuberculosis. J Assoc Physicians India. 1989;37:694–7.
65. Lin PL, Flynn JL. Understanding latent tuberculosis: a moving target. J Immunol. 2010;185:15–22.
66. Lin PL, Ford CB, Coleman MT, Myers AJ, Gawande R, Ioerger T, Sacchettini J, Fortune SM, Flynn JL. Sterilization of granulomas is common in active and latent tuberculosis despite within-host variability in bacterial killing. Nat Med. 2014;20:75–9.
67. Lin PL, Maiello P, Gideon HP, Coleman MT, Cadena AM, Rodgers MA, Gregg R, O'malley M, Tomko J, Fillmore D, Frye LJ, Rutledge T, Difazio RM, Janssen C, Klein E, Andersen PL, Fortune SM, Flynn JL. Pet CT identifies reactivation risk in cynomolgus macaques with latent *M. tuberculosis*. PLoS Pathog. 2016;12:e1005739.
68. Lin PL, Pawar S, Myers A, Pegu A, Fuhrman C, Reinhart TA, Capuano SV, Klein E, Flynn JL. Early events in *Mycobacterium tuberculosis* infection in cynomolgus macaques. Infect Immun. 2006;74:3790–803.
69. Lin PL, Rodgers M, Smith L, Bigbee M, Myers A, Bigbee C, Chiosea I, Capuano SV, Fuhrman C, Klein E, Flynn JL. Quantitative comparison of active and latent tuberculosis in the cynomolgus macaque model. Infect Immun. 2009;77:4631–42.
70. Jacobs WR Jr, Kalpana GV, Cirillo JD, Pascopella L, Udani RA, Jones WD Jr, Barletta RG, Bloom BR. Genetic systems for the mycobacteria. Methods Enzymol. 1991;204:537–55.
71. Jacobs WR Jr, Tuckman M, Bloom BR. Introduction of foreign DNA into mycobacteria using a shuttle phasmid. Nature. 1987;327:532–6.
72. Gautam US, McGillivray A, Mehra S, Didier PJ, Midkiff CC, Kissee RS, Golden NA, Alvarez X, Niu T, Rengarajan J, Sherman DR, Kaushal D. DosS is required for the complete virulence of *Mycobacterium tuberculosis* in mice with classical granulomatous lesions. Am J Respir Cell Mol Biol. 2015;52:708–16.
73. Stallings CL, Stephanou NC, Chu L, Hochschild A, Nickels BE, Glickman MS. CarD is an essential regulator of rRNA transcription required for *Mycobacterium tuberculosis* persistence. Cell. 2009;138:146–59.
74. Ryndak MB, Singh KK, Peng Z, Laal S. Transcriptional profile of *Mycobacterium tuberculosis* replicating in type II alveolar epithelial cells. PLoS One. 2015;10:e0123745.
75. Fang H, Yu D, Hong Y, Zhou X, Li C, Sun B. The LuxR family regulator Rv0195 modulates *Mycobacterium tuberculosis* dormancy and virulence. Tuberculosis (Edinb). 2013;93:425–31.

76. Converse PJ, Karakousis PC, Klinkenberg LG, Kesavan AK, Ly LH, Allen SS, Grosset JH, Jain SK, Lamichhane G, Manabe YC, McMurray DN, Nuermberger EL, Bishai WR. The role of the dosR/dosS two-component regulatory system in *Mycobacterium tuberculosis* virulence in three animal models. Infect Immun. 2009;77:1230–7.
77. Cirillo SL, Subbian S, Chen B, Weisbrod TR, Jacobs WR Jr, Cirillo JD. Protection of *Mycobacterium tuberculosis* from reactive oxygen species conferred by the mel2 locus impacts persistence and dissemination. Infect Immun. 2009;77:2557–67.
78. Modlin RL, Bloom BR. TB or not TB: that is no longer the question. Sci Transl Med. 2013;5:213sr6.
79. Turapov O, O'connor BD, Sarybaeva AA, Williams C, Patel H, Kadyrov AS, Sarybaev AS, Woltmann G, Barer MR, Mukamolova GV. Phenotypically adapted *Mycobacterium tuberculosis* populations from sputum are tolerant to first-line drugs. Antimicrob Agents Chemother. 2016;60:2476–83.
80. Garton NJ, Waddell SJ, Sherratt AL, Lee SM, Smith RJ, Senner C, Hinds J, Rajakumar K, Adegbola RA, Besra GS, Butcher PD, Barer MR. Cytological and transcript analyses reveal fat and lazy persister-like bacilli in tuberculous sputum. PLoS Med. 2008;5:e75.
81. Mukamolova GV, Murzin AG, Salina EG, Demina GR, Kell DB, Kaprelyants AS, Young M. Muralytic activity of *Micrococcus luteus* Rpf and its relationship to physiological activity in promoting bacterial growth and resuscitation. Mol Microbiol. 2006;59:84–98.
82. Telkov MV, Demina GR, Voloshin SA, Salina EG, Dudik TV, Stekhanova TN, Mukamolova GV, Kazaryan KA, Goncharenko AV, Young M, Kaprelyants AS. Proteins of the Rpf (resuscitation promoting factor) family are peptidoglycan hydrolases. Biochemistry (Mosc). 2006;71:414–22.
83. Downing KJ, Mischenko VV, Shleeva MO, Young DI, Young M, Kaprelyants AS, Apt AS, Mizrahi V. Mutants of Mycobacterium tuberculosis lacking three of the five rpf-like genes are defective for growth in vivo and for resuscitation in vitro. Infect Immun. 2005;73:3038–43.
84. Kaprelyants AS, Gottschal JC, Kell DB. Dormancy in non-sporulating bacteria. FEMS Microbiol Rev. 1993;10:271–85.
85. Mukamolova GV, Kaprelyants AS, Kell DB, Young M. Adoption of the transiently non-culturable state--a bacterial survival strategy? Adv Microb Physiol. 2003;47:65–129.
86. Mukamolova GV, Kaprelyants AS, Young DI, Young M, Kell DB. A bacterial cytokine. Proc Natl Acad Sci U S A. 1998;95:8916–21.
87. Mukamolova GV, Turapov OA, Kazarian K, Telkov M, Kaprelyants AS, Kell DB, Young M. The rpf gene of Micrococcus luteus encodes an essential secreted growth factor. Mol Microbiol. 2002;46:611–21.
88. Mukamolova GV, Yanopolskaya ND, Kell DB, Kaprelyants AS. On resuscitation from the dormant state of Micrococcus luteus. Antonie Van Leeuwenhoek. 1998;73:237–43.
89. Cohen-Gonsaud M, Barthe P, Bagneris C, Henderson B, Ward J, Roumestand C, Keep NH. The structure of a resuscitation-promoting factor domain from Mycobacterium tuberculosis shows homology to lysozymes. Nat Struct Mol Biol. 2005;12:270–3.
90. Cohen-Gonsaud M, Keep NH, Davies AP, Ward J, Henderson B, Labesse G. Resuscitation-promoting factors possess a lysozyme-like domain. Trends Biochem Sci. 2004;29:7–10.
91. Dziarski R, Gupta D. Review: mammalian peptidoglycan recognition proteins (PGRPs) in innate immunity. Innate Immun. 2010;16:168–74.
92. Gelius E, Persson C, Karlsson J, Steiner H. A mammalian peptidoglycan recognition protein with N-acetylmuramoyl-L-alanine amidase activity. Biochem Biophys Res Commun. 2003;306:988–94.
93. Long R, Gardam M. Tumour necrosis factor-alpha inhibitors and the reactivation of latent tuberculosis infection. CMAJ. 2003;168:1153–6.
94. Manabe YC, Kesavan AK, Lopez-Molina J, Hatem CL, Brooks M, Fujiwara R, Hochstein K, Pitt ML, Tufariello J, Chan J, McMurray DN, Bishai WR, Dannenberg AM Jr, Mendez S. The aerosol rabbit model of TB latency, reactivation and immune reconstitution inflammatory syndrome. Tuberculosis (Edinb). 2008;88:187–96.

95. Miller EA, Ernst JD. Anti-TNF immunotherapy and tuberculosis reactivation: another mechanism revealed. J Clin Invest. 2009;119:1079–82.
96. Tufariello JM, Mi K, Xu J, Manabe YC, Kesavan AK, Drumm J, Tanaka K, Jacobs WR Jr, Chan J. Deletion of the *Mycobacterium tuberculosis* resuscitation-promoting factor Rv1009 gene results in delayed reactivation from chronic tuberculosis. Infect Immun. 2006;74:2985–95.
97. Cheng Y, Xie H, Sule P, Hassounah H, Graviss EA, Kong Y, Cirillo JD, Rao J. Fluorogenic probes with substitutions at the 2 and 7 positions of cephalosporin are highly BlaC-specific for rapid *Mycobacterium tuberculosis* detection. Angew Chem Int Ed Engl. 2014;53:9360–4.
98. Kong Y, Yao H, REN H, Subbian S, Cirillo SL, Sacchettini JC, Rao J, Cirillo JD. Imaging tuberculosis with endogenous beta-lactamase reporter enzyme fluorescence in live mice. Proc Natl Acad Sci U S A. 2010;107:12239–44.
99. Xie H, Mire J, Kong Y, Chang M, Hassounah HA, Thornton CN, Sacchettini JC, Cirillo JD, Rao J. Rapid point-of-care detection of the tuberculosis pathogen using a BlaC-specific fluorogenic probe. Nat Chem. 2012;4:802–9.
100. Yang HJ, Kong Y, Cheng Y, Janagama H, Hassounah H, Xie H, Rao J, Cirillo JD. Real-time imaging of *Mycobacterium tuberculosis*, using a novel near-infrared fluorescent substrate. J Infect Dis. 2017;215:405–14.
101. Serra-Vidal MM, Latorre I, Franken KL, Diaz J, De Souza-Galvao ML, Casas I, Maldonado J, Mila C, Solsona J, Jimenez-Fuentes MA, Altet N, Lacoma A, Ruiz-Manzano J, Ausina V, Prat C, Ottenhoff TH, Dominguez J. Immunogenicity of 60 novel latency-related antigens of Mycobacterium tuberculosis. Front Microbiol. 2014;5:517.
102. Black GF, Thiel BA, Ota MO, Parida SK, Adegbola R, Boom WH, Dockrell HM, Franken KL, Friggen AH, Hill PC, Klein MR, Lalor MK, Mayanja H, Schoolnik G, Stanley K, Weldingh K, Kaufmann SH, Walzl G, Ottenhoff TH, GCGH Biomarkers for TB Consortium. Immunogenicity of novel DosR regulon-encoded candidate antigens of Mycobacterium tuberculosis in three high-burden populations in Africa. Clin Vaccine Immunol. 2009;16:1203–12.
103. Nooshabadi F, Yang HJ, Cheng Y, Durkee MS, Xie H, Rao J, Cirillo JD, Maitland KC. Intravital excitation increases detection sensitivity for pulmonary tuberculosis by whole-body imaging with beta-lactamase reporter enzyme fluorescence. J Biophotonics. 2016;10(6–7):821–9.
104. Sutherland JS, Lalor MK, Black GF, Ambrose LR, Loxton AG, Chegou NN, Kassa D, Mihret A, Howe R, Mayanja-Kizza H, Gomez MP, Donkor S, Franken K, Hanekom W, Klein MR, Parida SK, Boom WH, Thiel BA, Crampin AC, Ota M, Walzl G, Ottenhoff TH, Dockrell HM, Kaufmann SH, GCGH Biomarkers for TB consortium. Analysis of host responses to *Mycobacterium tuberculosis* antigens in a multi-site study of subjects with different TB and HIV infection states in sub-Saharan Africa. PLoS One. 2013;8:e74080.
105. Adekambi T, Ibegbu CC, Cagle S, Kalokhe AS, Wang YF, Hu Y, Day CL, Ray SM, Rengarajan J. Biomarkers on patient T cells diagnose active tuberculosis and monitor treatment response. J Clin Invest. 2015;125:1827–38.
106. Adekambi T, Ibegbu CC, Kalokhe AS, Yu T, Ray SM, Rengarajan J. Distinct effector memory CD4+ T cell signatures in latent Mycobacterium tuberculosis infection, Bcg vaccination and clinically resolved tuberculosis. PLoS One. 2012;7:e36046.
107. Schuetz A, Haule A, Reither K, Ngwenyama N, Rachow A, Meyerhans A, Maboko L, Koup RA, Hoelscher M, Geldmacher C. Monitoring CD27 expression to evaluate *Mycobacterium tuberculosis* activity in HIV-1 infected individuals in vivo. PLoS One. 2011;6:e27284.
108. Chegou NN, Black GF, Loxton AG, Stanley K, Essone PN, Klein MR, Parida SK, Kaufmann SH, Doherty TM, Friggen AH, Franken KL, Ottenhoff TH, Walzl G. Potential of novel *Mycobacterium tuberculosis* infection phase-dependent antigens in the diagnosis of Tb disease in a high burden setting. BMC Infect Dis. 2012;12:10.
109. Chegou NN, Essone PN, Loxton AG, Stanley K, Black GF, Van Der Spuy GD, Van Helden PD, Franken KL, Parida SK, Klein MR, Kaufmann SH, Ottenhoff TH, Walzl G. Potential of host markers produced by infection phase-dependent antigen-stimulated cells for the diagnosis of tuberculosis in a highly endemic area. PLoS One. 2012;7:e38501.

110. Kimuda SG, Nalwoga A, Levin J, Franken KL, Ottenhoff TH, Elliott AM, Cose S, Andia-Biraro I. Humoral responses to Rv1733c, Rv0081, Rv1735c, and Rv1737c DosR Regulon-encoded proteins of Mycobacterium tuberculosis in individuals with latent tuberculosis infection. J Immunol Res. 2017;2017:1593143.
111. Leyten EM, Lin MY, Franken KL, Friggen AH, Prins C, Van Meijgaarden KE, Voskuil MI, Weldingh K, Andersen P, Schoolnik GK, Arend SM, Ottenhoff TH, Klein MR. Human T-cell responses to 25 novel antigens encoded by genes of the dormancy regulon of Mycobacterium tuberculosis. Microbes Infect. 2006;8:2052–60.
112. Lin MY, Geluk A, Smith SG, Stewart AL, Friggen AH, Franken KL, Verduyn MJ, Van Meijgaarden KE, Voskuil MI, Dockrell HM, Huygen K, Ottenhoff TH, Klein MR. Lack of immune responses to Mycobacterium tuberculosis DosR regulon proteins following Mycobacterium bovis BCG vaccination. Infect Immun. 2007;75:3523–30.
113. Slavin RE, Walsh TJ, Pollack AD. Late generalized tuberculosis: a clinical pathologic analysis and comparison of 100 cases in the preantibiotic and antibiotic eras. Medicine (Baltimore). 1980;59:352–66.
114. Horsburgh CR, O'donnell M, Chamblee S, Moreland JL, Johnson J, Marsh BJ, Narita M, Johnson LS, Von Reyn CF. Revisiting rates of reactivation tuberculosis. Am J Respir Crit Care Med. 2010;182:420–5.
115. Anderson ST, Kaforou M, Brent AJ, Wright VJ, Banwell CM, Chagaluka G, Crampin AC, Dockrell HM, French N, Hamilton MS, Hibberd ML, Kern F, Langford PR, Ling L, Mlotha R, Ottenhoff THM, Pienaar S, Pillay V, Scott JAG, Twahir H, Wilkinson RJ, Coin LJ, Heyderman RS, Levin M, Eley B. Diagnosis of childhood tuberculosis and host Rna expression in Africa. N Engl J Med. 2014;370:1712–23.
116. Escalante P, Peikert T, Van Keulen VP, Erskine CL, Bornhorst CL, Andrist BR, McCoy K, Pease LR, Abraham RS, Knutson KL, Kita H, Schrum AG, Limper AH. Combinatorial immunoprofiling in latent tuberculosis infection. Toward better risk stratification. Am J Respir Crit Care Med. 2015;192:605–17.
117. Kaforou M, Wright VJ, Oni T, French N, Anderson ST, Bangani N, Banwell CM, Brent AJ, Crampin AC, Dockrell HM, Eley B, Heyderman RS, Hibberd ML, Kern F, Langford PR, Ling L, Mendelson M, Ottenhoff TH, Zgambo F, Wilkinson RJ, Coin LJ, Levin M. Detection of tuberculosis in HIV-infected and -uninfected African adults using whole blood RNA expression signatures: a case-control study. PLoS Med. 2013;10:e1001538.
118. Zak D, Scriba TJ, Hatherill M, Penn-Nicholson A, Hanekom W. Predicting tuberculosis risk – Authors' reply. Lancet. 2016;388:2233–4.
119. Zak DE, Penn-Nicholson A, Scriba TJ, Thompson E, Suliman S, Amon LM, Mahomed H, Erasmus M, Whatney W, Hussey GD, Abrahams D, Kafaar F, Hawkridge T, Verver S, Hughes EJ, Ota M, Sutherland J, Howe R, Dockrell HM, Boom WH, Thiel B, Ottenhoff TH, Mayanja-Kizza H, Crampin AC, Downing K, Hatherill M, Valvo J, Shankar S, Parida SK, Kaufmann SH, Walzl G, Aderem A, Hanekom WA, ACS and GC6-74 cohort study groups. A blood RNA signature for tuberculosis disease risk: a prospective cohort study. Lancet. 2016;387:2312–22.
120. Schubert OT, Ludwig C, Kogadeeva M, Zimmermann M, Rosenberger G, Gengenbacher M, Gillet LC, Collins BC, Rost HL, Kaufmann SH, Sauer U, Aebersold R. Absolute proteome composition and dynamics during dormancy and resuscitation of *Mycobacterium tuberculosis*. Cell Host Microbe. 2015;18:96–108.
121. Semu M, Fenta TG, Medhin G, Assefa D. Effectiveness of isoniazid preventative therapy in reducing incidence of active tuberculosis among people living with HIV/AIDS in public health facilities of Addis Ababa, Ethiopia: a historical cohort study. BMC Infect Dis. 2017;17:5.
122. International Union Against Tuberculosis Committee on Prophylaxis. Efficacy of various durations of isoniazid preventive therapy for tuberculosis: five years of follow-up in the IUAT trial. Bull World Health Organ. 1982;60:555–64.

123. Ai JW, Ruan QL, Liu QH, Zhang WH. Updates on the risk factors for latent tuberculosis reactivation and their managements. Emerg Microbes Infect. 2016;5:e10.
124. Comstock GW, Ferebee SH, Hammes LM. A controlled trial of community-wide isoniazid prophylaxis in Alaska. Am Rev Respir Dis. 1967;95:935–43.
125. Ferebee SH. Long-term effects of isoniazid prophylaxis. Bull Int Union Tuberc. 1968;41:161–6.
126. Ferebee SH. Controlled chemoprophylaxis trials in tuberculosis. A general review. Bibl Tuberc. 1970;26:28–106.
127. Churchyard GJ, Fielding KL, Grant AD. A trial of mass isoniazid preventive therapy for tuberculosis control. N Engl J Med. 2014;370:1662–3.

Trehalose Dimycolate (Cord Factor) as a Contributing Factor to Tuberculosis Pathogenesis

Jeffrey K. Actor

Abstract This chapter examines mycobacterial glycolipid trehalose 6,6′-dimycolate (TDM; cord factor) as it relates to the development of tuberculosis (TB) pathogenesis. TDM, a major surface glycolipid, is recognized as the most widely studied "virulence factor" of *Mycobacterium tuberculosis* (MTB). It is the most abundant glycolipid on the surface of mycobacterial species and contributes to organism morphology. Although it is known to play multiple roles in models of TB pathogenesis, direct understanding of how it leads to development of clinical disease states during tuberculosis disease is not yet clear. TDM induces the production of proinflammatory cytokines and chemokines from innate macrophages. It can also induce defined lung pathologies to mimic many aspects of primary MTB infection, including induction of activated foreign body granulomas and pneumonitis in naïve mice, and hypersensitive immune granulomas or hyper-coagulation in sensitized mice. Identification of numerous potential host receptors for this glycolipid has triggered renewed investigation into the importance of TDM in the clinical manifestation of disease. Here, a historical review is presented to support regulated innate and adaptive immune responses to cord factor which have potential to affect development of related pathologies. Examination of recent hypotheses that link its physical structure to development of post primary disease is also discussed.

Keywords Trehalose 6,6′-dimycolate · TDM · Cord factor · Mycobacterial glycolipid · Tuberculosis pathogenesis

J. K. Actor (✉)
Department of Pathology and Laboratory Medicine, University of Texas-Houston McGovern Medical School, Houston, TX, USA
e-mail: Jeffrey.K.Actor@uth.tmc.edu

J. D. Cirillo, Y. Kong (eds.), *Tuberculosis Host-Pathogen Interactions*,
https://doi.org/10.1007/978-3-030-25381-3_3

Introduction

The History of Cord Factor

In the 1880s Robert Koch released a series of published works detailing how microorganisms could be the cause of consumption and cavitary disease in humans [1–4]. The organisms were discovered to be mycobacteria, identified as rod-shaped "vibriones", which were responsible for purulent deposits leading to lung disorder. However, It was not until the mid-twentieth century that Hubert Bloch identified the surface extract of MTB as the cause of the observed cachexia following repeated administration [5–9]. The major components were eventually isolated, and defined as the lipid-rich constituents of the cell mycobacterial wall. One of those lipids was eventually discovered to be primarily responsible for organisms to interact with each other to form serpentine cords [10, 11]; thus identified descriptively as "cord factor". Kato and Meada were the first to isolate and prescribe the biochemical activities of cord factor, attributing activities to both the monomycolate and dimycolic acid forms [12, 13], with the dimycolate form having biological attributes responsible for directing pathology that mimics a form of primary tuberculosis lung disease [14].

Cord factor, officially trehalose 6,6′-dimycolate (TDM), may be considered the most studied and most prevalent virulence factor of MTB [6, 11, 15–17]. TDM is an external constituent of *Mycobacterium tuberculosis* (MTB). Over the course of 150 years, many studies have been completed to produce a deeper understanding of cord factor's value toward immune pathogenesis. The complexities of the physical nature of the molecule make it difficult to study. It is likely that the biological properties are dictated by cord factor's physical form and presence in unique microenvironments. Only recently have investigators appreciated this aspect of cord factor to speculate upon its physical state to influence bio-pathogenesis.

Lipids comprising the capsule of virulent MTB are varied. The most easily extractable of these lipids is TDM [18–20]. It has been known for nearly seven decades that modification of mycobacterial surface lipids greatly interferes with the organism's virulence [8]. More recently, it has been confirmed that MTB uses lipid products, such as TDM, to manipulate the local microenvironment to insure survival within macrophages and host cells [21–24].

Cord factor is a petroleum ether-soluble, surfactant extractable, lipid constituent component of virulent mycobacterial organisms [5–7, 15, 25]. Original observations attributed TDM with toxic properties [9, 26, 27]. It has since been discovered that TDM containing extracts also contained strong antigenic [28] and adjuvant properties [29, 30]. Many of the biological properties assigned to TDM appeared in contradiction with each other; it is now well accepted that function is strongly dependent upon the physical forms induced when different isolation techniques, formulation, and administration methodologies are used experimentally.

Trehalose 6,6'-dimycolate (TDM)

The mycobacterial surface lipids have been well described [31–35] and their physical localization in relation to each other on the cell membrane have been represented multiple times in the literature. The mycobacterium ssp. are characterized by the presence of a rich mycolic acid containing outer layer, which confers an efficient permeability barrier to therapeutics. The mycolic acids within the outermost layer of *M. tuberculosis* represent unique components with high antigenicity to stimulate innate (macrophage) activity [36]. The long mycolic acid chain in *M. tuberculosis* consists of 50–60 carbons, with an extended α-carbon branch. The total number of carbons in the mycolic acid methyl ester of TDM is reported to be between 74 and 90 carbons [37]. TDM is a cyclopropanated molecule [38], containing "kinks" in the carbon chain which are hypothesized to provide a distinctive molecular rigidity critical for regulating physical interactions and hydrophobic properties. TDM is synthesized both within and external to organisms; the pathways of mycolic acid production have been defined and described elsewhere [39–41]. The final step in TDM synthesis is the attachment of mycolic acids to trehalose by mycolyl transferases [42]. Disruption of the genes encoding enzymes responsible for the synthesis of TDM on *M. tuberculosis* directly affects growth in culture and within macrophages [43]. Of interest, TDM can be removed by gentle organic solvents or detergents without killing the organism, however its removal does affect overall virulence [8, 21, 24]; TDM will repopulate after removal, coinciding with recovery of organism virulence.

Physical Forms of TDM

The long chain mycolic acids that comprise TDM allow for non-covalent hydrophobic interaction with other surface lipids, such as lipoarabinomannan (LAM). The loose association has a benefit, in that TDM may be shed under appropriate conditions, such as during excess production or when organisms enter into conditions of environmental stress (e.g. the intracellular phagosome host compartment). While on the organism, it forms a protective coat, perhaps contributing through increased hydrophobicity. In 1993, Behling, et al. proposed a model by which cord factor allowed development of the cording properties [44]. This was followed by another monograph detailing the potential for TDM to form a rigid layer under immobilized and defined conditions [45]. Much of the structure could be explained through biophysical realization of the long-chain esterified mycolic acid arranged in a repeating lattice. That particular study suggested that the hydrophobic regions regulated "spreading" on a matrix, which resulted in exposure of the trehalose to the hydrophilic environment.

The biological properties of TDM are likely attributed to self-assembling physical forms [46, 47], hypothesized to be based in large part on biochemical/hydrophobic

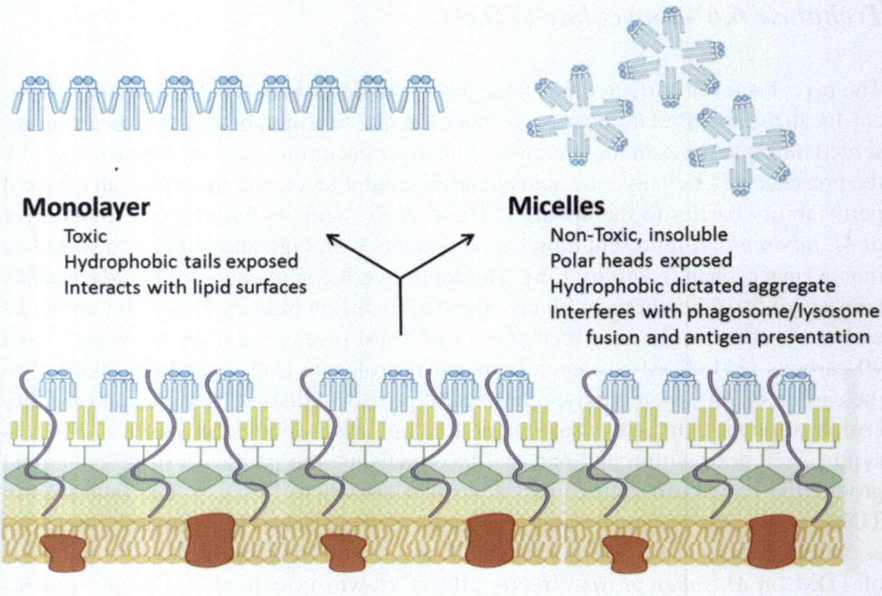

Fig. 1 Theoretical structure of TDM released from the mycobacterial surface. Two theoretical structures of TDM are depicted as released from virulent organisms. TDM can assume a toxic crystalline monolayer at the interface between the hydrophobic and aqueous surface, which likely happens when contact with lipids *in vivo* occurs, leaving trehalose exposed to bodily fluids or air when occurring in the lung (left). Alternatively, TDM can form a non-toxic micelles with the trehalose moieties exposed to aqueous solution and the hydrophobic esterified mycolic acid chains contained on the inside portion (right). Adapted in part from Hunter et al. [49]

features [48]. One structure is a cylindrical micelle, which can occur in aqueous media (Fig. 1). In this state, the TDM micelle is an insoluble, non-toxic amphiphile. This has the advantage of confining the trehalose in physical conformation that may be conducive for antigenicity. Here, the long carbon chain of the esterified mycolates interact in a way that compartmentalizes and sequesters their hydrophobic portions. The alternate form is a monolayer which is readily able to interact with hydrophobic interfaces. It is theorized that this form represents a potentially highly toxic crystalline monolayer-sheet, especially when it forms at a hydrophobe/aqueous interface [17, 44–46, 48, 49].

No direct animal experiments to date have demonstrated that TDM can be shed or excreted during *in vivo* infection. The physical conformation of TDM if it separates or leaves the organism's surface during *in vivo* infection would be difficult to determine. Yet antibodies reacting to mycobacterial antigens, TDM and other surface lipids, are able to detect these factors in lipid rich areas of lung tissue obtained from humans with post-primary disease. Of importance, these antibodies detect antigens in tissue regions lacking acid fast organisms [50]. Although speculative, this gives support to the notion that immunogenicity and physical structure are related in the host during late stage disease processes.

The potential for multiple physical formats helps to explain the different observations between scientists studying similar phenomena. Clearly differences in spreading onto a monolayer are dictated by the surface chemistry of the matrix support. Beads of different sizes have been used, as well as oil droplets [51–55], to deliver TDM *in vivo*. Many of these matrix/supports approximate the size of the mycobacteria, however, there is a wide variation (sometimes tenfold or greater in relative support structure size). This may explain difference in kinetics and overall immunoreactivity. When given a solid support of large relative size to that of the organism, monolayer formation is more likely to occur [53], thus influencing induction and attraction of cell phenotypes *in vivo*. This is expected to differ from results obtained using smaller (0.5–1.0 μm) TDM-coated polystyrene-divinylbenzene beads [56]. Oil-based emulsions also likely affect conformation, shown to be dependent on oil droplet size [57]; sometimes inducing primarily macrophage involvement [54] while other times inducing an accompanying neutrophilic contribution to pathology [58].

This nature of toxicity vs antigenicity as a function of TDM form may also explain the relative difference in binding to recently identified receptors; physical plasticity due to hydrophobic interactions may alter confirmation and thus relative binding to mammalian host cell receptors. For the organism, this may be considered as an evolutionary advantage, as recognition and internalization by innate cells is dictated through those surface receptors. Similarly, the reports of lysosome phagosome inhibition caused by TDM [21, 24] is probably dictated by the physical form of TDM available for intracellular interactions. The micelle is the most likely predicted intracellular form (R.L. Hunter, personal communication), however, this remains to be definitively proven.

The monolayer form of TDM has been reported to be one of the strongest biologic molecular monolayers ever described; certainly it is the most toxic lipid construct of MTB [46]. While this notion of TDM existing as a toxic monolayer was easily dismissed due to the structure being 'unphysiologic', revisiting of this concept led to hypotheses that the monolayer may indeed be a critical component of MTB virulence *in vivo* [48, 59]. Injection of TDM in the monolayer form, whether it is on beads or within an oil matrix, enhances chronic and reactivation TB in mice [60].

The toxic monolayer of TDM may be the form that induces multiple manifestations of clinical TB including coagulopathy and cachexia (consumption). Hunter and colleagues have theorized on its activity in this format to induce dissemination of MTB from granulomas, and as an agent of alveolitis resembling pathology during post-primary TB [16, 61, 62]. Only indirect evidence for these ideas exists, identified histologically from lung tissue of non-tuberculosis therapy treated patients. Antigen accumulation in these post primary patients is associated with cavitation, many times in the absence of overlap with high organism load in the region of pathology.

Immunogenicity of TDM

TDM has several sets of attributed biologic activities [63]. The organism has evolved multiple and complex utilities for TDM in addition to imparting a protective physical coat to permit the organism to survive outside of the host's cellular compartments. Interaction of TDM with host cells permits targeted engagement of immunological processes which are advantageous to survival of the host and to organism perpetuation.

Multiple studies have determined that mycobacterial mycolic acids are antigenic [28, 64, 65]. Kato et al. identified that antibodies directed against TDM containing fractions had an ability to modulate pathology in animal models [66]. Seggev et al. confirmed this observation when he identified a component that included both antibody reactivity and complement activation [67]; the link to complement was subsequently confirmed using deficient mice [68, 69]. In addition, a series of studies indicated that adaptive T lymphocytes were involved in higher order *in vivo* immune reactive responses. For example, our laboratory, as well as other investigative teams, identified a CD3+CD4+ defined cellular response [70–73] that is dictated in part through CD1 molecules [74, 75]. Furthermore, distinct epitopes unique to synthetic mycolic acids [76] as well as to TDM representing different mycobacterial species can be experimentally identified [77].

Receptors for TDM to Mediate Immune Function

The interactions of mycobacteria and its lipid components with cell surface antigens to elicit inflammatory responses have been well characterized [52], and is the subject of other papers and reviews [78–81]. TDM can specifically stimulate innate immune cells, culminating in initiation of cytokines to direct the granulomatous process. Identification of TDM receptors on host innate cells strengthens the observations that TDM modulates initial activities upon infection, and helps direct environments that control development of specific hypersensitive adaptive functionality. Much work has been done to identify specific innate cell receptors contributing to this process [82]. Even still, the direct link between receptors on innate cells and interaction of TDM which lead to a role in development of adaptive immunity remains unknown. This remains an on-going research goal to work towards understanding how this molecule can aid in clinical transition during development of post primary pathology.

The key to defining TDM's role in development of adaptive immunity must begin with a complete understanding of the initial events inherent in macrophage recognition of TDM while it resides on, and coats, the surface of organisms when initially encountered. It has been long known that TDM is involved in mediation of antigen presenting cells to allow production of secondary molecules involved in development of subsequent adaptive functions [83–85]. In this respect, TDM has been termed a "PAMP" [86]. Studies established a link with the C-type lectin Mincle

[87–89] as being a prime candidate for the TDM receptor. This is combined, in part, by additional interactions with the molecules MARCO and TLR2, and possibly CD14, which are also critical for activity mediation [79]. The recognition leads to internalized signaling events that likely function by way of Card9-dependent signaling mechanisms [90, 91]. Examples of infection of cells from mice deficient in these molecules show alteration of reactivity and inability to contain organism dissemination [92]. Following recognition, organisms are internalized. At this stage, *M. tuberculosis* blocks maturation of phagosomes [93–95], altering molecular events critical for organism destruction [96]. There is impediment of intra-phagosome events which are critical for antigen processing [22]. TDM is directly linked to this process [21, 24, 97]. Furthermore, the elimination of critical enzymes involved in TDM production (eg. attenuating fbpA) alters subsequent T cell immunity development [98, 99]. Indeed, the over expression of these and other related gene products can markedly increase protective T cell responses [100].

In reality, the physical form of TDM likely dictates which receptors are engaged at any given state of experimentally induced reactivity or infection. A novel hypothesis recently presented investigates TDM and other mycobacterial lipids to function as "immunostat" regulators of processes and outcomes of immune system engagement [101].

The TDM Granulomatous Response: Innate vs Hypersensitive

There is no perfect animal model that represents the complete spectrum of human tuberculosis. Primary tuberculosis begins as a pulmonary infection that spreads from the lymphatics, entering the blood stream before inducing a systemic immune response which is functional in containing organisms by way of a granulomatous pathology. Induction of the tuberculosis disease-induced granuloma is dependent on factors involved in response initiation and associated immune activity [102–107]. In an extreme simplification of the process, the underlying initiator is the existence of a poorly degradable persistent antigenic source within macrophages, exhibiting slow release of antigens to recruited cells. The net result of the granuloma is beneficial to both the host and the organism; the granuloma allows the host to control infection while at the same time providing a place for organisms to hide until an appropriate time for expansion with subsequent transmission to other individuals [108, 109]. The organism exhibits effects on tissues surrounding infected cells through released potent, bioactive cell wall constituents [110].

One of the accepted animal models that mimic aspects of the primary granulomatous response utilizes TDM to induce a transient pathology [54, 55, 57, 111–113]. This model is based on the non-infectious proinflammatory granuloma induced by the TDM from pathogenic organisms [46, 47, 55, 112]. These models have allowed confirmation that TDM plays a decisive role in MTB pathogenesis [48, 114], including a role in the formation of caseation in the lung post-infection [60]. TDM, whether formulated into an emulsion or placed on beads, injected intravenously into mice induces a transient pulmonary granulomatous response where focal cellular accumulation increases in complexity over a 7 day period, followed by resolution of pathology [54]. The molecular links have been defined for TDM to work as a mediator for innate molecular responses [68, 69, 115–117]; these mechanisms appear to be independent of interferon-γ [118]. Using knockout mice, our laboratory established patterns of cytokine production associated with pathology, allowing delineation of the major molecular events in innate establishment and maintenance of the TDM induced granuloma [16, 21, 24, 54, 56, 68, 69, 71, 119, 120] (Fig. 2).

Multiple investigators attribute properties to TDM as a T cell immunogen due to its potential to induce caseating granulomas in sensitized hosts [60, 70, 71, 86, 121, 122]. A direct link was established to adaptive (T cell mediated) hypersensitive responses critical for development of the pathological granuloma [70, 74] (Fig. 2). In this respect, TDM can experimentally induce an activated foreign-body type granulomas within naïve mice [54, 122], and immune hypersensitive granulomas in

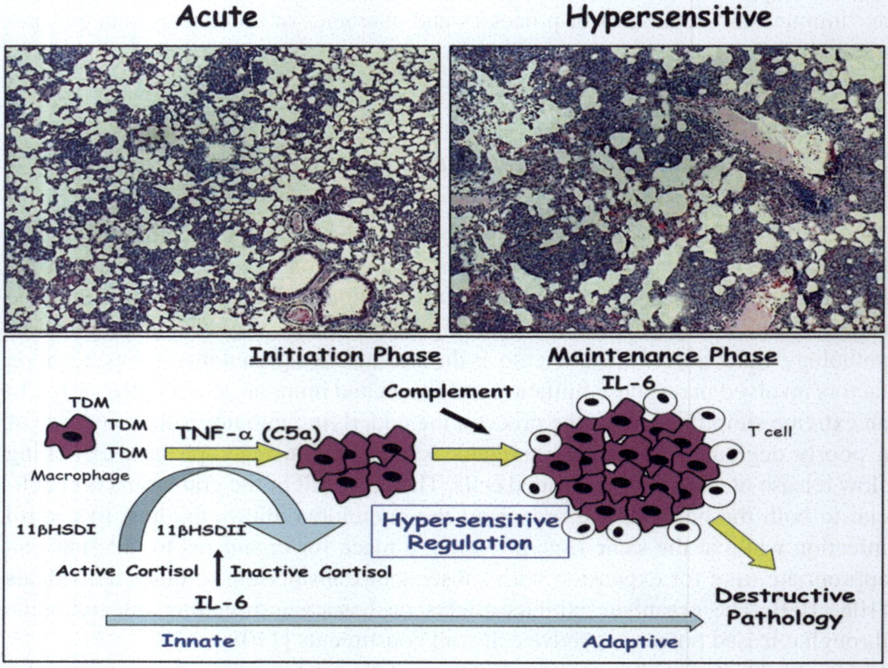

Fig. 2 Acute and Hypersensitive TDM-induced granulomas. TDM elicits an acute granulomatous response in C57BL/6 mice, comprised primarily of macrophages, at day 7 following administration in an emulsion formulation (top left). Mice pre-sensitized to TDM exhibit a markedly aggressive pathology, with additional influx of lymphocytes; vascular edema and perivascular cuffing are readily apparent (top right). As done by Guidry [71]. C57BL/6, day 7, 10x. Many of the molecular regulators of the granulomatous responses have been defined using knockout mice (bottom). Bottom Figure from Mediators Inflamm. 2015; PMID 26788020 [123]

appropriately sensitized (pre-exposed) mice [60, 71, 73]. Multiple investigative teams have identified a T cell defined hypersensitive response [70–73] that is dictated in part through CD1 related molecules [23, 56, 70, 74, 75]. Indeed, distinct epitopes unique to TDM from different mycobacterial species can be experimentally identified [11], some of which are unique to granulomatous pathology [111].

Overall, the studies cited above give credence that TDM exerts effective control over local microenvironments to provide multiple regulatory points that affect development of the innate and hypersensitive adaptive immune function. Cytokines and immune-regulatory factors induced by TDM play key roles in development of pathology induced during mycobacterial infection. These model systems using isolated TDM allow identification of host immune function to extrapolate findings of immune related pathology occurring during clinical manifestation of tuberculosis disease. It is further theorized that conformational restraints are required for TDM to elicit many of these higher order adaptive responses [44, 117, 124, 125]. These theories on structural requirements were in part validated by experimentation which proved that removal of the cyclopropane ring altered development of pathology during virulent *in vivo* infections [126–128]. More recently, a direct contribution of TDM to T cell responsiveness leading to development of pathology has been identified [70, 71, 73]; mechanisms have been detailed for how TDM can induce an antigen-specific adaptive response [72, 74]. This permits a foundation for models to study mediation of adaptive lymphocytes that contribute, directly or indirectly, to development of post primary tuberculosis and cavitary lesion pathology [129].

Hypotheses for TDM to Influence Clinical Tuberculosis Disease

TDM is known to play multiple roles in TB pathogenesis [11], yet a direct understanding of its role to modify development of clinical disease remains elusive. The histopathology which is associated with clinical primary tuberculosis is that of the granulomatous lesion. This includes development of granulomata comprised of activated epithelioid macrophages which are cuffed by lymphocytic cells [130, 131]. The described focal inflammation provides an environment where hosts can harbor the disease-causing organisms, permiting a functional sequestration of organisms. It is well appreciated that the surface glycolipid antigens, including all the mycolic acids, dictate inflammation that contributes to the pathological response [63, 117, 132, 133]. Primary disease in humans also includes an aspect of hemorrhagic pneumonia. Recent studies have re-confirmed the potential for TDM to induce similar pathologies in models with repeated intraperitoneal administrations of TDM [14, 134, 01]; in those models intraperitoneal pre-sensitization to TDM causes vascular occlusion upon subsequent intravascular challenge (Fig. 3).

Post primary tuberculosis disease differs from primary infection, as by definition it occurs in the presence of an established adaptive immune response generated towards MTB antigens. The lesions in post primary TB are likely preceded by an associated alveolitis with subsequent obstructive bronchial pneumonia. Paradigms

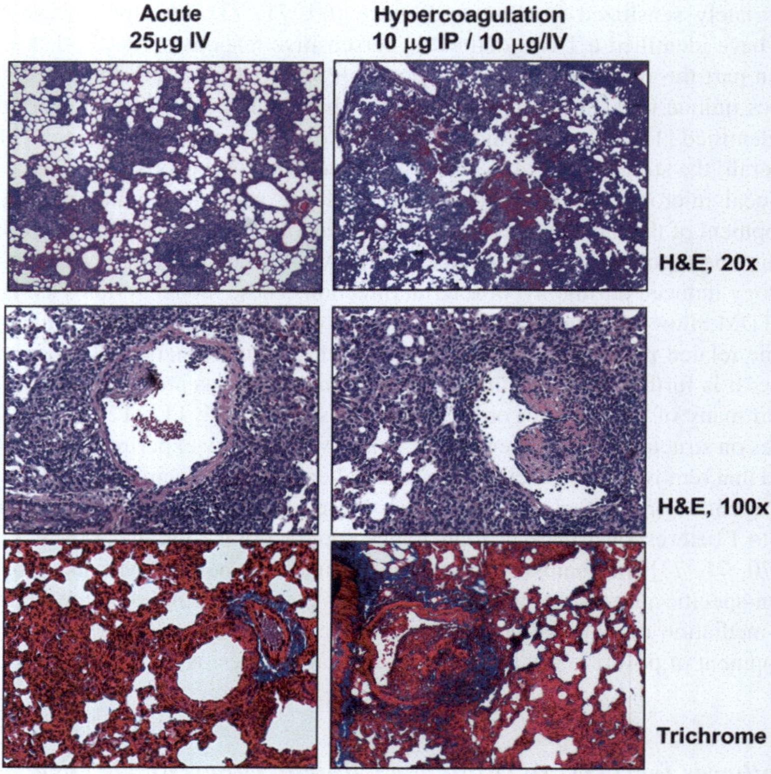

Fig. 3 TDM induced blood vessel occlusion. Naïve (left) or intraperitoneal pre-sensitized mice (right) were intravenous administered TDM emulsion, as described [134, 01] to induce hypercoagulation at day 7 (H&E at low and high power). Only the IP presensitized mice produced granulomatous inflammation with vascular remodeling and subepithelial deposition of collagen (blue) post treatment (H&E at 100x)

for post primary disease implicate inflammatory processes beginning with induction of that "lipid-like" necrotic pneumonia that transitions to a fibrocaseous disease [16, 61, 62, 129, 136–139]. Histopathologic evidence from non-antibiotic treated individuals implicates existence of a lipid pneumonia [129] preceding the caseating pathology. What is not particularly clear is the exact role of TDM in development of post primary tuberculosis pathology, especially disease pathology regulated through aggressive adaptive lymphocytic responses.

Reports suggest that a rapid necrosis occurring during tuberculous pneumonia could be the result of activation of both toxic and adaptive immunogenic properties after TDM comes into contact with host lipids [61, 129, 140–142]. The event is defined by accumulation of lipid and protein antigens, and presence of a strong and effective systemic specific adaptive immune response. This hypothesis diverges from the classical and broad acceptance that a growing granuloma forms the basis of the necrotizing lesion [130, 142]. It is supported by studies that show toxicity upon injection with TDM containing emulsions [143], and experiments showing relationship to TDM size and molecular composition [124]. The contribution of a lipid-based inflammatory process may also explain the histological observation that lesions appear to behave independently; at any given time, a defined lesion may progress toward cavitation while another appears to be in regression. A tipping point may be the accumulation of lipids, such as TDM, as well as other tuberculosis proteins and mycolic acids, in alveolar regions [50]. Perhaps TDM comes off organisms *in vivo* during a localized inflammation, and interacts with host lipids; the involvement of macrophages to accumulate lipid antigens has also been suggested, but has yet to be proven in humans or in non-human primates.

How a TDM-specific lymphocytic response could cause the pathological transition of lipid pneumonia to the status of a full cavitary disease state is in need of investigation. We may take clues from animal studies where it is known that classically defined CD4+ T helper lymphocytes greatly exacerbate the pathology during active acute infection. One idea could include involvement of NKT cells, which are adept at recognizing glycolipids. While there is theoretical support for this, Ryll and colleagues reported an opposite effect by elegantly demonstrating NKT cell depletion in response to TDM, rather than an expected proliferative response [144]. The involvement of NKT cells is still under investigation; that particular study only examined a model of acute infection. In humans, the development of post primary pathology occurs at a point well beyond the initial encounter with organisms, with ample time for regeneration of reactive and specific T cell phenotypic populations. It remains possible that neutrophils [58] or even γδ T cells [145] are required to initiate the response.

Summary

TDM remains an exciting molecule of research study, with an opportunity to address unanswered questions related to its function in development of both primary and post primary secondary clinical disease. Its associated biological properties appear to have defined polar extremes which need to be further examined. TDM is critical for generating environmental protection of organisms, both extracellularly and intracellularly. In addition, the unique physical properties of TDM likely dictate inflammatory responses to both initiate a protective granulomatous response, and to eventually develop long term hypersensitivity. Investigation of its function in regulating adaptive events, combined with understanding physical interactions with host lipids to generate toxic cues, will aid in our overall knowledge of necrosis and cavitation development during post primary clinical tuberculosis.

Acknowledgements A special note of appreciation goes to colleagues Shen-An Hwang, PhD, Chinnaswamy Jagannath, PhD, and Robert L. Hunter, MD, PhD, for their discussions and insights.

References

1. Koch R. The cure of consumption: further communications on a remedy for tuberculosis. London: W. Heinemann; 1890.
2. Koch Robert. 1880. Investigations into the etiology of traumatic infectious diseases. New Sydenham Society, London, United Kingdom; series v. 88. Translated by W. Watson Cheyne.
3. Koch R. Die Aetiologie der tuberculose. Berlin klin Wschschr Am Rev Tuberc 1932 Translation. 1882;25:298–323.
4. Sakula A. Robert koch: centenary of the discovery of the tubercle bacillus. Can Vet J. 1882;24(1983):127–31.
5. Bloch H. Studies on the virulence of tubercle bacilli; the relationship of the physiological state of the organisms to their pathogenicity. J Exp Med. 1950;92:507–26.
6. Bloch H. Studies on the virulence of tubercle bacilli; isolation and biological properties of a constituent of virulent organisms. J Exp Med. 1950;91:197–218.
7. Bloch H, Noll H. Studies on the virulence of tubercle bacilli; variations in virulence effected by tween 80 and thiosemicarbazone. J Exp Med. 1953;97:1–16.
8. Bloch H, Noll H. Studies on the virulence of tubercle bacilli. The effect of cord factor on murine tuberculosis. Br J Exp Path. 1955;36:8–17.
9. Bloch H, Sorkin E, Erlenmeyer H. A toxic lipid component of the tubercle bacillus (cord factor). I. Isolation from petroleum ether extracts of young bacterial cultures. Am Rev Tuberc. 1953;67:629–43.
10. Sorkin E, Erlenmeyer H, Bloch H. Purification of a lipid material ('cord factor') obtained from young cultures of tubercle bacilli. Nature. 1952;170:124.
11. Hunter RL, Venkataprasad N, Olsen MR. The role of trehalose dimycolate (cord factor) on morphology of virulent *M. tuberculosis* in vitro. Tuberculosis. 2006;86:349–56.
12. Kato M, Maeda J. Isolation and biochemical activities of trehalose-6-monomycolate of *Mycobacterium tuberculosis*. Infect Immun. 1974;9:8–14.
13. Kato M. Cord factor--its chemistry, biochemistry and immunochemistry. Nihon saikingaku zasshi. 1974;29:313–20.
14. Seggev J, Goren MB, Carr RI, Kirkpatrick CH. Interstitial and hemorrhagic pneumonitis induced by mycobacterial trehalose dimycolate. Am J Pathol. 1982;106:348–55.
15. Middlebrook G, Dubos RJ, Pierce C. Virulence and morphological characteristics of mammalian tubercle bacilli. J Exp Med. 1947;86:175–84.
16. Hunter RL. Tuberculosis as a three-act play: a new paradigm for the pathogenesis of pulmonary tuberculosis. Tuberculosis. 2016;97:8–17.
17. Hunter RL, Hwang SA, Jagannath C, Actor JK. Cord factor as an invisibility cloak? A hypothesis for asymptomatic TB persistence. Tuberculosis. 2016;101S:S2–8.
18. Youmans GP. Chapter 4. Mycobacterial lipids: chemistry and biologic activities. In: Youmans GP, editor. Tuberculosis. Philadelphia: W. B. Saunders Co.; 1979. p. 63–193.
19. Goren M. Cord factor revisited: a tribute to the late Hubert Bloch. Tubercle. 1975;56:65–71.
20. Behling CA, Nolte FS, Tinkley A, Hunter RL. The effect of tyloxapol on the surface lipids and biologic activities of BCG. Vaccine Res. 1994;3:1–14.
21. Indrigo J, Hunter RL Jr, Actor JK. Cord factor trehalose 6,6′-dimycolate (TDM) mediates trafficking events during mycobacterial infection of murine macrophages. Microbiology. 2003;149:2049–59.
22. Katti MK, Dai G, Armitige LY, Rivera Marrero C, Daniel S, Singh CR, Lindsey DR, Dhandayuthapani S, Hunter RL, Jagannath C. The Delta fbpA mutant derived from Mycobacterium tuberculosis H37Rv has an enhanced susceptibility to intracellular antimicrobial oxidative mechanisms, undergoes limited phagosome maturation and activates macrophages and dendritic cells. Cell Microbiol. 2008;10:1286–303.
23. Bakhru P, Sirisaengtaksin N, Soudani E, Mukherjee S, Khan A, Jagannath C. BCG vaccine mediated reduction in the MHC-II expression of macrophages and dendritic cells is reversed by activation of toll-like receptors 7 and 9. Cell Immunol. 2014;287:53–61.

24. Indrigo J, Hunter RL Jr, Actor JK. Influence of trehalose 6,6′-dimycolate (TDM) during mycobacterial infection of bone marrow macrophages. Microbiology. 2002;148:1991–8.
25. Bloch H, Noll H. Studies on the virulence of tubercle bacilli; the effect of cord factor on murine tuberculosis. Br J Exp Pathol. 1955;36:8–17.
26. Yarkoni E, Rapp HJ. Influence of oil and tween concentrations on enhanced endotoxin lethality in mice pretreated with emulsified trehalose-6,6′-dimycolate (cord factor). Infect Immun. 1979;24:571–2.
27. Sakurai T, Saiki I, Ishida H, Takeda K, Azuma I. Lethal toxicity and adjuvant activities of synthetic TDM and its related compounds in mice. Vaccine. 1989;7:269–74.
28. Brennan PJ, Goren MB. Mycobacterial glycolipids as bacterial antigens. Biochem Soc Trans. 1977;5:1687–93.
29. Bekierkunst A, Levij IS, Yarkoni E, Vilkas E, Adam A, Lederer E. Granuloma formation induced in mice by chemically defined mycobacterial fractions. J Bacteriol. 1969;100:95–102.
30. Saito R, Tanaka A, Sugiyama K, Azuma I, Yamamura Y. Adjuvant effect of cord factor, a mycobacterial lipid. Infect Immun. 1976;13:776–81.
31. Thanna S, Sucheck SJ. Targeting the trehalose utilization pathways of Mycobacterium tuberculosis. MedChemComm. 2016;7:69–85.
32. Jankute M, Cox JA, Harrison J, Besra GS. Assembly of the mycobacterial cell wall. Annu Rev Microbiol. 2015;69:405–23.
33. Torrelles JB, Schlesinger LS. Diversity in *Mycobacterium tuberculosis* mannosylated cell wall determinants impacts adaptation to the host. Tuberculosis. 2010;90:84–93.
34. Brennan PJ, Nikaido H. The envelope of mycobacteria. Annu Rev Biochem. 1995;64:29–63.
35. McNeil MR, Brennan PJ. Structure, function and biogenesis of the cell envelope of mycobacteria in relation to bacterial physiology, pathogenesis and drug resistance; some thoughts and possibilities arising from recent structural information. Res Microbiol. 1991;142:451–63.
36. Korf J, Stoltz A, Verschoor J, De Baetselier P, Grooten J. The *Mycobacterium tuberculosis* cell wall component mycolic acid elicits pathogen-associated host innate immune responses. Eur J Immunol. 2005;35:890–900.
37. Fujita Y, Naka T, McNeil MR, Yano I. Intact molecular characterization of cord factor (trehalose 6,6′-dimycolate) from nine species of mycobacteria by MALDI-TOF mass spectrometry. Microbiology. 2005;151:3403–16.
38. Noll H, Bloch H, Asselineau J, Lederer E. The chemical structure of the cord factor of *Mycobacterium tuberculosis*. Biochim Biophys Acta. 1956;20:299–309.
39. Takayama K, Wang C, Besra GS. Pathway to synthesis and processing of mycolic acids in *Mycobacterium tuberculosis*. Clin Microbiol Rev. 2005;18:81–101.
40. Veyron-Churlet R, Bigot S, Guerrini O, Verdoux S, Malaga W, Daffe M, Zerbib D. The biosynthesis of mycolic acids in *Mycobacterium tuberculosis* relies on multiple specialized elongation complexes interconnected by specific protein-protein interactions. J Mol Biol. 2005;353:847–58.
41. Chatterjee D. The mycobacterial cell wall: structure, biosynthesis and sites of drug action. Curr Opin Chem Biol. 1997;1:579–88.
42. Belisle JT, Vissa VD, Sievert T, Takayama K, Brennan PJ, Besra GS. Role of the major antigen of *Mycobacterium tuberculosis* in cell wall biogenesis. Science. 1997;276:1420–2.
43. Armitige LY, Jagannath C, Wanger AR, Norris SJ. Disruption of the genes encoding antigen 85A and antigen 85B of Mycobacterium tuberculosis H37Rv: effect on growth in culture and in macrophages. Infect Immun. 2000;68:767–78.
44. Behling CA, Bennett B, Takayama K, Hunter RL. Development of a trehalose 6,6′-dimycolate model which explains cord formation by Mycobacterium tuberculosis. Infect Immun. 1993;61:2296–303.
45. Schabbing RW, Garcia A, Hunter RL. Characterization of the trehalose 6,6′-dimycolate surface monolayer by scanning tunneling microscopy. Infect Immun. 1994;62:754–6.
46. Retzinger GS, Meredith SC, Hunter RL, Takayama K, Kezdy FJ. Identification of the physiologically active state of the mycobacterial glycolipid trehalose 6,6′-dimycolate and the role

of fibrinogen in the biologic activities of trehalose 6,6′-dimycolate monolayers. J Immunol. 1982;129:735–44.
47. Retzinger GS, Meredith SC, Takayama K, Hunter RL, Kezdy FJ. The role of surface in the biological activities of trehalose 6,6′-dimycolate. Surface properties and development of a model system. J Biol Chem. 1981;256:8208–16.
48. Hunter RL, Olsen MR, Jagannath C, Actor JK. Multiple roles of cord factor in the pathogenesis of primary, secondary, and cavitary tuberculosis, including a revised description of the pathology of secondary disease. Ann Clin Lab Sci. 2006;36:371–86.
49. Hunter RL, Armitige L, Jagannath C, Actor JK. TB research at UT-Houston--a review of cord factor: new approaches to drugs, vaccines and the pathogenesis of tuberculosis. Tuberculosis. 2009;89(Suppl 1):S18–25.
50. Mustafa T, Leversen NA, Sviland L, Wiker HG. Differential in vivo expression of mycobacterial antigens in *Mycobacterium tuberculosis* infected lungs and lymph node tissues. BMC Infect Dis. 2014;14:535.
51. Geisel RE, Sakamoto K, Russell DG, Rhoades ER. In vivo activity of released cell wall lipids of *Mycobacterium bovis* bacillus Calmette-Guerin is due principally to trehalose mycolates. J Immunol. 2005;174:5007–15.
52. Rhoades E, Hsu F, Torrelles JB, Turk J, Chatterjee D, Russell DG. Identification and macrophage-activating activity of glycolipids released from intracellular Mycobacterium bovis BCG. Mol Microbiol. 2003;48:875–88.
53. Rhoades ER, Geisel RE, Butcher BA, McDonough S, Russell DG. Cell wall lipids from *Mycobacterium bovis* BCG are inflammatory when inoculated within a gel matrix: characterization of a new model of the granulomatous response to mycobacterial components. Tuberculosis. 2005;85:159–76.
54. Perez RL, Roman J, Roser S, Little C, Olsen M, Indrigo J, Hunter RL, Actor JK. Cytokine message and protein expression during lung granuloma formation and resolution induced by the mycobacterial cord factor trehalose-6,6′-dimycolate. J Interf Cytokine Res. 2000;20:795–804.
55. Perez RL, Roman J, Staton GW Jr, Hunter RL. Extravascular coagulation and fibrinolysis in murine lung inflammation induced by the mycobacterial cord factor trehalose-6,6′-dimycolate. Am J Respir Crit Care Med. 1994;149:510–8.
56. Actor JK, Olsen M, Hunter RL Jr, Geng YJ. Dysregulated response to mycobacterial cord factor trehalose-6,6′-dimycolate in CD1D−/− mice. J Interf Cytokine Res. 2001;21:1089–96.
57. Yarkoni E, Rapp HJ. Granuloma formation in lungs of mice after intravenous administration of emulsified trehalose-6,6′-dimycolate (cord factor): reaction intensity depends on size distribution of the oil droplets. Infect Immun. 1977;18:552–4.
58. Lee WB, Kang JS, Yan JJ, Lee MS, Jeon BY, Cho SN, Kim YJ. Neutrophils promote mycobacterial trehalose dimycolate-induced lung inflammation via the Mincle pathway. PLoS Pathog. 2012;8:e1002614.
59. Arora R, Armitige L, Wanger A, Hunter RL, Hwang SA. Association of pellicle growth morphological characteristics and clinical presentation of Mycobacterium tuberculosis isolates. Tuberculosis. 2016;101S:S63–8.
60. Hunter RL, Olsen M, Jagannath C, Actor JK. Trehalose 6,6′-dimycolate and lipid in the pathogenesis of caseating granulomas of tuberculosis in mice. Am J Pathol. 2006;168:1249–61.
61. Hunter RL. Pathology of post primary tuberculosis of the lung: an illustrated critical review. Tuberculosis. 2011;91:497–509.
62. Hunter RL, Actor JK, Hwang SA, Karev V, Jagannath C. Pathogenesis of post primary tuberculosis: immunity and hypersensitivity in the development of cavities. Ann Clin Lab Sci. 2014;44:365–87.
63. Goren M, Brennan P. Mycobacterial lipids: chemistry and biologic activities. In: Youmans G, editor. Tuberculosis. Philadelphia: W.B. Saunders; 1979. p. 63–193.

64. Fujiwara N, Oka S, Ide M, Kashima K, Honda T, Yano I. Production and partial characterization of antibody to cord factor (trehalose 6,6′-dimycolate) in mice. Microbiol Immunol. 1999;43:785–93.
65. Kato M. Immunochemical properties of anti-cord factor antibody. Infect Immun. 1973;7:9–13.
66. Kato M. Effect of anti-cord factor antibody on experimental tuberculosis in mice. Infect Immun. 1973;7:14–21.
67. Seggev JS, Goren MB, Carr RI, Rubenstein E, Kirkpatrick CH. Pathogenesis of trehalose dimycolate-induced interstitial pneumonitis. IV. Evidence against roles for immunoglobulins and the complement system. Exp Lung Res. 1988;14:431–44.
68. Borders CW, Courtney A, Ronen K, Pilar Laborde-Lahoz M, Guidry TV, Hwang SA, Olsen M, Hunter RL Jr, Hollmann TJ, Wetsel RA, Actor JK. Requisite role for complement C5 and the C5a receptor in granulomatous response to mycobacterial glycolipid trehalose 6,6′-dimycolate. Scand J Immunol. 2005;62:123–30.
69. Welsh KJ, Abbott AN, Hwang SA, Indrigo J, Armitige LY, Blackburn MR, Hunter RL Jr, Actor JK. A role for tumour necrosis factor-alpha, complement C5 and interleukin-6 in the initiation and development of the mycobacterial cord factor trehalose 6,6′-dimycolate induced granulomatous response. Microbiology. 2008;154:1813–24.
70. Guidry TV, Hunter RL Jr, Actor JK. CD3+ cells transfer the hypersensitive granulomatous response to mycobacterial glycolipid trehalose 6,6′-dimycolate in mice. Microbiology. 2006;152:3765–75.
71. Guidry TV, Hunter RL Jr, Actor JK. Mycobacterial glycolipid trehalose 6,6′-dimycolate-induced hypersensitive granulomas: contribution of CD4+ lymphocytes. Microbiology. 2007;153:3360–9.
72. Oiso R, Fujiwara N, Yamagami H, Maeda S, Matsumoto S, Nakamura S, Oshitani N, Matsumoto T, Arakawa T, Kobayashi K. Mycobacterial trehalose 6,6′-dimycolate preferentially induces type 1 helper T cell responses through signal transducer and activator of transcription 4 protein. Microb Pathog. 2005;39:35–43.
73. Yamagami H, Matsumoto T, Fujiwara N, Arakawa T, Kaneda K, Yano I, Kobayashi K. Trehalose 6,6′-dimycolate (cord factor) of Mycobacterium tuberculosis induces foreign-body- and hypersensitivity-type granulomas in mice. Infect Immun. 2001;69:810–5.
74. Guidry TV, Olsen M, Kil KS, Hunter RL Jr, Geng YJ, Actor JK. Failure of CD1D−/− mice to elicit hypersensitive granulomas to mycobacterial cord factor trehalose 6,6′-dimycolate. J Interf Cytokine Res. 2004;24:362–71.
75. Otsuka A, Matsunaga I, Komori T, Tomita K, Toda Y, Manabe T, Miyachi Y, Sugita M. Trehalose dimycolate elicits eosinophilic skin hypersensitivity in mycobacteria-infected guinea pigs. J Immunol. 2008;181:8528–33.
76. Smet M, Pollard C, De Beuckelaer A, Van Hoecke L, Vander Beken S, De Koker S, Al Dulayymi JR, Huygen K, Verschoor J, Baird MS, Grooten J. Mycobacterium tuberculosis-associated synthetic mycolates differentially exert immune stimulatory adjuvant activity. Eur J Immunol. 2016;46:2149–54.
77. McMullen AM, Hwang SA, O'Shea K, Aliru ML, Actor JK. Evidence for a unique species-specific hypersensitive epitope in Mycobacterium tuberculosis derived cord factor. Tuberculosis. 2013;93(Suppl):S88–93.
78. Hossain MM, Norazmi MN. Pattern recognition receptors and cytokines in Mycobacterium tuberculosis infection--the double-edged sword? Biomed Res Int. 2013;2013:179174.
79. Bowdish DM, Sakamoto K, Kim MJ, Kroos M, Mukhopadhyay S, Leifer CA, Tryggvason K, Gordon S, Russell DG. MARCO, TLR2, and CD14 are required for macrophage cytokine responses to mycobacterial trehalose dimycolate and Mycobacterium tuberculosis. PLoS Pathog. 2009;5:e1000474.
80. Mortaz E, Adcock IM, Tabarsi P, Masjedi MR, Mansouri D, Velayati AA, Casanova JL, Barnes PJ. Interaction of pattern recognition receptors with Mycobacterium tuberculosis. J Clin Immunol. 2014;35(1):1–10.
81. Russell DG. Who puts the tubercle in tuberculosis? Nat Rev Microbiol. 2007;5:39–47.

82. Ishikawa E, Mori D, Yamasaki S. Recognition of mycobacterial lipids by immune receptors. Trends Immunol. 2017;38:66–76.
83. Oswald IP, Dozois CM, Fournout S, Petit JF, Lemaire G. Tumor necrosis factor is required for the priming of peritoneal macrophages by trehalose dimycolate. Eur Cytokine Netw. 1999;10:533–40.
84. Oswald IP, Dozois CM, Petit JF, Lemaire G. Interleukin-12 synthesis is a required step in trehalose dimycolate-induced activation of mouse peritoneal macrophages. Infect Immun. 1997;65:1364–9.
85. Afroun S, Oswald IP, Lantier F, Petit JF, Lemaire G. Stimulation of antimycobacterial activity in mouse peritoneal macrophages by priming with trehalose dimycolate (TDM). FEMS Microbiol Immunol. 1991;3:257–67.
86. Lang R. Recognition of the mycobacterial cord factor by Mincle: relevance for granuloma formation and resistance to tuberculosis. Front Immunol. 2013;4:5.
87. Schoenen H, Bodendorfer B, Hitchens K, Manzanero S, Werninghaus K, Nimmerjahn F, Agger EM, Stenger S, Andersen P, Ruland J, Brown GD, Wells C, Lang R. Cutting edge: Mincle is essential for recognition and adjuvanticity of the mycobacterial cord factor and its synthetic analog trehalose-dibehenate. J Immunol. 2010;184:2756–60.
88. Ishikawa E, Ishikawa T, Morita YS, Toyonaga K, Yamada H, Takeuchi O, Kinoshita T, Akira S, Yoshikai Y, Yamasaki S. Direct recognition of the mycobacterial glycolipid, trehalose dimycolate, by C-type lectin Mincle. J Exp Med. 2009;206:2879–88.
89. Matsunaga I, Moody DB. Mincle is a long sought receptor for mycobacterial cord factor. J Exp Med. 2009;206:2865–8.
90. Werninghaus K, Babiak A, Gross O, Holscher C, Dietrich H, Agger EM, Mages J, Mocsai A, Schoenen H, Finger K, Nimmerjahn F, Brown GD, Kirschning C, Heit A, Andersen P, Wagner H, Ruland J, Lang R. Adjuvanticity of a synthetic cord factor analogue for subunit Mycobacterium tuberculosis vaccination requires FcRgamma-Syk-Card9-dependent innate immune activation. J Exp Med. 2009;206:89–97.
91. LeibundGut-Landmann S, Gross O, Robinson MJ, Osorio F, Slack EC, Tsoni SV, Schweighoffer E, Tybulewicz V, Brown GD, Ruland J, e Sousa CR. Syk- and CARD9-dependent coupling of innate immunity to the induction of T helper cells that produce interleukin 17. Nat Immunol. 2007;8:630–8.
92. Martinez N, Ketheesan N, West K, Vallerskog T, Kornfeld H. Impaired recognition of Mycobacterium tuberculosis by alveolar macrophages from diabetic mice. J Infect Dis. 2016;214:1629–37.
93. Deretic V, Fratti RA. Mycobacterium tuberculosis phagosome. Mol Microbiol. 1999;31:1603–9.
94. Fratti RA, Vergne I, Chua J, Skidmore J, Deretic V. Regulators of membrane trafficking and Mycobacterium tuberculosis phagosome maturation block. Electrophoresis. 2000;21:3378–85.
95. Russell DG. Mycobacterium tuberculosis: here today, and here tomorrow. Nat Rev Mol Cell Biol. 2001;2:569–77.
96. Sturgill-Koszycki S, Schlesinger PH, Chakraborty P, Haddix PL, Collins HL, Fok AK, Allen RD, Gluck SL, Heuser J, Russell DG. Lack of acidification in Mycobacterium phagosomes produced by exclusion of the vesicular proton-ATPase. Science. 1994;263:678–81.
97. Patin EC, Geffken AC, Willcocks S, Leschczyk C, Haas A, Nimmerjahn F, Lang R, Ward TH, Schaible UE. Trehalose dimycolate interferes with FcgammaR-mediated phagosome maturation through Mincle, SHP-1 and FcgammaRIIB signalling. PLoS One. 2017;12:e0174973.
98. Roche CM, Smith A, Lindsey DR, Meher A, Schluns K, Arora A, Armitige LY, Jagannath C. The DeltafbpA attenuated candidate vaccine from Mycobacterium tuberculosis, H37Rv primes for a stronger T-bet dependent Th1 immunity in mice. Tuberculosis. 2011;91(Suppl 1):S96–S104.

99. Saikolappan S, Estrella J, Sasindran SJ, Khan A, Armitige LY, Jagannath C, Dhandayuthapani S. The fbpA/sapM double knock out strain of Mycobacterium tuberculosis is highly attenuated and immunogenic in macrophages. PLoS One. 2012;7:e36198.
100. Lindsey DR, Dhandayuthapani S, Jagannath C. Anti-tuberculosis immunity induced in mice by vaccination with Mycobacterium smegmatis over-expressing antigen 85B is due to the increased influx of IFNgamma-positive CD4 T cells into the lungs. Tuberculosis. 2009;89(Suppl 1):S46–8.
101. Queiroz A, Riley LW. Bacterial immunostat: Mycobacterium tuberculosis lipids and their role in the host immune response. Rev Soc Bras Med Trop. 2017;50:9–18.
102. Ramakrishnan L. Revisiting the role of the granuloma in tuberculosis. Nat Rev Immunol. 2012;12:352–66.
103. Silva Miranda M, Breiman A, Allain S, Deknuydt F, Altare F. The tuberculous granuloma: an unsuccessful host defence mechanism providing a safety shelter for the bacteria? Clin Dev Immunol. 2012;2012:139127.
104. Khader SA, Rangel-Moreno J, Fountain JJ, Martino CA, Reiley WW, Pearl JE, Winslow GM, Woodland DL, Randall TD, Cooper AM. In a murine tuberculosis model, the absence of homeostatic chemokines delays granuloma formation and protective immunity. J Immunol. 2009;183:8004–14.
105. Cooper AM, Khader SA. The role of cytokines in the initiation, expansion, and control of cellular immunity to tuberculosis. Immunol Rev. 2008;226:191–204.
106. Orme IM, Basaraba RJ. The formation of the granuloma in tuberculosis infection. Semin Immunol. 2014;26:601–9.
107. Orme IM, Robinson RT, Cooper AM. The balance between protective and pathogenic immune responses in the TB-infected lung. Nat Immunol. 2015;16:57–63.
108. Actor JK, Olsen M, Jagannath C, Hunter RL. Relationship of survival, organism containment, and granuloma formation in acute murine tuberculosis. J Interf Cytokine Res. 1999;19:1183–93.
109. Flynn JL, Chan J. What's good for the host is good for the bug. Trends Microbiol. 2005;13:98–102.
110. Russell DG. Mycobacterium tuberculosis and the intimate discourse of a chronic infection. Immunol Rev. 2011;240:252–68.
111. Baba T, Natsuhara Y, Kaneda K, Yano I. Granuloma formation activity and mycolic acid composition of mycobacterial cord factor. Cell Mol Life Sci. 1997;53:227–32.
112. Behling CA, Perez RL, Kidd MR, Staton GW Jr, Hunter RL. Induction of pulmonary granulomas, macrophage procoagulant activity, and tumor necrosis factor-alpha by trehalose glycolipids. Ann Clin Lab Sci. 1993;23:256–66.
113. Hamasaki N, Isowa K, Kamada K, Terano Y, Matsumoto T, Arakawa T, Kobayashi K, Yano I. In vivo administration of mycobacterial cord factor (Trehalose 6, 6′-dimycolate) can induce lung and liver granulomas and thymic atrophy in rabbits. Infect Immun. 2000;68:3704–9.
114. Actor JK. Mycobacterial TDM: a coat to modulate post primary pathogenesis? Mycobact Dis. 2012;2:e106.
115. Sakai Y, Uchida K, Nakayama H. Histopathological features and expression profiles of cytokines, chemokines and SOCS family proteins in trehalose 6,6′-dimycolate-induced granulomatous lesions. Inflamm Res. 2011;60:371–8.
116. Abbott AN, Guidry TV, Welsh KJ, Thomas AM, Kling MA, Hunter RL, Actor JK. 11beta-hydroxysteroid dehydrogenases are regulated during the pulmonary granulomatous response to the mycobacterial glycolipid trehalose-6,6′-dimycolate. Neuroimmunomodulation. 2009;16:147–54.
117. Ryll R, Kumazawa Y, Yano I. Immunological properties of trehalose dimycolate (cord factor) and other mycolic acid-containing glycolipids--a review. Microbiol Immunol. 2001;45:801–11.
118. Takimoto H, Maruyama H, Shimada KI, Yakabe R, Yano I, Kumazawa Y. Interferon-gamma independent formation of pulmonary granuloma in mice by injections with trehalose

dimycolate (cord factor), lipoarabinomannan and phosphatidylinositol mannosides isolated from Mycobacterium tuberculosis. Clin Exp Immunol. 2006;144:134–41.
119. Actor JK, Indrigo J, Beachdel CM, Olsen M, Wells A, Hunter RL Jr, Dasgupta A. Mycobacterial glycolipid cord factor trehalose 6,6′-dimycolate causes a decrease in serum cortisol during the granulomatous response. Neuroimmunomodulation. 2002;10:270–82.
120. Abbott AN, Welsh KJ, Hwang SA, Ploszaj P, Choudhury T, Boyd S, Blackburn MR, Hunter RL Jr, Actor JK. IL-6 mediates 11betaHSD type 2 to effect progression of the mycobacterial cord factor trehalose 6,6′-dimycolate-induced granulomatous response. Neuroimmunomodulation. 2011;18:212–25.
121. Feinberg H, Jegouzo SA, Rowntree TJ, Guan Y, Brash MA, Taylor ME, Weis WI, Drickamer K. Mechanism for recognition of an unusual mycobacterial glycolipid by the macrophage receptor mincle. J Biol Chem. 2013;288:28457–65.
122. Bekierkunst A, Yarkoni E. Granulomatous hypersensitivity to trehalose 6,6′-dimycolate (cord factor) in mice infected with BCG. Infect Immun. 1973;7:631–8.
123. Actor JK. Lactoferrin: A modulator for immunity against tuberculosis related granulomatous pathology. Mediators Inflamm. 2015;2015:409596. PMID: 26788020.
124. Fujita Y, Okamoto Y, Uenishi Y, Sunagawa M, Uchiyama T, Yano I. Molecular and supramolecular structure related differences in toxicity and granulomatogenic activity of mycobacterial cord factor in mice. Microb Pathog. 2007;43:10–21.
125. Yarkoni E, Rapp HJ. Toxicity of emulsified trehalose-6,6′-dimycolate (cord factor) in mice depends on size distribution of mineral oil droplets. Infect Immun. 1978;20:856–60.
126. Glickman MS, Cox JS, Jacobs WR Jr. A novel mycolic acid cyclopropane synthetase is required for cording, persistence, and virulence of Mycobacterium tuberculosis. Mol Cell. 2000;5:717–27.
127. Rao V, Gao F, Chen B, Jacobs WR Jr, Glickman MS. Trans-cyclopropanation of mycolic acids on trehalose dimycolate suppresses Mycobacterium tuberculosis -induced inflammation and virulence. J Clin Invest. 2006;116:1660–7.
128. Rao V, Fujiwara N, Porcelli SA, Glickman MS. Mycobacterium tuberculosis controls host innate immune activation through cyclopropane modification of a glycolipid effector molecule. J Exp Med. 2005;201:535–43.
129. Hunter RL, Jagannath C, Actor JK. Pathology of postprimary tuberculosis in humans and mice: contradiction of long-held beliefs. Tuberculosis. 2007;87:267–78.
130. Dannenberg A. Tuberculosis and nontuberculosis mycobacterial infections. In: Schlossberg D, editor. Pathophysiology: basic aspects. Philadelphia: W. B. Saunders; 1999. p. 26–7.
131. Paige C, Bishai WR. Penitentiary or penthouse condo: the tuberculous granuloma from the microbe's point of view. Cell Microbiol. 2010;12:301–9.
132. Kallenius G, Correia-Neves M, Buteme H, Hamasur B, Svenson SB. Lipoarabinomannan, and its related glycolipids, induce divergent and opposing immune responses to Mycobacterium tuberculosis depending on structural diversity and experimental variations. Tuberculosis. 2016;96:120–30.
133. Fukuda T, Matsumura T, Ato M, Hamasaki M, Nishiuchi Y, Murakami Y, Maeda Y, Yoshimori T, Matsumoto S, Kobayashi K, Kinoshita T, Morita YS. Critical roles for lipomannan and lipoarabinomannan in cell wall integrity of mycobacteria and pathogenesis of tuberculosis. MBio. 2013;4:e00472–12.
134. Donnachie E, Fedotova EP, Hwang SA. Trehalose 6,6-Dimycolate from Mycobacterium tuberculosis induces hypercoagulation. Am J Pathol. 2016;186:1221–33.
135. Hwang SA, Byerly CD, Actor JK. Mycobacterial trehalose 6,6'-dimycolate induced vascular occlusion is accompanied by subendothelial inflammation. Tuberculosis (Edinb). 2019:116S:S118-S122. PMID: 31072690.
136. Hunter RL. On the pathogenesis of post primary tuberculosis: the role of bronchial obstruction in the pathogenesis of cavities. Tuberculosis. 2011;91(Suppl 1):S6–10.
137. Hunter RL, Hwang SA, Jagannath C, Actor JK. Cord factor as an invisibility cloak? A hypothesis for asymptomatic TB persistence. Tuberculosis (Edinb). 2016;101:S2–8.

138. Welsh KJ, Hunter RL, Actor JK. Trehalose 6,6′-dimycolate--a coat to regulate tuberculosis immunopathogenesis. Tuberculosis. 2013;93(Suppl):S3–9.
139. Kim MJ, Wainwright HC, Locketz M, Bekker LG, Walther GB, Dittrich C, Visser A, Wang W, Hsu FF, Wiehart U, Tsenova L, Kaplan G, Russell DG. Caseation of human tuberculosis granulomas correlates with elevated host lipid metabolism. EMBO Mol Med. 2010;2:258–74.
140. Gideon HP, Flynn JL. Latent tuberculosis: what the host "sees"? Immunol Res. 2011;50:202–12.
141. Hunter RL. On the pathogenesis of post primary tuberculosis: the role of bronchial obstruction in the pathogenesis of cavities. Tuberculosis (Edinb). 2011;91(Suppl 1):S6–S10.
142. Syed SS, Hunter RL Jr. Studies on the toxic effects of quartz and a mycobacterial glycolipid, trehalose 6,6′-dimycolate. Ann Clin Lab Sci. 1997;27:375–83.
143. Rich A. The pathogenesis of tuberculosis, Charles C. Sringfield: Thomas; 1951.
144. Ozeki Y, Kaneda K, Fujiwara N, Morimoto M, Oka S, Yano I. In vivo induction of apoptosis in the thymus by administration of mycobacterial cord factor (trehalose 6,6′-dimycolate). Infect Immun. 1997;65:1793–9.
145. Ryll R, Watanabe K, Fujiwara N, Takimoto H, Hasunuma R, Kumazawa Y, Okada M, Yano I. Mycobacterial cord factor, but not sulfolipid, causes depletion of NKT cells and upregulation of CD1d1 on murine macrophages. Microbes Infect. 2001;3:611–9.
146. Saitoh T, Yano I, Kumazawa Y, Takimoto H. Pulmonary TCR gammadelta T cells induce the early inflammation of granuloma formation by a glycolipid trehalose 6,6′-dimycolate (TDM) isolated from Mycobacterium tuberculosis. Immunopharmacol Immunotoxicol. 2012;34:815–23.

Role of Myeloid-Derived Suppressor Cells and Regulatory T-Cells in the Tuberculous Granuloma

Laurene S. Cheung, Geetha Srikrishna, and William R. Bishai

Abstract In the course of *Mycobacterium tuberculosis* (*M.tb*) infection, while a robust immune response is required for containment and clearance of the pathogen, immune-mediated tissue damage may also occur. Immune suppressive cells, such as regulatory T cells (Tregs) and myeloid-derived suppressor cells (MDSCs) are recruited to the site of infection, but in the process of controlling immune responses can promote pathogen survival. Tregs are known to be elevated in tuberculosis (TB) patients with active disease and studies in animal models demonstrate that Tregs inhibit effector T cell function through multiple mechanisms during *M.tb* infection (Guyot-Revol et al., Am J Respir Crit Care Med 173:803–10, 2006). More recently, increased levels of MDSCs have been found in patients with active TB and although less is known about their role in infection, it has become clear that MDSCs are very effective in suppressing T cell responses in tumors (El Daker et al., PLoS One 10:e0123772, 2015). In this chapter, we will give a brief overview of the early immune response to *M.tb.* infection and the host's attempt to contain infection through the formation of granulomas in the lung. We will then review the function of MDSCs and Tregs and what is known about their role during TB infection. Finally, we will discuss currently available drugs that can target these cell populations and their potential use for the treatment of TB.

Keywords Tuberculosis · Regulatory T cells · Myeloid-derived suppressor cells · Granuloma · Host-directed therapy · Immune checkpoint inhibition · Effector T cells · Immune suppression · Immunotherapy · Inflammation

L. S. Cheung · G. Srikrishna · W. R. Bishai (✉)
Center for Tuberculosis Research, Department of Medicine, Division of Infectious Diseases, Johns Hopkins School of Medicine, Baltimore, MD, USA
e-mail: wbishai@jhmi.edu

J. D. Cirillo, Y. Kong (eds.), *Tuberculosis Host-Pathogen Interactions*,
https://doi.org/10.1007/978-3-030-25381-3_4

Introduction

> Now, here, you see, it takes all the running you can do, to keep in the same place
> (Red Queen to Alice in Lewis Carroll's *Through the Looking-Glass*)

The Red Queen hypothesis, an evolutionary theory proposed by biologist Leigh Van Valen, suggests that reciprocal coevolution of hosts and pathogens selects for discrete molecular events that lead to continued survival of both. Tuberculosis (TB) is an ancient human disease, estimated to have originated and evolved for over many thousands of years alongside the modern human population [1]. This reciprocal co-evolution has made *Mycobacterium tuberculosis* (*M.tb*) one of humanity's most successful obligate pathogens, with the mycobacterial niche so fine-tuned within this primordial host-pathogen relationship, that today it is estimated that one-fourth of the world's population harbors *M.tb* [2]. According to the CDC, there were 10.4 million incident cases of TB worldwide in 2015, associated with 1.8 million deaths, making TB one of the world's most significant medical challenges. The emergence of multi-drug-resistant and extensively-drug resistant (MDR and XDR) *M.tb* strains, combined with limited resources in developing communities, and the lack of quality diagnostics and effective chemotherapy regimens, critically hinder control of this disease. Failure to contain the disease globally has led to increased and targeted efforts towards identification of novel therapeutic targets. While many bacterial pathogens have devised multiple strategies to avoid phagocytic engulfment and killing, invading *M.tb* has adopted a highly successful strategy, wherein following recognition and phagocytosis by host pulmonary alveolar macrophages, the bacteria use these cells as sanctuary sites for persistence and propagation. Active or primary TB, characterized by symptomatic disease, is manifest only in a small percentage of infected individuals. In a majority of infected individuals however, latency is established even in the presence of a fully competent host immune system that helps to contain, but not eliminate, the infection, though the individual remains asympotmatic. Lifetime risk of reactivation or post-primary TB in individuals with latent infection (LTBI, Latent Tuberculosis Infection) is about 5–10%, with the risk being higher in immunosuppressed individuals, as seen with HIV co-infection or following treatment with immunosuppressive drugs. Bacillus Calmette–Guérin (BCG), the only available vaccine against TB for the last 90 years, has an efficacy ranging from 0–80% in adults. This variation has been attributed to geographical differences and pre-exposure to endemic mycobacteria among others [3]. The inadequacy of the vaccine to protect all young and adult populations has intensified global efforts to improve its efficacy and to develop newer vaccines.

A highly evolved and coordinated sequence of immune evasion strategies, involving both innate and adaptive immunity, allows *M.tb* to avoid immune-mediated clearance by the host [4]. For example, inside pulmonary alveolar macrophages, *M.tb* arrests phagosome maturation and modulates cell death pathways that allow replication in the early endosomal compartment [5]. Bacteria are sheltered and sequestered within organized lung structures called granulomas which consist of a dynamic population of immunologically altered macrophages and other cells of myeloid and lymphoid origin [6–8]. Host adaptive immunity is triggered by the processing of mycobacterial antigens by antigen-presenting cells that activate T lymphocytes, and is further enhanced by pro- and anti-inflammatory cytokines released during infection. Multiple effects mediated by the cells within the granuloma, while limiting bacterial growth, also suppress immune responses, and provide a survival niche from which the bacteria may ultimately disseminate [6, 9]. The functional outcome of this dynamic cell recruitment by the host and manipulation of adaptive immunity by *M.tb* is a fine-tuning of the balance between pro- and anti-inflammatory networks [4, 10] that dictates the outcome of disease, akin to immune events of a tumor microenvironment. Understanding of this dynamic host-pathogen interaction is therefore of major importance in the development of novel host-directed therapies (HDTs) against TB, and to improve vaccine efficacy.

Strategies developed by *M.tb* for evading host defense include manipulation of the immune system towards immunosuppression and tolerance. Recent studies in patients and animal models show that among the host cell populations that promote immune evasion and suppression during *M.tb* infection are myeloid-derived suppressor cells (MDSC) and regulatory T-cells (Tregs). MDSCs exhibit immune-regulatory potential in both adaptive and innate immunity. They have been shown to accumulate in lungs during pulmonary TB, and they not only dampen anti-mycobacterial T-cell responses, but also phagocytose and shelter *M.tb* intracellularly. In addition, MDSCs promote the development of $CD4^{+}CD25^{+}FOXP3^{+}$ Tregs, which are known to play an important role in the prevention of autoimmunity and in the control of pro-inflammatory immune responses. Concomitant with increase in MDSC, the numbers of Tregs in the lung have also been shown to increase dramatically during *M.tb* infection in both animal models and in human patients. Skewing host immunity by selectively targeting cells that promote bacterial persistence and mediators that either promote their accumulation or lead to suppression of effector responses, might therefore prove highly valuable in reducing *M.tb* persistence and disease. This chapter focuses on the role played by MDSC and Tregs in TB pathogenesis and on possible new therapeutic avenues for targeting these cells in TB management.

The Tuberculous Granuloma: Host Immune Quarantine of *M. tb.*

Innate Immune Recognition of M.tb.

The lung serves as the predominant site of entry, containment, long-term persistence, disease manifestation, and ultimate spread of the pathogen. The most characteristic lesion of TB is the tuberculous granuloma (Fig. 1), which serves as an immune quarantine where the infection can be contained and controlled, but not altogether eliminated [8, 11]. After aerosol inhalation, the bacteria are deposited in

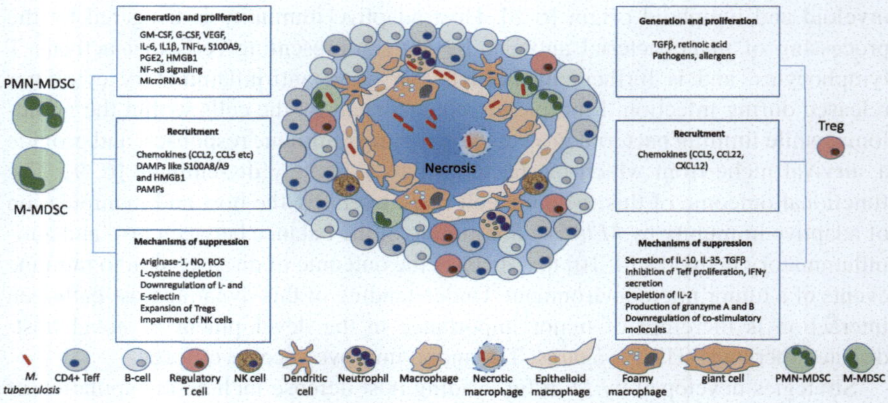

Fig. 1 Cellular composition of the necrotic granuloma: factors promoting immunosuppressive cells and their known mechanism of action. Upon *M.tb* infection, bacteria are phagocytosed by macrophages and recruitment of additional macrophages, neutrophils, dendritic cells, and lymphocytes leads to the formation of a granuloma in an attempt to contain the infection. In addition to alveolar macrophages, epithelioid macrophages, foamy macrophages, neutrophils, and myeloid derived suppresor cells (MDSCs) support intracellular replication of bacilli. Bacilli are found in these cell types as well as the central necrotic region of the granuloma. T cells, B cells, Tregs and MDSCs migrate to the granuloma as well. While Tregs and MDSCs may prevent destructive hyper-inflammation, these suppressive cells also inhibit T effector responses during TB infection, leading to pathogen persistence

the alveoli. An initial innate immune response ensues when *M.tb* is engulfed by alveolar and interstitial macrophages, as well as local dendritic cells (DCs), following recognition by pattern recognition receptors (PRRs) present on these cells [12]. Several classes of germline-encoded PRRs associated with myeloid cells, either on the cell surface or cytosolic, including Toll-like receptors such as TLR2 and TLR9, C-type lectin receptors, mannose receptor and scavenger receptors, NOD2 and NLRP3, members of the NOD-like receptor family, AIM-2 like receptors (absent in myeloma, ALRs), nucleic acid sensors such as cyclic GMP-AMP synthase (cGAS) and stimulator of IFN genes, recognize specific mycobacterial pathogen-associated molecular patterns (PAMPs) and promote innate immune responses including the activation of NF-κB, the Type I interferon (IFN) response, and inflammasome activation, collectively known as the cytosolic surveillance pathway (CSP) [13]. On human DCs, the major receptor involved in *M.tb* recognition appears to be DC-SIGN [13]. This innate immune response serves a critical role as the first line of defense against the invading pathogen. However, *M.tb* has evolved several mechanisms to survive within the hostile environment of the macrophage. Despite sequestration within a membrane-bound phagosome, *M.tb* components also gain access to the macrophage cytosol via the bacterial secretion system ESX [14]. This allows for host recognition of the *M.tb*-derived nucleic acids, dsDNA and c-di-AMP, triggering CSP and autophagy. Our recent studies for example, show that secreted

M.tb-derived c-di-AMP functions as a PAMP to activate the host CSP and autophagy during infection [15].

Type I interferons (IFNα/β) activated during *M.tb* infection of macrophages promote downstream signaling pathways leading to induction of a large number of IFN-stimulated genes (ISGs). Studies in mouse models of infection and human patients with active TB have now clearly established that Type I interferons promote the progression of disease [16, 17]. Patients with active TB have a prominent whole blood IFNα/β-inducible transcriptional signature that correlates with the extent of disease [18]. On the other hand, signaling pathways activated by *M.tb* infection of macrophages lead to the production of IL-1α and IL-1β and other key pro-inflammatory mediators TNFα, and IL-6, all of which stimulate vigorous anti-microbial responses [19]. There also appears to be a significant cross-talk between these pro- and anti-microbial responses. While IFNα/β suppress the production of host-protective cytokines, IL-1α and IL-1β inhibit IFNα/β induction. This counter-regulation of IL-1 and Type I IFN signaling appears to provide a balanced host response that helps to keep the infection contained [20, 21]. Additionally, in certain contexts, Type I IFNs may play a protective role during TB infection. Studies in mice demonstrate that in the absence of IFNγ signaling, loss of Type I IFN signaling led to increased lung bacterial burden and pathology, due to increased frequency of alternatively activated macrophages and impaired recruitment and differentiation of macrophages and myeloid DCs in the lungs of infected mice [22, 23].

Immune Cell Recruitment and Initiation of an Adaptive Immune Response to M.tb

Following *M.tb* infection, chemokines and many related mediators produced by activated macrophages lead to additional recruitment of monocytes, neutrophils and dendritic cells to the site of infection, leading to a focal accumulation of mononuclear cells [24]. This initial innate response is followed by initiation of adaptive immunity when dendritic cells that have phagocytosed *M.tb* migrate to lymph nodes and present antigen and principally prime CD4+ and CD8+ T-helper lymphocytes [24, 25]. The adaptive immune response to *M.tb* is delayed, however, relative to responses to other pathogens. Infected humans do not become tuberculin positive until six weeks after exposure, and mice infected with low dose *M.tb* show delayed T cell response (3–4 weeks) in comparison to responses to other acute bacterial and viral infections such as to *Listeria monocytogenes* and influenza virus, which typically peak between 7 and 10 days after infection [26]. This delay has been attributed in part to regulatory T-cells [27]. In *M.tb* infection, DC-derived IL-12 is essential for development of Th1 cells [28]. Primed *M.tb* antigen-specific CD4+ effector Th1-cells migrate to infection sites and promote strong anti-mycobacterial effects through the secretion of IFN-γ, TNF-α, and IL-2 [29]. Mice that lack IL-12 or IL-12 receptor, which show defective Th1 responses, are highly susceptible to *M.tb* infection, as are individuals with mutations in IL-12 or its signaling components [30]. Antigen-primed CD8+ T cells also produce IFN-γ, and TNFα, although to a lesser extent than CD4+ T cells [31]. In addition, CD8+ T cells perform cytolytic functions capable of killing *M.tb* infected cells. Although evidence for a role of CD8+ T cells in control of *M.tb* infection in humans has not yet been well established, infection in humans is known to induce generation of both MHC Class I restricted classical CD8+ T cells as well as non-classically restricted CD8+ T cells, which include CD1-restricted and MHC I-related (MR1) restricted T cells, such as mucosal associated invariant T cells (MAIT) [32]. These cells are classified as innate lymphoid cells (ILCs), which function as early responders similar to innate immune cells but exhibit functional overlap with adaptive immune cells. Unlike adaptive lymphocytes, ILCs do not express antigen-specific receptors that have undergone somatic recombination and generally respond to cytokines and engagement of activating receptors on their cell surface. Other ILCs recruited to the site of infection include NKT cells and γδ T cells, and adaptive immune cells like B-lymphocytes [33–35]. γδ T cells secreting IL-17, and NKT cells expressing TCR and NK cell markers serve as intermediaries between the innate and adaptive immune responses [36]. In mice, Th17 cells promote neutrophil accumulation and tissue damage, but also promote recruitment of IFN-γ producing cells and granuloma formation [37, 38]. Th2 cells, which counter-regulate Th1 cells, likely impair protective immunity against TB, but this has not been fully established. Prolonged *M.tb*-induced TLR-2 signaling also promotes recruitment to the granulomas of $CD4^+$ $CD25^+$ $FoxP3^+$ regulatory T cells that dampen immune responses [39]. As discussed in detail later in this chapter, they are a major source of anti-inflammatory cytokine IL-10 and contribute to the down modulation of the immune response to the pathogen [6]. The infiltrating leukocytes ultimately remodel the infection site to form a granuloma, which helps to seal off the infection by creating a cellular and cytokine microenvironment of optimal immune response, but does not completely eradicate bacterial replication and persistence [40]. This is because *M.tb* continues to survive and proliferate in the mononuclear cells by (1) interfering with phagosome-lysosome fusion (2) inducing anti-inflammatory responses and (3) infecting newly recruited uninfected macrophages after exiting dying cells. Macrophages within granulomas have a high turnover rate and also demonstrate considerable phenotypic heterogeneity and functional plasticity [7]. Besides classically activated M1 macrophages, which inhibit *M.tb* replication, granulomas contain alternatively activated M2 macrophages, and transformed macrophages such as epithelioid, foamy, and multinucleated giant cells, which promote *M.tb* persistence by exhibiting anti-inflammatory phenotypes. Myeloid cell populations in TB granulomas has been recently expanded to include MDSCs, which are well known inhibitors of T-cell responses [7]. In addition, other recruited immune cells also aid in *M.tb* persistence and ultimate spread. Polymorphonuclear leukocytes (PMN) are recruited early to the lungs primarily in response to CXCL5 produced by pneumocytes and macrophages during *M.tb* infection [41]. Although they exhibit early anti-bacterial effects, and contribute to granuloma assembly [42], they secrete matrix metalloproteinases that are important drivers of cavitation preceding release and spread of *M.tb* [43]. A study in CXCL5 deficient mice demonstrated that decreased PMN recruitment to the lungs during *M.tb* infection due to lack of CXCL5-mediated signaling led to enhanced survival [44].

TB Granuloma Morphology and Heterogeneity

Three distinct types of granulomas have been observed in human disease [8, 45, 46]. The early stage of disease is characterized by a solid non-necrotic granuloma with a central area containing *M.tb* infected macrophages, surrounded by non-infected macrophages, neutrophils and CD4+ and CD8+ T cells, B-cells, and further by a layer of fibroblasts, collagen and extracellular matrix components [47, 48]. In early stages, a pronounced pro-angiogenic vascular endothelial growth factor response leads to neovascularization promoting a dynamic influx of cells. Studies in *M.tb* infected macaques suggest that early granulomas can harbor bacterium that replicate rapidly followed by either bacterial killing and control or progression of the lesion [49]. In situations when the granulomatous immune response becomes ineffective, active post-primary TB disease ensues. The lungs of such individuals contain enlarging granulomas that differentiate with time. Extensive neutrophilic infiltrates lead to a central core of suppuration and necrosis, forming the necrotic granuloma that expands and causes tissue damage [50]. Liquefaction of dead immune cells in the core allows for the development of the caseous granuloma, which is highly permissive for bacterial replication. Matrix degradation and dysfunctional tissue remodeling cause fibrosis, leading to the development of cavitary pulmonary disease that allows access of *M.tb* into alveoli and outward spread [51]. Cavity formation involves breakdown of extracellular lung matrix by specific hydrolytic enzymes, including proteinases, nucleases, and lipases. Collagen fibrils, specifically type I, III, and IV collagen, are the major structural components of the human lung extracellular matrix. They are highly resistant to enzymatic breakdown and can only be degraded by specific matrix metalloproteinases which are activated by signaling pathways involving mitogen-activated protein (MAP) kinase, PI3-kinase/Akt pathway, and transcription factors NF-κB and AP-1 macrophage infection, [52–54]. Cavitation correlates with bacterial abundance in the sputum [55, 56]. TB transmission is therefore highly increased by cavitary disease. Clinically, cavitation impairs the efficacy of antibiotics, contributing to treatment failure and the emergence of antibiotic resistance [57, 58].

Although pulmonary TB is the most common presentation, *M.tb* can also disseminate into other organs causing extrapulmonary TB [59]. Frequent sites of extrapulmonary infection include the pleura, lymph nodes, bones and joints, meninges in the central nervous system, larynx, skeleton especially the spine, eyes, gastrointestinal and genitourinary tracts, adrenal gland, and skin. Dissemination from initial infection site indicates spread from an unprotected pulmonary granuloma or bacterial dissemination into the sites via regional lymph nodes.

Myeloid-Derived Suppressor Cells: Serving Up a Double Whammy in the Tuberculous Granuloma

MDSCs: Discovery and Characterization in Disease

While latent *M.tb* infection is characterized by a balance of *M.tb* specific cellular and cytokine immune responses as discussed above, development of active disease is known to correlate with impaired immune cell responses [60, 61]. Reduced polyfunctional IFN-γ^+IL-2^+TNFα^+ CD4+ T cells, increased TNFα single-positive CD4+ T cells, progressive T cell dysfunction, and impaired proliferation of *M.tb*-specific CD4+ and CD8+ T cells correlating with high bacterial burden have been found in patients with smear-positive TB, relative to patients with smear-negative TB and latent TB [62]. However, the underlying mechanisms leading to impaired T-cell responses in active TB are not completely understood. Recent research has begun to focus attention on immune cells and mediators that actively promote bacterial growth by suppressing anti-mycobacterial immune responses in TB. Among the immune cells that face scrutiny are a heterogeneous group of suppressive myeloid cells, which have developed evolutionarily to prevent excessive tissue damage in the host during infections and to promote wound healing and tissue remodeling, but also found to be co-opted by tumors and pathogens to support immune evasion and growth in a suppressive niche amidst host immunosurveillance [63–65]. Interestingly, they were first identified in 1978 as a suppressive population activated in the spleens and bone marrow of mice after the administration of BCG [66]. Further studies of immune tolerance demonstrated a population of "natural suppressor" cells in the neonatal spleen [67]. Studies in the late 1990s and early in the last decade identified the cells to accumulate in lymphoid organs, blood, liver, lungs and tumors in many mouse models of cancers, and to be phenotypically similar to neutrophils and monocytes, but functionally distinct [68, 69]. The suppressor cells have now also been identified in many different human tumors, including head and neck cancers, gliomas, renal, prostate, pancreatic, hepatocellular and non-small lung carcinomas among others [70, 71]. Their phenotypic heterogeneity had rendered their characterization and terminology contentious, and in 2007, leading cancer investigators suggested naming the cells as myeloid-derived suppressor cells or MDSCs, a terminology that defines both their origin and their functional nature [72]. Their characterization has been revisited more recently [73]. Accumulating evidence of their clinical significance has rendered them an integral part of the field of tumor immunology and a promising target for cancer immunotherapy, as well as infectious diseases [74].

MDSC Markers and Mechanisms of Suppression

MDSCs are classified as monocytic or M-MDSCs, and polymorphonuclear or PMN-MDSCs [73]. In cancers more than 80% of MDSCs are PMN-MDSCs, but both populations induce host-driven T cell tolerance that promotes immune evasion, thus limiting the efficacy of immune-based therapies. In mice, PMN-MDSCs are defined as $CD11b^{+}Ly6G^{+}Ly6C^{low}$, and M-MDSCs as $CD11b^{+}Ly6G^{-}Ly6C^{high}$ cells. In humans, MDSCs have been mostly identified in blood and tumors described as $CD11b^{+}CD33^{+}HLA\text{-}DR^{low/neg}$ cells. Human PMN-MDSCs are $CD14^{-}$ and $CD15^{+}$, while M-MDSCs are $CD14^{+}$ and $CD15^{-}$. Some of the $CD33^{+}HLA\text{-}DR^{low/neg}$ cells are myeloid progenitors (or early MDSCs). Newer markers that have been identified to characterize MDSCs include CD124 (IL-4Rα), CD40, CD80, CD115 and S100A9. These markers do not however, define any specific subpopulations, and since none of the markers are unique to MDSCs, their identification requires further evidence of immune-suppressive properties.

The most important functional characteristic of MDSCs is their ability to inhibit antigen-specific and non-specific activation and proliferation of $CD4^{+}$ and $CD8^{+}$ T cells. While PMNs and monocytes/macrophages are recruited early in an attempt to control infection by phagocytosing bacteria and facilitating activation of T cells [75], PMN-MDSCs and M-MDSCs directly inhibit T-cell-driven immune responses [65]. MDSCs utilize multiple mechanisms to inhibit T cells that include depletion of amino acids, generation of NO and reactive oxygen species (ROS), inhibition of T-cell migration, induction of Tregs and Th17 cells, and impairment of NK-cell mediated cytotoxicity [63, 76].

L-arginine is required for functional T-cell responses. MDSCs express arginase-1, which degrades L-arginine into urea and ornithine, thereby depleting it from the environment. MDSCs also express the inducible NO-synthase, which catalyzes the production of citrulline and NO from L-arginine, further contributing to L-arginine depletion [77]. Cysteine, an essential amino acid required for T cell activation, is normally obtained from cystine exported from macrophages because T cells lack cystathionase, which converts methionine to cysteine. By sequestering cystine, MDSCs limit its availability for T-cell proliferation [78]. NO also inhibits JAK3, STAT5, ERK, and AKT, blocking IL-2R mediated signaling pathways, thereby impairing the generation of effector and memory T cells [79]. In addition, MDSCs generate reactive oxygen species (ROS) through isoforms of superoxide-generating NADPH oxidase [80], which disrupt the T-cell function by modifying its TCR-ζ-chain [81]. The nature of suppression depends on the subpopulation of MDSC. While M-MDSCs mainly generate NO, PMN-MDSCs produce higher levels of ROS [82]. MDSCs also prevent the homing of T cells to draining lymph nodes and tumor sites by downregulating L-selectin on naïve T cells and E-selectin on vasculature [83, 84].

MDSCs have been shown to induce the expansion and activation of Tregs [85–87]. Expansion of Tregs is mediated through secretion of IL-10 and TGFβ, and requires the expression of CD40 on MDSCs [85, 88, 89]. More recently, it has been shown that MDSCs induce Th17 ($CD4^{+}$ $ROR\gamma t^{+}$ $IL\text{-}17^{+}$) cells through secreted IL-6 and TGFβ [90]. In addition, IFNγ and TNFα can promote survival and accumulation of MDSCs and MDSCs treated with these cytokines have been found to produce CCL4, a Th17 chemoattractant that facilitates recruitment of Th17 cells [80, 91, 92]. IL-17, in turn, has been found to activate the ERK1/2 pathway in MDSCs and promote survival and accumulation of MDSCs in animal models of cancer [93, 94].

MDSCs have also been shown to impair the function of NK cells. TGFβ and H_2O_2 produced by MDSCs decrease the expression of NK cell activating receptors NKG2D, NKp46, and NKp44 [95, 96]. MDSCs also decrease the ability of NK cells to induce apoptosis of target cells by down-regulating their production of perforin and by limiting their response to growth factor IL-2 [97].

MDSCs are normally present at low or undetectable levels in healthy individuals, but their numbers dramatically increase in chronic inflammatory states, likely as a compensatory mechanism to limit bystander tissue damage, and in cancers [70]. Tumors appear to have co-opted the cells to facilitate immune escape and consequently their growth and dissemination and initial studies in animal models suggest *M.tb* and other bacteria do the same.

Induction of MDSCs and Their Involvement in Disease

During tumor progression, MDSC are generated from a common myeloid progenitor, promoted by tumor-derived GM-CSF, G-CSF, VEGF, IL-6, IL1β and TNFα, prostaglandin E2 and damage-associated molecular pattern (DAMP) molecules S100A8/A9 [98]. A two-step model was proposed to describe their generation: inhibition of terminal differentiation of progenitors, and conversion of immature myeloid cells to MDSC. A major transcription factor involved in growth factor and cytokine-mediated MDSC expansion is signal transducer and activator of transcription STAT3. Activated STAT3 also induces the expression of S100A8 and S100A9, which block differentiation of immature myeloid cells into dendritic cells and macrophages and promote MDSC expansion [99, 100]. More recently, another DAMP molecule, HMGB1, has been shown to promote the expansion of MDSCs from bone marrow progenitor cells in vitro. Neutralization of HMGB1 in tumor-bearing mice reduces MDSC levels in the tumor, spleen, and blood [101]. In addition, MDSC themselves secrete pro-inflammatory mediators IL-6 and S100A8/A9, which leads to an autocrine feedback loop that amplifies MDSC accumulation in the tumor microenvironment [100]. Other related transcription factors of the STAT family, STAT1 and STAT6, activated by Th1 cytokine IFN-γ and Th2 cytokines IL-4 and IL-13 respectively, have been implicated in MDSC activation and function [102, 103]. Activation of NF-κB, which is downstream of TLR, IL-1R and TNFR signaling is known to lead to MDSC expansion, as do RAS and PI3K/Akt signaling [104].

MicroRNAs (miRNAs), endogenous ~22 nt long non-coding RNAs, which have significantly advanced our understanding of gene regulation, modulate host immune responses by regulating the expression of important genes involved in the differentiation of immune cells. Several miRNAs have been implicated in the accumulation and function of MDSC [105], but discrepancies exist. For example, miR-155 has been shown to both promote and negatively regulate accumulation of MDSC [106, 107]. In this regard, it is interesting to note that infection of human macrophages with *M.tb* decreased the expression of miR-155 [108], and that miR-155 is significantly reduced in the serum of TB patients [109].

Chronic inflammatory states occur during TB infection and also precede tumor development. Many important cytokines, myeloid differentiation factors, as well as DAMP molecules such as S100A8/A9 and HMGB1, all of which promote MDSC expansion in tumors as described above, are also elevated during infections and acute and chronic inflammation. MDSCs have in fact been implicated in immune regulation of chronic inflammation, in asthma, and in autoimmune diseases such as autoimmune enterocolitis and encephalomyelitis [110, 111]. Microbial factors and PAMPs also induce MDSCs. For example, *Pseudomonas aeruginosa* induces MDSC generation through flagellin [112]. An increase in MDSC frequency has been observed in *H. pylori* infected mice and humans [113]. Fungal infections (*Aspergillus fumigatus* and *Candida albicans*) induce a subset of MDSCs through pattern recognition receptor Dectin-1 [114]. Cystic fibrosis patients with chronic *P. aeruginosa* infections demonstrate a higher MDSC frequency in blood compared to patients without *P. aeruginosa* infections or healthy control subjects [112]. Mice infected with *K. pneumoniae* show MDSC expansion and increased levels of IL-10 [115]. Immunosuppressive subsets of MDSC have also been demonstrated in *S. aureus* skin infection models [116]. Elevated levels of MDSCs are found in the serum of patients with sepsis, although in sepsis they can be both pro-inflammatory and immunosuppressive [117]. Such paradoxical dual roles are evident in the early and late phases of infections. Since many of the factors leading to MDSC expansion are elevated during host immune response to *M.tb* and formation of the granuloma, it seems only logical to speculate that MDSCs would also accumulate in TB, and may play a pathophysiological role.

Evidence for MDSC Involvement During TB Infection

In support of this hypothesis, Gr-1 (Ly-6G/C) positive cells, which appear to modulate T cell expansion through production of NO and superoxide anion, were identified in the spleen mice primed with heat-killed Mycobacterium [118]. BCG vaccination of mice was found to increase the levels of myeloid cells, which impaired T cell priming in the draining lymph node in a MyD88-dependent manner [119]. Subsequently, MDSCs were found to be induced not only in patients with TB, but also in individuals recently exposed to *M.tb* (household exposure) [120]. These cells inhibited activation and proliferation of CD4+ and CD8+ T cells, altered T-cell trafficking, and were associated with increased production of IL-1β, IL-6, IL-8, G-CSF, and MCP-1. Another study showed that in patients with active TB, the frequency of $CD244^{high}$ cells with MDSC phenotypes were significantly higher, and negatively correlated with the activation and function of $CD4^{+}$ and $CD8^{+}$ T-cells [121]. MDSC accumulation has also been observed in both lungs and blood of patients with active TB and anti-TB therapy appeared to reduce MDSC accumulation in the blood [122]. In mouse models of TB, accumulation of MDSC was found to correlate with increased TB lethality [123]. Knaul et al. showed that MDSCs expressing *Arg-1* and *Nos2*, comprising a heterogeneous population of PMN-MDSC and M-MDSC with immunosuppressive properties and elevated IL-4R expression, accumulated in the lungs at the site of infection. Excessive MDSC accumulation in lungs correlated with increased TB lethality [124]. Treatment with all-trans-retinoic acid (ATRA), which is known to reduce MDSC in vivo, decreased the frequency of lung $CD11b^{+}Gr1^{+}$ MDSCs in *M.tb* infected mice. ATRA treatment significantly reduced bacterial loads and ameliorated pathology suggesting that MDSCs are potential targets for host-directed therapies [124]. In addition, the study demonstrated the presence of *M.tb* in purified MDSC subsets, strongly indicating that the role of MDSCs in pathogenesis is multifactorial; that in addition to providing immune suppression and evasion from host immune responses, they also phagocytose and harbor *M.tb*, thus offering a newly defined physical niche for *M.tb* survival within the lungs.

S100A8/A9 are secreted by MDSCs, and they promote differentiation of myeloid progenitors into MDSC in the bone marrow as well as autocrine accumulation and activation of MDSCs in tumors [99, 100]. They are calcium-binding protein molecules that are constitutively expressed by myeloid cells, and contribute to intracellular homeostatic processes. However, during infections, inflammation, and in tumors, they are also secreted into the extracellular medium, and serve as endogenous danger signals or DAMP, promoting immune responses and repair mechanisms through binding to cell surface receptors such as the Receptor for Advanced Glycation End Products (RAGE) and Toll-like Receptor 4 (TLR4) [125, 126]. It has been shown that in human patients with active TB and in nonhuman primate models and mouse models of *M.tb* infection, myeloid cells producing S100A8/A9 proteins dominate within the inflammatory lung granulomas and exacerbate inflammation [127]. In fact, recent proteomic studies suggest that S100A9 could serve a serum diagnostic biomarker for pulmonary TB and to discriminate pulmonary TB from other lung diseases such as pneumonia and lung cancer [128]. In BCG-challenged guinea pig lungs, administration of tasquinimod, which binds to S100A9 and blocks its interaction with cell surface receptors, impaired the formation of granulomas indicating that S100A9 plays an important role in the organization of the tuberculous granuloma [129]. All the above studies suggest that MDSCs may play a pathological role in the progression of TB and could therefore be targeted for anti-mycobacterial therapy.

Regulatory T Cells: Amplifying the Immunosuppressive Microenvironment Within the Tuberculous Granuloma

Tregs: Essential Mediators of Immune Homeostasis

As mentioned earlier, *M.tb* elicits both innate and adaptive immune responses in the host. While MDSCs straddle both the innate and adaptive systems in the immune hierarchy, another set of immunosuppressive cells found in the tuberculous granuloma, the regulatory T-cells or Tregs, serve as an integral part of the adaptive immune system. Tregs were initially discovered as a specialized subset of CD4+ T cells expressing IL-2 receptor a chain (CD25), that play a pivotal role in maintaining self-tolerance and preventing autoimmune diseases [130]. They provide tolerance to both self-antigens and to commensal flora and innocuous environmental antigens and allergens [131]. Tregs express a specific marker, the transcription factor forkhead box P3 (FOXP3), which regulates expression of genes responsible both for the differentiation of Tregs, and for the suppression of immune response [132, 133]. In humans, FOXP3 deficiency results in the development of a multi-organ lymphoproliferative autoimmune disease, also known as immune dysregulation, polyendocrinopathy, enteropathy and X-linked (IPEX) syndrome [134, 135]. Tregs play a critical role in the induction and maintenance of peripheral tolerance in allogeneic stem cell transplantation [136]. Studies using graft-versus-host disease (GvHD) model systems have shown the adoptive transfer of Tregs inhibits the allogeneic immune response [137, 138]. In the periphery, it is now well established that Tregs also regulate host immune responses to pathogens by preventing uncontrolled immunopathology and collateral tissue damage associated with hyper-inflammatory reactions [139]. MDSCs have been shown to promote the expansion of Tregs, thus helping to maintain and amplify an immune tolerant microenvironment [85–87]. As with MDSCs however, Tregs can also be co-opted by pathogens such as *M.tb* to subvert effector immune responses, allowing their survival in the host [140, 141].

Based on their origin and function, two major populations of Tregs have been described: natural (nTreg) and induced (iTreg) cells. It has also been recently recommended that Treg populations be denoted by place of induction: "thymus derived" (tTregs) or "peripherally derived" (pTregs) [142]. nTregs or tTregs arising in the thymus form the major population of $CD4^+FOXP3^+$ Tregs, and they mediate tolerance to self-antigens [143]. iTregs ($CD4^+FOXP3^+$) or pTregs arise in peripheral lymphoid tissues from naive conventional $CD4^+FOXP3^-$ T cells after exposure to antigens. They are especially abundant in the gastrointestinal tract and in lungs and exhibit specificities against microbial antigens or environmental allergens, and also restrain immune responses to exogenous pathogens [144]. Their induction from naive $CD4^+$ T cells requires TGF-β and retinoic acid that are secreted by dendritic cells and resident macrophages [145]. Specific markers on human Tregs are lacking and therefore are defined by multiple regulatory markers and/or by demonstrating suppressive activity.

Mechanisms of Treg-Mediated Suppression of Immune Responses

Tregs produce immunosuppressive cytokines IL-10, TGFβ and IL-35 [146–148]. IL-35 is a recently identified member of the IL-12 family of heterodimeric cytokines. However, unlike other members of the IL-12 family, IL-35 is not produced by antigen-presenting cells, but primarily by Tregs and B-regulatory cells [149]. IL-35 can directly suppress the proliferation and function of effector T-cells and increasingly being considered as a key mediator of immune suppression.

It is now recognized that Tregs are in fact heterogeneous and include several subpopulations that are able to suppress immune reactions, maintain self-tolerance and restore homeostasis after immune response. Recently, a unique population of iTregs expressing the marker CD39 has been identified. $CD8^+CD25^+FOXP3^+$ T cells and $CD8^+CD25^+CD39^+FOXP3^+$ T cells, both referred to as $CD8^+$ Tregs, are a small subset of an immunosuppressive population of $CD8^+$ suppressor T cells, which have been identified in *M.tb* and *M.bovis* infections [150]. IL-35 further promotes tolerance to infections by generating a potent population of IL-35-producing inducible Tregs called iTr35, which in turn produce IL-35, but not IL-10 or TGFβ [149]. $CD4^+$ type 1 regulatory T (T_R1) cells represent another subset of Treg cells defined by the expression of IL-10, a master regulator of inflammation, but do not express FOXP3 and CD25 [151]. The T_R1 cells express a number of transcription factors, such as c-MAF and IRF1, which are common to other T-cell populations.

Tregs suppress both innate immune responses, as well as induction of T-cell responses at the activation, proliferation, and differentiation stages and at the effector stages in tissues. Their suppressive activity targets dendritic cells, macrophages, NK cells, CD4+ and CD8+ T-cells, B-cells, and NKT cells and are mediated primarily through the secretion of inhibitory cytokines IL-10, TGFβ and IL-35 [152]. These cytokines directly inhibit effector T-cell (Teff) proliferation, and also the expression of MHC class II and co-stimulatory molecules on antigen-presenting cells, thus indirectly suppressing Teff activation. IL-2 is a major trophic cytokine for various T-cell subsets and expression of IL-2Rα chain (CD25) on the surface of Tregs allows them to bind and deplete IL-2 from the environment, which leads to inhibition of proliferation and apoptosis of effector T-cells [152]. Tregs also release granzymes A and B, which promote T-cell cytolysis. Granzyme A-induced cytolysis is perforin-dependent, FAS-FASL-independent, and requires cell-contact [153]. Treg cells derived from the tumor environment induce NK and CD8+ T cell death in a granzyme B- and perforin-dependent fashion [154]. Activated Tregs also express galectin-1 on the surface, which binds to relevant carbohydrate ligands on effector T-cells, inhibiting their proliferation and decreasing the production of IFNγ [155]. Tregs also function through down-modulation of antigen-presenting cells through interactions of CTLA-4-CD80/CD86 and LAG-3-MHC class II interactions [156, 157]. CTLA-4 is a Foxp3-dependent protein expressed on Tregs. Mice with Tregs that lack CTLA-4 protein expression develop lethal autoimmunity [156]. CTLA-4 on Tregs binds to costimulatory molecules CD80 and CD86 on dendritic cells reducing their availability for naive T-cells and hindering co-stimulation during antigen presentation. This is followed by development of anergy and apoptosis in antigen-specific T cells. Indoleamine 2,3-dioxygenase (IDO), induced by CTLA-4, depletes tryptophan in local tissue microenvironment, leading to reduced proliferation and apoptosis of Teff cells [158]. Recently, lymphocyte-activation gene 3 (LAG-3), homologous to CD4, has emerged as another important molecule that regulates T cell function [157]. It is expressed on different subsets of T cells and also on B cells, NK cells and plasmacytoid DC. Lag-3 binds to MHC class II with high affinity, and negatively regulates cellular proliferation, activation, and homeostasis of T cells.

Role of Treg Suppression in Disease

A wide range of human pathologies has been associated with altered Treg function. These include pathologies associated with loss of tolerance, such as in immune dysregulation of genetic origin leading to autoimmunity, and allergic responses to food and environmental allergens [159, 160]. Mutations of *FOXP3* lead to the development of dysfunctional thymic Treg cells resulting in severe autoimmunity in the early-onset and life-threatening IPEX syndrome, manifesting with severe eczema, intractable diarrhea, and type I diabetes in the first months of life [134, 135]. Tregs have been implicated in suppressing effector responses in other autoimmune disorders such as myasthenia gravis and rheumatoid arthritis [159].

Tumors and pathogens exploit Tregs to suppress host immune responses for proliferation and survival. Tregs suppress anti-tumor immune responses, and along with MDSCs, contribute to the development of an immunosuppressive tumor microenvironment that facilitates immune evasion and cancer progression. An accumulation of $FOXP3^{+}$ Tregs is associated with unfavorable prognoses in many human cancers, including ovarian, pancreatic, lung cancers, and other malignancies [161, 162]. Tregs are also induced by a wide range of viral, bacterial and parasitic pathogens and play a dual role during infections: during acute infections, they benefit the host by limiting immune-mediated pathology and excessive inflammation. However, in the long-term, they also promote chronic pathogen persistence [140, 141]. Studies in mouse models of persistent *Salmonella enterica* infections show that after acute infection Tregs are elevated, but failure to completely eradicate the pathogen leads to a carrier state of persistent asymptomatic infection. Several studies have shown that *Helicobacter pylori* induce Tregs as well. Pathogen persistence during chronic *H. pylori* infection leads to chronic inflammation and gastric tumor induction. The role of Tregs has also been extensively studied in *M.tb* infections both in the latent and active disease states.

Treg Suppression of Immune Responses During TB Infection

Being an efficient manipulator of host immunity, *M.tb* elicits expansion of Tregs to support its persistence. Studies in mouse models show that Tregs act as checkpoint in three stages of *M.tb* infection: blocking effector cell responses in the lung, inhibiting priming and differentiation of T cells in the lymph node and inhibiting migration of activated T cells to the lung. In mouse models of *M.tb* infection, Tregs were found in granulomas in the lung, and were shown to prevent pathogen clearance

[163, 164]. Pathogen-specific Tregs induced by *M.tb* delayed priming of $CD4^+$ and $CD8^+$ T-cells in the pulmonary lymph nodes, thereby delaying migration of these cells to the lung [27]. Delayed onset of adaptive immunity allows initial establishment of infection. Depletion of $CD25^+$ cells early after *M.tb* infection decreased bacterial load and granuloma formation [165]. In macaques, an increasing frequency of Tregs in lungs and blood was found in animals developing active disease after challenge with *M.tb*. Tregs and IFNγ-producing effector T-cells expanded early after pulmonary TB infection, yet in vivo depletion of both T-effector cells and Tregs led to decreased resistance against granuloma progression [150]. These studies in animal models showed that Tregs aggravated the pathology of tuberculosis by blunting Th1 responses and thereby inhibiting *M.tb* clearance.

Treg cells are known to accumulate in human TB. Increased frequencies of $CD4^+CD25^{+/HI}$ cells and $CD4^+CD25^{HI}CD39^+$ cells have been identified in the peripheral blood and bronchoalvelolar lavage fluids in TB patients compared to healthy controls [166–170]. Frequencies of Tregs and levels of TGFβ have also been shown to be significantly higher in cavitary TB patients than in non-cavitary TB patients [171]. Circulatory $CD4^+CD25^+$ and $CD4^+CD25^+$ $FoxP3^+$ Treg cells were elevated in patients with cavitary MDR-TB and decreased after pulmonary resection [172]. The frequencies of Tregs in blood of TB patients declined after successful chemotherapy, but remained high in patients with emerging drug-resistant TB [173].

Increased frequencies of $CD4^+Foxp3^+CD25^+$ Tregs have also been found in peripheral blood and in broncho-alveolar lavage fluid in patients with active TB compared to individuals with latent disease [174, 175]. *M.tb* is known to migrate to and establish infection in extra-pulmonary sites. Treg cell frequency is higher in pleural fluid than in circulation in tuberculous pleurisy [176]. Patients with miliary TB also show increased frequencies of Tregs in peripheral blood, pleural fluid and bronchoalveolar lavage [177].

The presence of Tregs through granuloma evolution and increased frequency in cavitary disease suggests that they could play important roles in dissemination of TB. Increased frequencies during active disease compared to latent stages, and decline after therapy also indicate that functional signatures of Tregs can serve as biomarkers for disease progression and response to therapy.

Therapeutic Targeting of MDSCs and Tregs in TB

Studies from animal models of TB show that blocking the recruitment or functions of MDSC and Tregs impede progress of disease, suggesting that they can serve as valid targets for HDT (Table 1). Pre-exposure to mycobacterial antigens in endemic regions is believed to induce immune-regulatory cells in the host, which are further stimulated by BCG vaccination, and could partly account for the reduction in vaccine efficacy. Induction of Tregs has in fact been demonstrated in several TB-vaccine candidate trials [141]. Preventing induction of MDSCs and Tregs are therefore powerful new approaches to improving the efficacy of BCG and other novel anti-TB

Table 1 Therapeutic targeting of MDSCs and Tregs

Target cell effect	Therapy	Mechanism of action	Treatment outcome	Reference
Treg depletion	Anti-CD25	Antibody mediated depletion of CD25+ cells	Treg depletion in *M.tb* infected mice led to transient decrease in lung bacterial load	[165]
	Denileukin diftitox	Recombinant diphtheria fusion toxin targeting IL-2 receptor bearing cells	Treg depletion in *M.tb* infected mice resulted in decreased bacterial burden in lung and spleen	[178]
	Anti CTLA-4, ipilimumab	Antibody mediated depletion of CTLA-4+ cells	Treatment resulted in lower frequency of Tregs in tumors of bladder cancer patients. Treatment of BCG infected mice does not decrease bacterial burden	[179, 180]
Inhibition of Treg suppressive activity	Anti PD-1	Antibody blockade of PD-1	PD-1 blockade of Tregs from TB patients decreases suppressive activity in vitro	[173]
MDSC depletion	Sunitinib, sorafenib	Receptor tyrosine kinase inhibitor	Sunitinib treatment depleted MDSCs in a murine model of breast cancer	[181]
	Gemcitabine	Nucleoside analog	Gemcitabine treatment depleted G-MDSCs in patients with pancreatic cancer	[182, 183]
Promotion of MDSC differentiation	ATRA	Binds RAR nuclear receptors	ATRA treatment leads to decreased lung bacterial burden in *M.tb* infected mice	[124]
Inhibition of MDSC infiltration	Tasquinimod	Binds S100A9 and blocks interaction with its receptors	Tasquinimod treatment reduces infiltration of MDSCs into tumors in a murine model of breast cancer. Treatment of BCG-infected guinea pigs decreases lung granuloma formation	[129, 184, 185]
Inhibition of MDSC suppressive activity and reduction in MDSC numbers	Sildenafil, tadalafil, vardenafil	PDE-5 inhibitors	Tadalafil treatment lowers MDSCs in patients with head and neck cancer	[186, 187]

vaccines [188]. Vast literature on therapeutic targeting of MDSCs and Tregs in tumors show that they can be targeted by interfering with either their production, or blocking their trafficking to sites of infection, or inhibiting their immunosuppressive function.

Among major factors regulating MDSC generation in the bone marrow are stem cell factor receptor c-kit, and its downstream effector signaling that involves STAT3. Blocking of c-kit and STAT3 signaling using tyrosine-kinase inhibitors such as sunitinib and sorafenib have been shown to effectively reduce MDSC populations in both tumor-bearing mice and cancer patients [181, 189]. Gemcitabine, a nucleoside analog, is used as a chemotherapeutic in many cancers. Gemcitabine administration depletes MDSCs from spleens and tumors of tumor-bearing mice [182]. It has been shown to reduce MDSC and Tregs in patients with pancreatic cancer [183]. Since MDSCs are immature myeloid cells, an attractive therapeutic approach would also be to promote differentiation of MDSCs toward fully mature myeloid cells. Such an effect can be achieved by using ATRA (all-trans-retinoic acid). Treatment with ATRA substantially decreases the presence of MDSC in spleens of tumor-bearing mice and in peripheral blood of patients with renal cell carcinoma [190, 191]. In fact, in a rat model of *M.tb* infection, retinoic acid administration has been shown to reduce disease pathology and promote expression of TNFα and IL1β in alveolar macrophages [192]. Treatment with ATRA decreased the frequency of lung MDSCs, reduced bacterial loads and pathology in a mouse model of TB [124].

Another drug that targets MDSCs is tasquinimod, a second generation quinoline-3-carboxamide analogue. This analogue has shown anti-angiogenic, antitumor and immune-modulatory properties in preclinical models of prostate cancer and other solid tumors [193, 194] and has been found to inhibit the accumulation of immunosuppressive MDSC in tumors and premetastatic niches [193, 195]. Quinoline-3-caboxamides show high affinity binding to S100A9 protein [196]. Tasquinimod binds S100A9 protein on MDSCs and inhibits its interaction with cell surface receptors TLR4 and RAGE, thus reducing the infiltration of MDSC. Large randomized phase II trials of tasquinimod in men with chemotherapy-naïve metastatic castration-resistant prostate cancer (mCRPC) has demonstrated a significant prolongation in radiographic and symptomatic progression-free survival compared with placebo [184, 185]. Incidentally, in BCG-challenged guinea pig lungs, tasquinimod impairs the formation of granulomas, the organization of which is regulated by S100A9 [129].

The immunosuppressive function of MDSCs depends on their production of NO and ARG-1. Phosphodiesterase-5 (PDE5) inhibitors such as sildenafil, tadalafil, and vardenafil that are currently in clinical use, down-regulate ARG-1 and NO production. Preclinical studies in tumor models have shown that phosphodiesterase-5 (PDE5) inhibition is able to not only reverse MDSC suppression, but also Treg accumulation, thereby promoting antitumor immunity [86, 197]. In patients with head and neck squamous cell carcinoma (HNSCC) tadalafil administration has been shown to lower MDSCs and Tregs and increase tumor-specific $CD8^+$ T cells in a dose-dependent fashion [186, 187]. It has to be noted that human PDE inhibitors have emerged as an attractive strategy for adjunctive HDTs against TB. We have found that in mouse models, addition of the FDA-approved cAMP phosphodiesterase inhibitors cilostazol (Type III PDE-I) as an adjunctive drug, either alone or with sildenafil (Type V PDE-I) to the standard TB treatment regimen, reduces tissue pathology, leads to faster bacterial clearance and shortens the time to lung sterilization by one month, compared to standard treatment alone [198].

Recently FDA-approved immune checkpoint inhibitors (ICI) for cancer treatment aim to re-establish anti-tumor immune responses by blocking inhibitory immune checkpoint molecules or their ligands, thereby enhancing Teff and cytotoxic T-cell (CTL) functionality. As mentioned earlier, Tregs highly upregulate expression of various immune checkpoint molecules (CTLA-4, PD-1, LAG-3), making them attractive targets for ICI. Monoclonal antibodies (mAbs) against CTLA-4 (ipilimumab) and PD-1 (nivolumab/pembrolizumab) have been used for the treatment of metastatic melanoma, non-small-cell lung cancer, advanced renal carcinoma and Hodgkin's lymphoma. Pre-clinical murine models have shown that anti-CTLA-4 mAbs activate Teff and CTLs, and promote ADCC (antibody-dependent cell-mediated cytotoxicity)-mediated depletion of intra-tumoral Tregs [199]. Intra-tumoral $FoxP3^+$ Tregs were depleted by ADCC-mediated lysis following ipilimumab treatment in metastatic lesions of melanoma patients, although this observation remains controversial [179]. CTLA-4 blockade has not been thoroughly explored in the context of *M.tb* infection. BCG-infected mice treated with anti-CTLA-4 had increased lymphocyte recruitment to the lungs, however bacterial burden remained unchanged [180]. Further work must be done to determine whether CTLA-4 blockade changes Treg frequency or function and can alter the adaptive immune response to infection. Studies examining the effect of PD-1 blockade for treatment of *M.tb* have produced mixed results. PD-1 is highly upregulated on "exhausted" T cells, and inhibits T cell proliferation and IFN-γ and IL-2 production [200]. Preclinical studies show that nivolumab impairs Treg suppressive activity, possibly by downregulating intracellular expression of FoxP3, and promotes CTL proliferation [201]. Blockade of PD-1 on Tregs from patients with pulmonary TB decreased their suppressive activity in vitro, however loss of PD-1 in mice leads to increased susceptibility to *M.tb* [173, 202]. These data suggest that the effects of PD-1 blockade on immune response to infection are likely to be target cell-dependent.

Ontak® (denileukin diftitox; DAB389IL-2), is a FDA-approved biologic that specifically targets cells expressing the high affinity IL-2 receptor. It is a fusion protein comprised of the diphtheria toxin catalytic- and transmembrane domains fused to human IL-2 [203]. The cytotoxic potency of diphtheria toxin is selectively targeted to those eukaryotic cells that display high-affinity receptor for IL-2 [204–207]. The relative sensitivity of a given IL-2 receptor-positive cell line to Ontak® is dependent upon the pattern of expression of each of the three subunits of IL-2R. The high-affinity receptor (αβγ chains) is found on Tregs and activated T cells, while the intermediate affinity receptor (βγ chains) is found on resting memory T cells and NK cells. Expression of the α chain, also known as CD25, is used to identify Tregs expressing high-affinity IL-2 receptor. In 1999, Ontak® was approved by the FDA under the accelerated program for the treatment of refractory cutaneous T cell lymphoma

CTCL, based on durable objective responses [208], and used off-label for patients presenting with chronic lymphocytic leukemia, non-Hodgkin's lymphoma, and human T cell lymphotropic virus-1 [209]. The drug has also been used off-label to successfully treat steroid-resistant graft-versus-host disease [210], methotrexate-resistant psoriasis [211] and as an immunotherapeutic agent for the transient depletion of Tregs in patients with unresectable stage IV malignant melanoma [212, 213]. Ontak® treatment of *M.tb* infected mice resulted in decreased Treg frequency and bacterial burden in the lungs [178]. In addition, another Ontak®-related fusion protein DAB389mIL-4 is selectively toxic for eukaryotic cells that display the IL-4R on their cell surface, and the cytotoxic potency of this fusion protein toxin is directly proportional to the number of IL-4Rs on the cell surface [214]. Both fusion proteins therefore provide a unique and novel opportunity for the development of a new HDT for TB by targeting $CD25^+$ Tregs and $IL\text{-}4R^+$ MDSC which have engulfed *M.tb*.

Although current therapies for targeting MDSCs and Tregs have proven to be promising, there are impediments that need to be considered. Specifically, the heterogeneity of MDSC and Tregs highlights the need for specific markers to be identified to categorize subsets of immunosuppressive populations depleted. In addition, compounds targeting MDSC and Treg accumulation or function could also lead to systemic depletion of immune cells and generalized immunosuppression. In addition, for therapeutic success, it is critical that not only are MDSCs and Tregs depleted, but that Teff and CTLs are activated or released from T cell exhaustion. Also, as part of combination therapies with first and second line TB regimens, there is the likelihood compounds targeting MDSCs or Tregs or both will have unfavorable interactions with other drugs in the regimens. Therefore, further studies are required to achieve the goal of specific targeting of MDSCs and Tregs as HDT for TB.

Conclusions and Future Perspectives

Recent studies have provided new insights into the roles played by MDSCs and Tregs in the progression of TB. Although *M.tb* infection promotes antigen-specific T cell responses, robust immunosuppression provided by MDSCs and Tregs in the tuberculous granuloma may partly account for the persistence of *M.tb* and the limited efficacy of vaccines. They provide new therapeutic opportunities for shifting the immune system in favor of potent anti-mycobacterial responses. MDSCs serve multiple functions, from harboring *M.tb*, to promoting expansion of Tregs, to attenuating pro-mycobacterial host immune responses. In humans infected with *M.tb*, the adaptive immune response is delayed and bacteria specific T cells are only detectable 6 weeks after infection [26]. Tregs appear to play an important role in mediating this delay and facilitating establishment of infection. Tregs induced by viral, bacterial and parasitic pathogens may account for the reduced efficacy of BCG vaccine, particularly in settings endemic for helminths, malaria, HIV etc. Many aspects of immune suppression mediated by MDSCs and Tregs in TB still remain unexplored. Deciphering of mechanisms and molecules used by suppressive networks that lead to pathogen persistence and disease progression is of paramount importance for the design of successful HDT and for boosting vaccine-induced protective immunity. Murine studies need to be translated to relevant aspects of human pathology. Establishing Tregs and MDSCs or their mediators as biomarkers for treatment monitoring also deserves further attention.

Acknowledgements The support of NIH grants AI37856, HL133190, AI 130595, and AI135280 is gratefully acknowledged.

References

1. Wirth T, Hildebrand F, Allix-Beguec C, et al. Origin, spread and demography of the Mycobacterium tuberculosis complex. PLoS Pathog. 2008;4:e1000160.
2. WHO. Global tuberculosis report. 2018.
3. Singh VK, Srivastava R, Srivastava BS. Manipulation of BCG vaccine: a double-edged sword. Eur J Clin Microbiol Infect Dis. 2016;35:535–43.
4. Cambier CJ, Falkow S, Ramakrishnan L. Host evasion and exploitation schemes of Mycobacterium tuberculosis. Cell. 2014;159:1497–509.
5. Dorhoi A, Reece ST, Kaufmann SH. For better or for worse: the immune response against Mycobacterium tuberculosis balances pathology and protection. Immunol Rev. 2011;240:235–51.
6. Dorhoi A, Kaufmann SH. Pathology and immune reactivity: understanding multidimensionality in pulmonary tuberculosis. Semin Immunopathol. 2016;38:153–66.
7. Dorhoi A, Kaufmann SH. Versatile myeloid cell subsets contribute to tuberculosis-associated inflammation. Eur J Immunol. 2015;45:2191–202.
8. Ehlers S, Schaible UE. The granuloma in tuberculosis: dynamics of a host-pathogen collusion. Front Immunol. 2012;3:411.
9. Guirado E, Schlesinger LS. Modeling the Mycobacterium tuberculosis granuloma - the critical battlefield in host immunity and disease. Front Immunol. 2013;4:98.
10. Kaufmann SH, Dorhoi A. Inflammation in tuberculosis: interactions, imbalances and interventions. Curr Opin Immunol. 2013;25:441–9.
11. Martin CJ, Carey AF, Fortune SM. A bug's life in the granuloma. Semin Immunopathol. 2016;38:213–20.
12. Stamm CE, Collins AC, Shiloh MU. Sensing of Mycobacterium tuberculosis and consequences to both host and bacillus. Immunol Rev. 2015;264:204–19.
13. Mishra A, Akhtar S, Jagannath C, Khan A. Pattern recognition receptors and coordinated cellular pathways involved in tuberculosis immunopathogenesis: emerging concepts and perspectives. Mol Immunol. 2017;87:240–8.
14. Groschel MI, Sayes F, Simeone R, Majlessi L, Brosch R. ESX secretion systems: mycobacterial evolution to counter host immunity. Nat Rev Microbiol. 2016;14:677–91.
15. Dey B, Dey RJ, Cheung LS, et al. A bacterial cyclic dinucleotide activates the cytosolic surveillance pathway and mediates innate resistance to tuberculosis. Nat Med. 2015;21:401–6.
16. Travar M, Petkovic M, Verhaz A. Type I, II, and III interferons: regulating immunity to *Mycobacterium tuberculosis* infection. Arch Immunol Ther Exp. 2016;64:19–31.
17. McNab F, Mayer-Barber K, Sher A, Wack A, O'Garra A. Type I interferons in infectious disease. Nat Rev Immunol. 2015;15:87–103.
18. Cliff JM, Kaufmann SH, McShane H, van Helden P, O'Garra A. The human immune response to tuberculosis and its treatment: a view from the blood. Immunol Rev. 2015;264:88–102.

19. Matucci A, Maggi E, Vultaggio A. Cellular and humoral immune responses during tuberculosis infection: useful knowledge in the era of biological agents. J Rheumatol Suppl. 2014;91:17–23.
20. Mayer-Barber KD, Andrade BB, Oland SD, et al. Host-directed therapy of tuberculosis based on interleukin-1 and type I interferon crosstalk. Nature. 2014;511:99–103.
21. Mayer-Barber KD, Yan B. Clash of the Cytokine Titans: counter-regulation of interleukin-1 and type I interferon-mediated inflammatory responses. Cell Mol Immunol. 2017;14:22–35.
22. Desvignes L, Wolf AJ, Ernst JD. Dynamic roles of type I and type II IFNs in early infection with *Mycobacterium tuberculosis*. J Immunol. 2012;188:6205–15.
23. Moreira-Teixeira L, Sousa J, McNab FW, et al. Type I IFN inhibits alternative macrophage activation during Mycobacterium tuberculosis infection and leads to enhanced protection in the absence of IFN-gamma signaling. J Immunol. 2016;197:4714–26.
24. Domingo-Gonzalez R, Prince O, Cooper A, Khader SA. Cytokines and chemokines in mycobacterium tuberculosis infection. Microbiol Spectr. 2016;4. https://doi.org/10.1128/microbiolspec.TBTB2-0018-2016.
25. Mayer-Barber KD, Barber DL. Innate and adaptive cellular immune responses to *Mycobacterium tuberculosis* infection. Cold Spring Harb Perspect Med. 2015;5:a018424.
26. Cooper AM. Cell-mediated immune responses in tuberculosis. Annu Rev Immunol. 2009;27:393–422.
27. Shafiani S, Tucker-Heard G, Kariyone A, Takatsu K, Urdahl KB. Pathogen-specific regulatory T cells delay the arrival of effector T cells in the lung during early tuberculosis. J Exp Med. 2010;207:1409–20.
28. Prendergast KA, Kirman JR. Dendritic cell subsets in mycobacterial infection: control of bacterial growth and T cell responses. Tuberculosis (Edinb). 2013;93:115–22.
29. Prezzemolo T, Guggino G, La Manna MP, Di Liberto D, Dieli F, Caccamo N. Functional signatures of human CD4 and CD8 T cell responses to Mycobacterium tuberculosis. Front Immunol. 2014;5:180.
30. Cooper AM, Solache A, Khader SA. Interleukin-12 and tuberculosis: an old story revisited. Curr Opin Immunol. 2007;19:441–7.
31. Woodworth JS, Behar SM. *Mycobacterium tuberculosis*-specific CD8+ T cells and their role in immunity. Crit Rev Immunol. 2006;26:317–52.
32. Lin PL, Flynn JL. CD8 T cells and *Mycobacterium tuberculosis* infection. Semin Immunopathol. 2015;37:239–49.
33. Arora P, Foster EL, Porcelli SA. CD1d and natural killer T cells in immunity to *Mycobacterium tuberculosis*. Adv Exp Med Biol. 2013;783:199–223.
34. Chen ZW. Immune regulation of gammadelta T cell responses in mycobacterial infections. Clin Immunol. 2005;116:202–7.
35. du Plessis WJ, Walzl G, Loxton AG. B cells as multi-functional players during *Mycobacterium tuberculosis* infection and disease. Tuberculosis (Edinb). 2016;97:118–25.
36. Meraviglia S, El Daker S, Dieli F, Martini F, Martino A. Gammadelta T cells cross-link innate and adaptive immunity in *Mycobacterium tuberculosis* infection. Clin Dev Immunol. 2011;2011:587315.
37. Okamoto Yoshida Y, Umemura M, Yahagi A, et al. Essential role of IL-17A in the formation of a mycobacterial infection-induced granuloma in the lung. J Immunol. 2010;184:4414–22.
38. Cruz A, Khader SA, Torrado E, et al. Cutting edge: IFN-gamma regulates the induction and expansion of IL-17-producing CD4 T cells during mycobacterial infection. J Immunol. 2006;177:1416–20.
39. McBride A, Konowich J, Salgame P. Host defense and recruitment of Foxp3(+) T regulatory cells to the lungs in chronic Mycobacterium tuberculosis infection requires toll-like receptor 2. PLoS Pathog. 2013;9:e1003397.
40. Shaler CR, Horvath CN, Jeyanathan M, Xing Z. Within the Enemy's Camp: contribution of the granuloma to the dissemination, persistence and transmission of Mycobacterium tuberculosis. Front Immunol. 2013;4:30.

41. Kang DD, Lin Y, Moreno JR, Randall TD, Khader SA. Profiling early lung immune responses in the mouse model of tuberculosis. PLoS One. 2011;6:e16161.
42. Seiler P, Aichele P, Bandermann S, et al. Early granuloma formation after aerosol *Mycobacterium tuberculosis* infection is regulated by neutrophils via CXCR3-signaling chemokines. Eur J Immunol. 2003;33:2676–86.
43. Ong CW, Elkington PT, Brilha S, et al. Neutrophil-derived MMP-8 drives AMPK-dependent matrix destruction in human pulmonary tuberculosis. PLoS Pathog. 2015;11:e1004917.
44. Nouailles G, Dorhoi A, Koch M, et al. CXCL5-secreting pulmonary epithelial cells drive destructive neutrophilic inflammation in tuberculosis. J Clin Invest. 2014;124:1268–82.
45. Reece ST, Kaufmann SH. Floating between the poles of pathology and protection: can we pin down the granuloma in tuberculosis? Curr Opin Microbiol. 2012;15:63–70.
46. Silva Miranda M, Breiman A, Allain S, Deknuydt F, Altare F. The tuberculous granuloma: an unsuccessful host defence mechanism providing a safety shelter for the bacteria? Clin Dev Immunol. 2012;2012:139127.
47. Davis JM, Ramakrishnan L. The role of the granuloma in expansion and dissemination of early tuberculous infection. Cell. 2009;136:37–49.
48. Egen JG, Rothfuchs AG, Feng CG, Winter N, Sher A, Germain RN. Macrophage and T cell dynamics during the development and disintegration of mycobacterial granulomas. Immunity. 2008;28:271–84.
49. Lin PL, Ford CB, Coleman MT, et al. Sterilization of granulomas is common in active and latent tuberculosis despite within-host variability in bacterial killing. Nat Med. 2014;20:75–9.
50. Berry MP, Graham CM, McNab FW, et al. An interferon-inducible neutrophil-driven blood transcriptional signature in human tuberculosis. Nature. 2010;466:973–7.
51. Al Shammari B, Shiomi T, Tezera L, et al. The extracellular matrix regulates granuloma necrosis in tuberculosis. J Infect Dis. 2015;212:463–73.
52. Bateman ED, Turner-Warwick M, Adelmann-Grill BC. Immunohistochemical study of collagen types in human foetal lung and fibrotic lung disease. Thorax. 1981;36:645–53.
53. Davidson JM. Biochemistry and turnover of lung interstitium. Eur Respir J. 1990;3:1048–63.
54. Clark IM, Swingler TE, Sampieri CL, Edwards DR. The regulation of matrix metalloproteinases and their inhibitors. Int J Biochem Cell Biol. 2008;40:1362–78.
55. Matsuoka S, Uchiyama K, Shima H, et al. Relationship between CT findings of pulmonary tuberculosis and the number of acid-fast bacilli on sputum smears. Clin Imaging. 2004;28:119–23.
56. Gomes M, Saad Junior R, Stirbulov R. Pulmonary tuberculosis: relationship between sputum bacilloscopy and radiological lesions. Rev Inst Med Trop Sao Paulo. 2003;45:275–81.
57. Kempker RR, Rabin AS, Nikolaishvili K, et al. Additional drug resistance in *Mycobacterium tuberculosis* isolates from resected cavities among patients with multidrug-resistant or extensively drug-resistant pulmonary tuberculosis. Clin Infect Dis. 2012;54:e51–4.
58. Chatterjee A, D'Souza D, Vira T, et al. Strains of Mycobacterium tuberculosis from western Maharashtra, India, exhibit a high degree of diversity and strain-specific associations with drug resistance, cavitary disease, and treatment failure. J Clin Microbiol. 2010;48:3593–9.
59. Yang D, Kong Y. The bacterial and host factors associated with extrapulmonary dissemination of *Mycobacterium tuberculosis*. Front Biol. 2015;10:252–61.
60. Jurado JO, Alvarez IB, Pasquinelli V, et al. Programmed death (PD)-1:PD-ligand 1/PD-ligand 2 pathway inhibits T cell effector functions during human tuberculosis. J Immunol. 2008;181:116–25.
61. Wang X, Cao Z, Jiang J, et al. Elevated expression of Tim-3 on CD8 T cells correlates with disease severity of pulmonary tuberculosis. J Infect. 2011;62:292–300.
62. Qiu Z, Zhang M, Zhu Y, et al. Multifunctional CD4 T cell responses in patients with active tuberculosis. Sci Rep. 2012;2:216.
63. Parker KH, Beury DW, Ostrand-Rosenberg S. Myeloid-derived suppressor cells: critical cells driving immune suppression in the tumor microenvironment. Adv Cancer Res. 2015;128:95–139.

64. Condamine T, Ramachandran I, Youn JI, Gabrilovich DI. Regulation of tumor metastasis by myeloid-derived suppressor cells. Annu Rev Med. 2015;66:97–110.
65. Gabrilovich DI. Myeloid-derived suppressor cells. Cancer Immunol Res. 2017;5:3–8.
66. Bennett JA, Rao VS, Mitchell MS. Systemic bacillus Calmette-Guerin (BCG) activates natural suppressor cells. Proc Natl Acad Sci U S A. 1978;75:5142–4.
67. Strober S. Natural suppressor (NS) cells, neonatal tolerance, and total lymphoid irradiation: exploring obscure relationships. Annu Rev Immunol. 1984;2:219–37.
68. Gabrilovich DI, Nagaraj S. Myeloid-derived suppressor cells as regulators of the immune system. Nat Rev Immunol. 2009;9:162–74.
69. Ostrand-Rosenberg S, Sinha P. Myeloid-derived suppressor cells: linking inflammation and cancer. J Immunol. 2009;182:4499–506.
70. Shipp C, Speigl L, Janssen N, Martens A, Pawelec G. A clinical and biological perspective of human myeloid-derived suppressor cells in cancer. Cell Mol Life Sci. 2016;73:4043–61.
71. Tobin RP, Davis D, Jordan KR, McCarter MD. The clinical evidence for targeting human myeloid-derived suppressor cells in cancer patients. J Leukoc Biol. 2017;102:381.
72. Gabrilovich DI, Bronte V, Chen SH, et al. The terminology issue for myeloid-derived suppressor cells. Cancer Res. 2007;67:425; author reply 6
73. Bronte V, Brandau S, Chen SH, et al. Recommendations for myeloid-derived suppressor cell nomenclature and characterization standards. Nat Commun. 2016;7:12150.
74. De Sanctis F, Solito S, Ugel S, Molon B, Bronte V, Marigo I. MDSCs in cancer: conceiving new prognostic and therapeutic targets. Biochim Biophys Acta. 2016;1865:35–48.
75. Blomgran R, Ernst JD. Lung neutrophils facilitate activation of naive antigen-specific CD4+ T cells during Mycobacterium tuberculosis infection. J Immunol. 2011;186:7110–9.
76. Dilek N, Vuillefroy de Silly R, Blancho G, Vanhove B. Myeloid-derived suppressor cells: mechanisms of action and recent advances in their role in transplant tolerance. Front Immunol. 2012;3:208.
77. Raber P, Ochoa AC, Rodriguez PC. Metabolism of L-arginine by myeloid-derived suppressor cells in cancer: mechanisms of T cell suppression and therapeutic perspectives. Immunol Investig. 2012;41:614–34.
78. Srivastava MK, Sinha P, Clements VK, Rodriguez P, Ostrand-Rosenberg S. Myeloid-derived suppressor cells inhibit T-cell activation by depleting cystine and cysteine. Cancer Res. 2010;70:68–77.
79. Mazzoni A, Bronte V, Visintin A, et al. Myeloid suppressor lines inhibit T cell responses by an NO-dependent mechanism. J Immunol. 2002;168:689–95.
80. Ortiz ML, Kumar V, Martner A, et al. Immature myeloid cells directly contribute to skin tumor development by recruiting IL-17-producing CD4+ T cells. J Exp Med. 2015;212:351–67.
81. Corzo CA, Cotter MJ, Cheng P, et al. Mechanism regulating reactive oxygen species in tumor-induced myeloid-derived suppressor cells. J Immunol. 2009;182:5693–701.
82. Raber PL, Thevenot P, Sierra R, et al. Subpopulations of myeloid-derived suppressor cells impair T cell responses through independent nitric oxide-related pathways. Int J Cancer. 2014;134:2853–64.
83. Hanson EM, Clements VK, Sinha P, Ilkovitch D, Ostrand-Rosenberg S. Myeloid-derived suppressor cells down-regulate L-selectin expression on CD4+ and CD8+ T cells. J Immunol. 2009;183:937–44.
84. Gehad AE, Lichtman MK, Schmults CD, et al. Nitric oxide-producing myeloid-derived suppressor cells inhibit vascular E-selectin expression in human squamous cell carcinomas. J Invest Dermatol. 2012;132:2642–51.
85. Huang B, Pan PY, Li Q, et al. Gr-1+CD115+ immature myeloid suppressor cells mediate the development of tumor-induced T regulatory cells and T-cell anergy in tumor-bearing host. Cancer Res. 2006;66:1123–31.
86. Serafini P, Mgebroff S, Noonan K, Borrello I. Myeloid-derived suppressor cells promote cross-tolerance in B-cell lymphoma by expanding regulatory T cells. Cancer Res. 2008;68:5439–49.

87. Zoso A, Mazza EM, Bicciato S, et al. Human fibrocytic myeloid-derived suppressor cells express IDO and promote tolerance via Treg-cell expansion. Eur J Immunol. 2014;44:3307–19.
88. Hoechst B, Ormandy LA, Ballmaier M, et al. A new population of myeloid-derived suppressor cells in hepatocellular carcinoma patients induces CD4(+)CD25(+)Foxp3(+) T cells. Gastroenterology. 2008;135:234–43.
89. Pan PY, Ma G, Weber KJ, et al. Immune stimulatory receptor CD40 is required for T-cell suppression and T regulatory cell activation mediated by myeloid-derived suppressor cells in cancer. Cancer Res. 2010;70:99–108.
90. Chatterjee S, Das S, Chakraborty P, Manna A, Chatterjee M, Choudhuri SK. Myeloid derived suppressor cells (MDSCs) can induce the generation of Th17 response from naive CD4+ T cells. Immunobiology. 2013;218:718–24.
91. Medina-Echeverz J, Haile LA, Zhao F, et al. IFN-gamma regulates survival and function of tumor-induced CD11b+ Gr-1high myeloid derived suppressor cells by modulating the anti-apoptotic molecule Bcl2a1. Eur J Immunol. 2014;44:2457–67.
92. Zhao X, Rong L, Zhao X, et al. TNF signaling drives myeloid-derived suppressor cell accumulation. J Clin Invest. 2012;122:4094–104.
93. He D, Li H, Yusuf N, et al. IL-17 promotes tumor development through the induction of tumor promoting microenvironments at tumor sites and myeloid-derived suppressor cells. J Immunol. 2010;184:2281–8.
94. Wang J, Zhang Y, Yin K, et al. IL-17A weakens the antitumor immuity by inhibiting apoptosis of MDSCs in Lewis lung carcinoma bearing mice. Oncotarget. 2017;8:4814–25.
95. Elkabets M, Ribeiro VS, Dinarello CA, et al. IL-1beta regulates a novel myeloid-derived suppressor cell subset that impairs NK cell development and function. Eur J Immunol. 2010;40:3347–57.
96. Mao Y, Sarhan D, Steven A, Seliger B, Kiessling R, Lundqvist A. Inhibition of tumor-derived prostaglandin-e2 blocks the induction of myeloid-derived suppressor cells and recovers natural killer cell activity. Clin Cancer Res. 2014;20:4096–106.
97. Liu C, Yu S, Kappes J, et al. Expansion of spleen myeloid suppressor cells represses NK cell cytotoxicity in tumor-bearing host. Blood. 2007;109:4336–42.
98. Condamine T, Mastio J, Gabrilovich DI. Transcriptional regulation of myeloid-derived suppressor cells. J Leukoc Biol. 2015;98:913–22.
99. Cheng P, Corzo CA, Luetteke N, et al. Inhibition of dendritic cell differentiation and accumulation of myeloid-derived suppressor cells in cancer is regulated by S100A9 protein. J Exp Med. 2008;205:2235–49.
100. Sinha P, Okoro C, Foell D, Freeze HH, Ostrand-Rosenberg S, Srikrishna G. Proinflammatory S100 proteins regulate the accumulation of myeloid-derived suppressor cells. J Immunol. 2008;181:4666–75.
101. Parker KH, Sinha P, Horn LA, et al. HMGB1 enhances immune suppression by facilitating the differentiation and suppressive activity of myeloid-derived suppressor cells. Cancer Res. 2014;74:5723–33.
102. Movahedi K, Guilliams M, Van den Bossche J, et al. Identification of discrete tumor-induced myeloid-derived suppressor cell subpopulations with distinct T cell-suppressive activity. Blood. 2008;111:4233–44.
103. Munera V, Popovic PJ, Bryk J, et al. Stat 6-dependent induction of myeloid derived suppressor cells after physical injury regulates nitric oxide response to endotoxin. Ann Surg. 2010;251:120–6.
104. Bao B, Thakur A, Li Y, et al. The immunological contribution of NF-kappaB within the tumor microenvironment: a potential protective role of zinc as an anti-tumor agent. Biochim Biophys Acta. 2012;1825:160–72.
105. Chen S, Zhang Y, Kuzel TM, Zhang B. Regulating tumor myeloid-derived suppressor cells by microRNAs. Cancer Cell Microenviron. 2015;2:e637.
106. Chen S, Wang L, Fan J, et al. Host miR155 promotes tumor growth through a myeloid-derived suppressor cell-dependent mechanism. Cancer Res. 2015;75:519–31.

107. Kim S, Song JH, Kim S, et al. Loss of oncogenic miR-155 in tumor cells promotes tumor growth by enhancing C/EBP-beta-mediated MDSC infiltration. Oncotarget. 2016;7:11094–112.
108. Rajaram MV, Ni B, Morris JD, et al. *Mycobacterium tuberculosis* lipomannan blocks TNF biosynthesis by regulating macrophage MAPK-activated protein kinase 2 (MK2) and microRNA miR-125b. Proc Natl Acad Sci U S A. 2011;108:17408–13.
109. Wagh V, Urhekar A, Modi D. Levels of microRNA miR-16 and miR-155 are altered in serum of patients with tuberculosis and associate with responses to therapy. Tuberculosis (Edinb). 2017;102:24–30.
110. Yang H, Bi Y, Han F, et al. Myeloid-derived suppressor cells in immunity and autoimmunity. Expert Rev Clin Immunol. 2015;11:911–9.
111. Kwak Y, Kim HE, Park SG. Insights into myeloid-derived suppressor cells in inflammatory diseases. Arch Immunol Ther Exp. 2015;63:269–85.
112. Rieber N, Brand A, Hector A, et al. Flagellin induces myeloid-derived suppressor cells: implications for Pseudomonas aeruginosa infection in cystic fibrosis lung disease. J Immunol. 2013;190:1276–84.
113. Zhuang Y, Cheng P, Liu XF, et al. A pro-inflammatory role for Th22 cells in Helicobacter pylori-associated gastritis. Gut. 2015;64:1368–78.
114. Rieber N, Singh A, Oz H, et al. Pathogenic fungi regulate immunity by inducing neutrophilic myeloid-derived suppressor cells. Cell Host Microbe. 2015;17:507–14.
115. Poe SL, Arora M, Oriss TB, et al. STAT1-regulated lung MDSC-like cells produce IL-10 and efferocytose apoptotic neutrophils with relevance in resolution of bacterial pneumonia. Mucosal Immunol. 2013;6:189–99.
116. Skabytska Y, Wolbing F, Gunther C, et al. Cutaneous innate immune sensing of Toll-like receptor 2-6 ligands suppresses T cell immunity by inducing myeloid-derived suppressor cells. Immunity. 2014;41:762–75.
117. Cuenca AG, Delano MJ, Kelly-Scumpia KM, et al. A paradoxical role for myeloid-derived suppressor cells in sepsis and trauma. Mol Med. 2011;17:281–92.
118. Dietlin TA, Hofman FM, Lund BT, Gilmore W, Stohlman SA, van der Veen RC. Mycobacteria-induced Gr-1+ subsets from distinct myeloid lineages have opposite effects on T cell expansion. J Leukoc Biol. 2007;81:1205–12.
119. Martino A, Badell E, Abadie V, et al. Mycobacterium bovis bacillus Calmette-Guerin vaccination mobilizes innate myeloid-derived suppressor cells restraining in vivo T cell priming via IL-1R-dependent nitric oxide production. J Immunol. 2010;184:2038–47.
120. du Plessis N, Loebenberg L, Kriel M, et al. Increased frequency of myeloid-derived suppressor cells during active tuberculosis and after recent mycobacterium tuberculosis infection suppresses T-cell function. Am J Respir Crit Care Med. 2013;188:724–32.
121. Yang B, Wang X, Jiang J, Zhai F, Cheng X. Identification of CD244-expressing myeloid-derived suppressor cells in patients with active tuberculosis. Immunol Lett. 2014;158:66–72.
122. El Daker S, Sacchi A, Tempestilli M, et al. Granulocytic myeloid derived suppressor cells expansion during active pulmonary tuberculosis is associated with high nitric oxide plasma level. PLoS One. 2015;10:e0123772.
123. Tsiganov EN, Verbina EM, Radaeva TV, et al. Gr-1dimCD11b+ immature myeloid-derived suppressor cells but not neutrophils are markers of lethal tuberculosis infection in mice. J Immunol. 2014;192:4718–27.
124. Knaul JK, Jorg S, Oberbeck-Mueller D, et al. Lung-residing myeloid-derived suppressors display dual functionality in murine pulmonary tuberculosis. Am J Respir Crit Care Med. 2014;190:1053–66.
125. Srikrishna G. S100A8 and S100A9: new insights into their roles in malignancy. J Innate Immun. 2012;4:31–40.
126. Srikrishna G, Freeze HH. Endogenous damage-associated molecular pattern molecules at the crossroads of inflammation and cancer. Neoplasia. 2009;11:615–28.
127. Gopal R, Monin L, Torres D, et al. S100A8/A9 proteins mediate neutrophilic inflammation and lung pathology during tuberculosis. Am J Respir Crit Care Med. 2013;188:1137–46.

128. Xu D, Li Y, Li X, et al. Serum protein S100A9, SOD3, and MMP9 as new diagnostic biomarkers for pulmonary tuberculosis by iTRAQ-coupled two-dimensional LC-MS/MS. Proteomics. 2015;15:58–67.
129. Yoshioka Y, Mizutani T, Mizuta S, et al. Neutrophils and the S100A9 protein critically regulate granuloma formation. Blood Adv. 2016;1:184–92.
130. Sakaguchi S, Sakaguchi N, Asano M, Itoh M, Toda M. Immunologic self-tolerance maintained by activated T cells expressing IL-2 receptor alpha-chains (CD25). Breakdown of a single mechanism of self-tolerance causes various autoimmune diseases. J Immunol. 1995;155:1151–64.
131. Plitas G, Rudensky AY. Regulatory T cells: differentiation and function. Cancer Immunol Res. 2016;4:721–5.
132. Fontenot JD, Gavin MA, Rudensky AY. Foxp3 programs the development and function of CD4+CD25+ regulatory T cells. Nat Immunol. 2003;4:330–6.
133. Hori S, Nomura T, Sakaguchi S. Control of regulatory T cell development by the transcription factor Foxp3. Science. 2003;299:1057–61.
134. Bennett CL, Christie J, Ramsdell F, et al. The immune dysregulation, polyendocrinopathy, enteropathy, X-linked syndrome (IPEX) is caused by mutations of FOXP3. Nat Genet. 2001;27:20–1.
135. Wildin RS, Ramsdell F, Peake J, et al. X-linked neonatal diabetes mellitus, enteropathy and endocrinopathy syndrome is the human equivalent of mouse scurfy. Nat Genet. 2001;27:18–20.
136. Ukena SN, Velaga S, Geffers R, et al. Human regulatory T cells in allogeneic stem cell transplantation. Blood. 2011;118:e82–92.
137. Hoffmann P, Ermann J, Edinger M, Fathman CG, Strober S. Donor-type CD4(+)CD25(+) regulatory T cells suppress lethal acute graft-versus-host disease after allogeneic bone marrow transplantation. J Exp Med. 2002;196:389–99.
138. Cohen JL, Trenado A, Vasey D, Klatzmann D, Salomon BL. CD4(+)CD25(+) immunoregulatory T Cells: new therapeutics for graft-versus-host disease. J Exp Med. 2002;196:401–6.
139. Teh PP, Vasanthakumar A, Kallies A. Development and function of effector regulatory T cells. Prog Mol Biol Transl Sci. 2015;136:155–74.
140. Garib FY, Rizopulu AP. T-regulatory cells as part of strategy of immune evasion by pathogens. Biochemistry. 2015;80:957–71.
141. Boer MC, Joosten SA, Ottenhoff TH. Regulatory T-cells at the interface between human host and pathogens in infectious diseases and vaccination. Front Immunol. 2015;6:217.
142. Abbas AK, Benoist C, Bluestone JA, et al. Regulatory T cells: recommendations to simplify the nomenclature. Nat Immunol. 2013;14:307–8.
143. Lio CW, Hsieh CS. Becoming self-aware: the thymic education of regulatory T cells. Curr Opin Immunol. 2011;23:213–9.
144. Bilate AM, Lafaille JJ. Induced CD4+Foxp3+ regulatory T cells in immune tolerance. Annu Rev Immunol. 2012;30:733–58.
145. Coombes JL, Siddiqui KR, Arancibia-Carcamo CV, et al. A functionally specialized population of mucosal CD103+ DCs induces Foxp3+ regulatory T cells via a TGF-beta and retinoic acid-dependent mechanism. J Exp Med. 2007;204:1757–64.
146. Kitani A, Fuss I, Nakamura K, Kumaki F, Usui T, Strober W. Transforming growth factor (TGF)-beta1-producing regulatory T cells induce Smad-mediated interleukin 10 secretion that facilitates coordinated immunoregulatory activity and amelioration of TGF-beta1-mediated fibrosis. J Exp Med. 2003;198:1179–88.
147. Nakamura K, Kitani A, Fuss I, et al. TGF-beta 1 plays an important role in the mechanism of CD4+CD25+ regulatory T cell activity in both humans and mice. J Immunol. 2004;172:834–42.
148. Collison LW, Workman CJ, Kuo TT, et al. The inhibitory cytokine IL-35 contributes to regulatory T-cell function. Nature. 2007;450:566–9.

149. Egwuagu CE, Yu CR, Sun L, Wang R. Interleukin 35: critical regulator of immunity and lymphocyte-mediated diseases. Cytokine Growth Factor Rev. 2015;26:587–93.
150. Chen CY, Huang D, Yao S, et al. IL-2 simultaneously expands Foxp3+ T regulatory and T effector cells and confers resistance to severe tuberculosis (TB): implicative Treg-T effector cooperation in immunity to TB. J Immunol. 2012;188:4278–88.
151. Roncarolo MG, Gregori S, Battaglia M, Bacchetta R, Fleischhauer K, Levings MK. Interleukin-10-secreting type 1 regulatory T cells in rodents and humans. Immunol Rev. 2006;212:28–50.
152. Shevach EM. Mechanisms of foxp3+ T regulatory cell-mediated suppression. Immunity. 2009;30:636–45.
153. Grossman WJ, Verbsky JW, Barchet W, Colonna M, Atkinson JP, Ley TJ. Human T regulatory cells can use the perforin pathway to cause autologous target cell death. Immunity. 2004;21:589–601.
154. Cao X, Cai SF, Fehniger TA, et al. Granzyme B and perforin are important for regulatory T cell-mediated suppression of tumor clearance. Immunity. 2007;27:635–46.
155. Garin MI, Chu CC, Golshayan D, Cernuda-Morollon E, Wait R, Lechler RI. Galectin-1: a key effector of regulation mediated by CD4+CD25+ T cells. Blood. 2007;109:2058–65.
156. Wing K, Onishi Y, Prieto-Martin P, et al. CTLA-4 control over Foxp3+ regulatory T cell function. Science. 2008;322:271–5.
157. Liang B, Workman C, Lee J, et al. Regulatory T cells inhibit dendritic cells by lymphocyte activation gene-3 engagement of MHC class II. J Immunol. 2008;180:5916–26.
158. Grohmann U, Orabona C, Fallarino F, et al. CTLA-4-Ig regulates tryptophan catabolism in vivo. Nat Immunol. 2002;3:1097–101.
159. Tao JH, Cheng M, Tang JP, Liu Q, Pan F, Li XP. Foxp3, regulatory T cell, and autoimmune diseases. Inflammation. 2017;40:328–39.
160. Noval Rivas M, Chatila TA. Regulatory T cells in allergic diseases. J Allergy Clin Immunol. 2016;138:639–52.
161. Nishikawa H, Sakaguchi S. Regulatory T cells in cancer immunotherapy. Curr Opin Immunol. 2014;27:1–7.
162. Hatziioannou A, Alissafi T, Verginis P. Myeloid-derived suppressor cells and T regulatory cells in tumors: unraveling the dark side of the force. J Leukoc Biol. 2017;102:407.
163. Scott-Browne JP, Shafiani S, Tucker-Heard G, et al. Expansion and function of Foxp3-expressing T regulatory cells during tuberculosis. J Exp Med. 2007;204:2159–69.
164. Kursar M, Koch M, Mittrucker HW, et al. Cutting edge: regulatory T cells prevent efficient clearance of Mycobacterium tuberculosis. J Immunol. 2007;178:2661–5.
165. Ozeki Y, Sugawara I, Udagawa T, et al. Transient role of CD4+CD25+ regulatory T cells in mycobacterial infection in mice. Int Immunol. 2010;22:179–89.
166. Guyot-Revol V, Innes JA, Hackforth S, Hinks T, Lalvani A. Regulatory T cells are expanded in blood and disease sites in patients with tuberculosis. Am J Respir Crit Care Med. 2006;173:803–10.
167. Ribeiro-Rodrigues R, Resende Co T, Rojas R, et al. A role for CD4+CD25+ T cells in regulation of the immune response during human tuberculosis. Clin Exp Immunol. 2006;144:25–34.
168. Chiacchio T, Casetti R, Butera O, et al. Characterization of regulatory T cells identified as CD4(+)CD25(high)CD39(+) in patients with active tuberculosis. Clin Exp Immunol. 2009;156:463–70.
169. Semple PL, Binder AB, Davids M, Maredza A, van Zyl-Smit RN, Dheda K. Regulatory T cells attenuate mycobacterial stasis in alveolar and blood-derived macrophages from patients with tuberculosis. Am J Respir Crit Care Med. 2013;187:1249–58.
170. Geffner L, Yokobori N, Basile J, et al. Patients with multidrug-resistant tuberculosis display impaired Th1 responses and enhanced regulatory T-cell levels in response to an outbreak of multidrug-resistant Mycobacterium tuberculosis M and Ra strains. Infect Immun. 2009;77:5025–34.

171. Pang H, Yu Q, Guo B, et al. Frequency of regulatory T-cells in the peripheral blood of patients with pulmonary tuberculosis from Shanxi province, China. PLoS One. 2013;8:e65496.
172. Wu YE, Peng WG, Cai YM, et al. Decrease in CD4+CD25+FoxP3+ Treg cells after pulmonary resection in the treatment of cavity multidrug-resistant tuberculosis. Int J Infect Dis. 2010;14:e815–22.
173. Singh A, Dey AB, Mohan A, Sharma PK, Mitra DK. Foxp3+ regulatory T cells among tuberculosis patients: impact on prognosis and restoration of antigen specific IFN-gamma producing T cells. PLoS One. 2012;7:e44728.
174. Marin ND, Paris SC, Velez VM, Rojas CA, Rojas M, Garcia LF. Regulatory T cell frequency and modulation of IFN-gamma and IL-17 in active and latent tuberculosis. Tuberculosis (Edinb). 2010;90:252–61.
175. Kim K, Perera R, Tan DB, et al. Circulating mycobacterial-reactive CD4+ T cells with an immunosuppressive phenotype are higher in active tuberculosis than latent tuberculosis infection. Tuberculosis (Edinb). 2014;94:494–501.
176. Geffner L, Basile JI, Yokobori N, et al. CD4(+) CD25(high) forkhead box protein 3(+) regulatory T lymphocytes suppress interferon-gamma and CD107 expression in CD4(+) and CD8(+) T cells from tuberculous pleural effusions. Clin Exp Immunol. 2014;175:235–45.
177. Sharma PK, Saha PK, Singh A, Sharma SK, Ghosh B, Mitra DK. FoxP3+ regulatory T cells suppress effector T-cell function at pathologic site in miliary tuberculosis. Am J Respir Crit Care Med. 2009;179:1061–70.
178. Gupta S, Cheung L, Pokkali S, et al. Suppressor cell-depleting immunotherapy with denileukin diftitox is an effective host-directed therapy for tuberculosis. J Infect Dis. 2017;215:1883–7.
179. Romano E, Kusio-Kobialka M, Foukas PG, et al. Ipilimumab-dependent cell-mediated cytotoxicity of regulatory T cells ex vivo by nonclassical monocytes in melanoma patients. Proc Natl Acad Sci U S A. 2015;112:6140–5.
180. Kirman J, McCoy K, Hook S, et al. CTLA-4 blockade enhances the immune response induced by mycobacterial infection but does not lead to increased protection. Infect Immun. 1999;67:3786–92.
181. Draghiciu O, Nijman HW, Hoogeboom BN, Meijerhof T, Daemen T. Sunitinib depletes myeloid-derived suppressor cells and synergizes with a cancer vaccine to enhance antigen-specific immune responses and tumor eradication. Oncoimmunology. 2015;4:e989764.
182. Suzuki E, Kapoor V, Jassar AS, Kaiser LR, Albelda SM. Gemcitabine selectively eliminates splenic Gr-1+/CD11b+ myeloid suppressor cells in tumor-bearing animals and enhances antitumor immune activity. Clin Cancer Res. 2005;11:6713–21.
183. Eriksson E, Wenthe J, Irenaeus S, Loskog A, Ullenhag G. Gemcitabine reduces MDSCs, tregs and TGFbeta-1 while restoring the teff/treg ratio in patients with pancreatic cancer. J Transl Med. 2016;14:282.
184. Pili R, Haggman M, Stadler WM, et al. Phase II randomized, double-blind, placebo-controlled study of tasquinimod in men with minimally symptomatic metastatic castrate-resistant prostate cancer. J Clin Oncol. 2011;29:4022–8.
185. Armstrong AJ, Haggman M, Stadler WM, et al. Long-term survival and biomarker correlates of tasquinimod efficacy in a multicenter randomized study of men with minimally symptomatic metastatic castration-resistant prostate cancer. Clin Cancer Res. 2013;19:6891–901.
186. Califano JA, Khan Z, Noonan KA, et al. Tadalafil augments tumor specific immunity in patients with head and neck squamous cell carcinoma. Clin Cancer Res. 2015;21:30–8.
187. Weed DT, Vella JL, Reis IM, et al. Tadalafil reduces myeloid-derived suppressor cells and regulatory T cells and promotes tumor immunity in patients with head and neck squamous cell carcinoma. Clin Cancer Res. 2015;21:39–48.
188. Jayashankar L, Hafner R. Adjunct strategies for tuberculosis vaccines: modulating key immune cell regulatory mechanisms to potentiate vaccination. Front Immunol. 2016;7:577.
189. Kao J, Ko EC, Eisenstein S, Sikora AG, Fu S, Chen SH. Targeting immune suppressing myeloid-derived suppressor cells in oncology. Crit Rev Oncol Hematol. 2011;77:12–9.

190. Kusmartsev S, Cheng F, Yu B, et al. All-trans-retinoic acid eliminates immature myeloid cells from tumor-bearing mice and improves the effect of vaccination. Cancer Res. 2003;63:4441–9.
191. Mirza N, Fishman M, Fricke I, et al. All-trans-retinoic acid improves differentiation of myeloid cells and immune response in cancer patients. Cancer Res. 2006;66:9299–307.
192. Yamada H, Mizuno S, Ross AC, Sugawara I. Retinoic acid therapy attenuates the severity of tuberculosis while altering lymphocyte and macrophage numbers and cytokine expression in rats infected with Mycobacterium tuberculosis. J Nutr. 2007;137:2696–700.
193. Shen L, Sundstedt A, Ciesielski M, et al. Tasquinimod modulates suppressive myeloid cells and enhances cancer immunotherapies in murine models. Cancer Immunol Res. 2015;3:136–48.
194. Raymond E, Dalgleish A, Damber JE, Smith M, Pili R. Mechanisms of action of tasquinimod on the tumour microenvironment. Cancer Chemother Pharmacol. 2014;73:1–8.
195. Deronic A, Leanderson T, Ivars F. The anti-tumor effect of the quinoline-3-carboxamide tasquinimod: blockade of recruitment of CD11b(+) Ly6C(hi) cells to tumor tissue reduces tumor growth. BMC Cancer. 2016;16:440.
196. Bjork P, Bjork A, Vogl T, et al. Identification of human S100A9 as a novel target for treatment of autoimmune disease via binding to quinoline-3-carboxamides. PLoS Biol. 2009;7:e97.
197. Serafini P, Meckel K, Kelso M, et al. Phosphodiesterase-5 inhibition augments endogenous antitumor immunity by reducing myeloid-derived suppressor cell function. J Exp Med. 2006;203:2691–702.
198. Maiga M, Ammerman NC, Maiga MC, et al. Adjuvant host-directed therapy with types 3 and 5 but not type 4 phosphodiesterase inhibitors shortens the duration of tuberculosis treatment. J Infect Dis. 2013;208:512–9.
199. Smyth MJ, Ngiow SF, Teng MW. Targeting regulatory T cells in tumor immunotherapy. Immunol Cell Biol. 2014;92:473–4.
200. Buchbinder EI, Desai A. CTLA-4 and PD-1 pathways: similarities, differences, and implications of their inhibition. Am J Clin Oncol. 2016;39:98–106.
201. Wang W, Lau R, Yu D, Zhu W, Korman A, Weber J. PD1 blockade reverses the suppression of melanoma antigen-specific CTL by CD4+ CD25(Hi) regulatory T cells. Int Immunol. 2009;21:1065–77.
202. Barber DL, Mayer-Barber KD, Feng CG, Sharpe AH, Sher A. CD4 T cells promote rather than control tuberculosis in the absence of PD-1-mediated inhibition. J Immunol. 2011;186:1598–607.
203. Williams DP, Parker K, Bacha P, et al. Diphtheria toxin receptor binding domain substitution with interleukin-2: genetic construction and properties of a diphtheria toxin-related interleukin-2 fusion protein. Protein Eng. 1987;1:493–8.
204. Bacha P, Williams DP, Waters C, Williams JM, Murphy JR, Strom TB. Interleukin 2 receptor-targeted cytotoxicity. Interleukin 2 receptor-mediated action of a diphtheria toxin-related interleukin 2 fusion protein. J Exp Med. 1988;167:612–22.
205. Waters CA, Schimke PA, Snider CE, et al. Interleukin 2 receptor-targeted cytotoxicity. Receptor binding requirements for entry of a diphtheria toxin-related interleukin 2 fusion protein into cells. Eur J Immunol. 1990;20:785–91.
206. Re GG, Waters C, Poisson L, Willingham MC, Sugamura K, Frankel AE. Interleukin 2 (IL-2) receptor expression and sensitivity to diphteria fusion toxin DAB389IL-2 in cultured hematopoietic cells. Cancer Res. 1996;56:2590–5.
207. Kochi SK, Collier RJ. DNA fragmentation and cytolysis in U937 cells treated with diphtheria toxin or other inhibitors of protein synthesis. Exp Cell Res. 1993;208:296–302.
208. Foss FM. DAB(389)IL-2 (ONTAK): a novel fusion toxin therapy for lymphoma. Clin Lymphoma. 2000;1:110–6; discussion 7
209. Manoukian G, Hagemeister F. Denileukin diftitox: a novel immunotoxin. Expert Opin Biol Ther. 2009;9:1445–51.

210. Ho VT, Zahrieh D, Hochberg E, et al. Safety and efficacy of denileukin diftitox in patients with steroid-refractory acute graft-versus-host disease after allogeneic hematopoietic stem cell transplantation. Blood. 2004;104:1224–6.
211. Gottlieb SL, Gilleaudeau P, Johnson R, et al. Response of psoriasis to a lymphocyte-selective toxin (DAB389IL-2) suggests a primary immune, but not keratinocyte, pathogenic basis. Nat Med. 1995;1:442–7.
212. Rasku MA, Clem AL, Telang S, et al. Transient T cell depletion causes regression of melanoma metastases. J Transl Med. 2008;6:12.
213. Telang S, Rasku MA, Clem AL, et al. Phase II trial of the regulatory T cell-depleting agent, denileukin diftitox, in patients with unresectable stage IV melanoma. BMC Cancer. 2011;11:515.
214. Lakkis F, Steele A, Pacheco-Silva A, Rubin-Kelley V, Strom TB, Murphy JR. Interleukin 4 receptor targeted cytotoxicity: genetic construction and in vivo immunosuppressive activity of a diphtheria toxin-related murine interleukin 4 fusion protein. Eur J Immunol. 1991;21:2253–8.

Interactions of *Mycobacterium tuberculosis* with Human Mesenchymal Stem Cells

Arshad Khan and Chinnaswamy Jagannath

Abstract Tuberculosis is a leading cause of death due to infections in mankind. The causative pathogen *Mycobacterium tuberculosis* (Mtb) infects macrophages but also many other mammalian cells including hematopoietic and mesenchymal stem cells (MSCs). MSCs are multipotent and can differentiate into multiple cell phenotypes including macrophage like cells that express scavenger receptor-A (SR-A), mannose receptor, TLR-2/4 and contain NOD1/2 receptors in the cytosol. They express very low levels of HLA-DR (MHC-II) and HLA-ABC (MHC-I) because of which, they can be transplanted without adverse reactions. MSCs have self-renewal and regenerative properties, and secrete cytokines and chemokines; growth factors to reduce inflammation, repair and remodel tissues and maintain homeostasis. Thus, they have been used to treat human diseases including tuberculosis. Mtb infects MSCs from both humans and mice and persists within them for prolonged periods. We illustrate here that naïve MSCs interact with Mtb by phagocytosing them through SR-A, and killing them through intrinsic autophagy and nitric oxide. Persisting organisms then become dormant, and thus MSCs provide a niche for latent tuberculosis. Naive MSCs usually exert immunosuppressive properties on macrophages, T cells and DCs although they can be immune-enhancing depending on environmental milieu, and prior activation with cytokines like IFN-γ. Therefore, MSCs can play a dual role during the pathogenesis of tuberculosis. First, MSCs internalize Mtb either during primary aerosol infection or during progressive disease and migrate to bone marrow, where, they provide a niche, and secrete cytokines to dampen immune cell function. Secondly, they can kill replicating Mtb through autophagy and NO but seem to require additional activation or drugs for complete elimination of dormant Mtb. Since MSCs can be grown in vitro into large numbers for transplantation, and can be either pharmacologically or genetically modified, we discuss emerging stem cell based immunotherapeutic strategies for tuberculosis.

A. Khan · C. Jagannath (✉)
Department of Pathology and Genomic Medicine, Houston Methodist Research Institute, Houston, TX, USA
e-mail: akhan@houstonmethodist.org; cjagannath@houstonmethodist.org

J. D. Cirillo, Y. Kong (eds.), *Tuberculosis Host-Pathogen Interactions*,
https://doi.org/10.1007/978-3-030-25381-3_5

Keywords Mesenchymal stem cells · *Mycobacterium tuberculosis* · Dormancy · Tuberculosis · Immunotherapy · Immunosuppression · Autophagy · Nitric oxide · Hypoxia · Mouse · Human · Macrophages · Dendritic cells · CD4 · CD8 · Neutrophils · Granuloma

Abbreviations

AM	Alveolar macrophages
Bcl-2	B cell lymphoma proteins
EGF	Epithelial growth factor
FGF-2	Fibroblast growth factor
HGF	Hepatocyte growth factor
HLA-DR	Human Leukocyte Antigen–D Related
HSCs	Hematopoietic stem cells
IDO	Indoleamine 2,3-Dioxygenase (IDO)
IGF-1	Insulin-like growth factor-1
LTBI	Latent tuberculosis Infection
M1, M2	Macrophage phenotypes
MDR	Multi drug resistant
MHC	Major histocompatibility complex
MNGC	Multinucleate giant cells
MSCs	Mesenchymal stem cells
Mtb	Mycobacterium tuberculosis
NO	Nitric oxide
NOD-1/2	Nuclear oligomerization domain
PGE-2	Prostaglandin E2
ROS	Reactive oxygen species
SR-A	Scavenger receptor-A
TGF-α/β	Transforming growth factor-α/β
TLR	Toll-like receptor
VEGF	Vascular endothelial growth factor

Introduction

Mycobacterium tuberculosis (Mtb), the pathogen that causes tuberculosis (TB), is a leading cause of death due to infections claiming 1.4 million lives worldwide in 2016 [1]. Although active disease following aerosol infection occurs only in one out of ten individuals, about eight to nine million active tuberculosis cases are reported each year worldwide (WHO Global Tuberculosis report 2017). Mtb is unique in being able to persist among humans for prolonged periods of time and this phase is referred to as latent tuberculosis infection (LTBI). Compounding this problem, Mtb persists even after completion of chemotherapy [2–5]. Interestingly, nearly a third of mankind appears to be latently infected with Mtb from which active cases occur, usually after immune-senescence, and immunosuppressive drug treatment or anti-TNFα antibody therapy. It is well established that Mtb persists within macrophages, and many studies document the emergence of a latent state in Mtb, and its regulation through *dosR* mediated genes. However, Mtb can also infect, multiply or persist in a variety of mammalian cells including respiratory epithelial cells. More recent studies show that Mtb infects and persist in mouse and human mesenchymal (MSCs) and hematopoietic stem cells (HSCs). Herein, we describe the cell biology of MSCs and how it relates to the persistence of dormant Mtb organisms.

Tuberculosis occurs as an aerosol infection in humans, and after alveolar macrophages (AMs) ingest Mtb, they are either killed within AMs which prevents exacerbation of infection or AMs with infected Mtb infiltrate into lung parenchyma. Cytokine and chemokine signaling mediated signaling by Mtb infected AMs recruits peripheral blood derived monocytes, neutrophils, dendritic cells, and NK, CD4 and CD8 T cells thereby initiating adaptive immunity [6–8]. A key feature of adaptive immunity is the formation of an organized structure called granuloma around a central core of infected macrophages [9–11]. Although, granulomas play an important role in preventing the spread of infection as well as inflammation that can damage the tissues, they may not successfully kill Mtb. Immunological and pathological studies in non-human primate models of tuberculosis now support the alternative notion that granulomas are much more dynamic with a wide spectrum of heterogeneity [12]. While some granulomas can successfully contain the infection, others may facilitate the dissemination of organisms from cavitary lesions. Thus, it is now widely believed that mature granulomas represent an equilibrium between host and pathogen, characterized by adaptive immunity sufficient to arrest progressive infection but insufficient to kill the intracellular mycobacteria [13].

Since LTBI presents a major reservoir from which active tuberculosis occurs, efforts have been made to understand the mechanisms through which Mtb can persist in a dormant/latent state. Mtb are thought to survive in a dormant stage within multinucleated giant cells (MNGCs), epithelioid cells and foamy macrophages, which usually occur in the center of the granulomas, surrounded by a rim of macrophages, dendritic cells, lymphocytes and neutrophils [14, 15]. Macrophages can transform into epithelioid cells which then fuse to become Langhans' type of multinucleate giant cells (MNGCs), which occur at the center of a typical lung tuberculosis granuloma, and contain acid fact bacilli. The lipid rich 'foam cells' are also derived from Mtb infected macrophages and are either a transitional or terminal stage providing a niche for latent Mtb. Paradoxically, MNGCs and foamy macrophages can also contribute to tissue pathology. Although Mtb containing MNGCs and foamy macrophages can persist for prolonged periods, life time persistence of Mtb may require that additional macrophages are infected in vivo for the duration of latency. Interestingly, live Mtb, Mtb DNA and mRNA transcripts can be demonstrated in a variety of mammalian cells. Thus, it appears that multiple mammalian cells can provide a niche for the persistence of Mtb; Mtb may either transfer from one niche to another in vivo or Mtb can infect multiple cell types during the initial or progressive infection.

Mesenchymal Stem Cells Provide a Novel Niche for Dormant *Mycobacterium tuberculosis*

Recent studies report an intriguing observation that Mtb infects both $CD34^+$ hematopoietic stem cells (HSCs), and $CD271^+$ mesenchymal stem cells (MSCs) of mice and humans [16–18]. Unlike highly differentiated cells like macrophages, DCs and various subsets of T cells, multipotent MSCs can further differentiate into various mammalian cell phenotypes. Importantly, pathogenesis of tuberculosis begins with the aerosol mediated infection within alveolar lumen where macrophages internalize Mtb, and subsequently within the lung parenchyma, blood derived monocytes, T cells, DCs and neutrophils are recruited to form the granuloma. Granulomas in turn either heal or exacerbate into necrotic lesions, facilitating dissemination of Mtb through the air ways, associated with extensive inflammation. Hematogenous dissemination of Mtb can also occur, as evident from tuberculous meningitis of children and military tuberculosis of adults. Tuberculosis is therefore a complex disease involving either activation or selective suppression of multiple immune cell types, stage specific inflammation and tissue damage indicating a need for interventional and therapeutic strategies (Fig. 1).

Unlike HSCs, MSCs can be grown to large numbers from bone marrow or other tissues enabling transplantation and indeed more than 400 clinical trials have evaluated their functional significance. Since MSCs can home to lungs and alveoli during inflammation and infection, they are likely to play an immunomodulatory role during tuberculosis pathogenesis [19]. Indeed, clinical trials indicate the beneficial effects following transplantation of MSCs among in MDR-tuberculosis patients. Stem cell properties which could be beneficial or antagonistic for immunotherapy of tuberculosis are discussed below.

Mesenchymal Stem Cells Differentiate into Multiple Cellular Phenotypes, Show Regenerative Capacity and May Help to Mitigate Tissue Damage During Tuberculosis

MSCs, are non-hematopoietic cells (aka. Multipotent stromal cells), which retain stem cell-like characteristics of self-renewal and differentiation [20–22]. The bone marrow is a major source of MSCs, which can home to various tissues and differentiate into many phenotypes. However, MSCs can also be enriched from many tissues including adipose tissue, umbilical cord, Whartons' jelly and placenta [23].

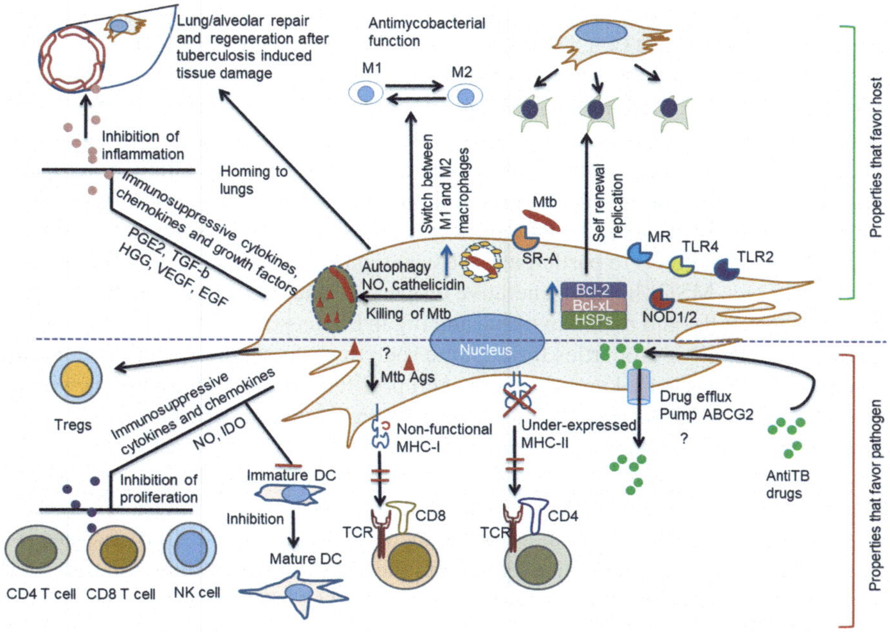

Fig. 1 Immunomodulating and immunosuppressive properties of Mesenchymal stem cells which allow *Mycobacterium tuberculosis* to persist as dormant organisms. *Upper panel* demonstrates the molecular mechanisms of MSCs which favor the host in combating tuberculosis through its direct effects and through programming of macrophages. MSCs from bone marrow migrate to tuberculosis affected lungs and release a number of anti-inflammatory cytokines and growth factors including PGE2, TGF-β, HGG, VEGF and EGF that attenuate inflammation, and promote tissue regeneration and repair. MSCs secrete cytokines like IL-6, IL-10 and IL-13 to skew macrophages between M1 and M2 although prior activation with IFN-γ may reverse the switch. M1 and M2 macrophages differentially control intracellular growth of Mtb. MSCs retain anti-apoptotic properties through an increased expression of Bcl-2, Bcl-xL, and heat shock proteins (HSPs), which protects against infection-induced cell death, concurrently supporting self-renewal and regeneration. MSCs express scavenger receptor-A (SR-A) and phagocytose *Mycobacterium tuberculosis* (Mtb), and inhibit their growth through intrinsic autophagy and nitric oxide (NO). They also express a functional mannose receptor (MR), Toll-like receptors (TLR) 2 and 4 on the surface, and Nuclear Oligomerization Domain (NOD) like receptors 1 and 2 in the cytosol. Mtb bacilli which survive autophagy, NO and cathelicidin mediated killing by MSCs persist as dormant organisms. *Lower panel* illustrates putative mechanisms which can exacerbate tuberculosis infection. MSCs secrete NO, Indoleamine 2,3-Dioxygenase (IDO) and PGE2 to inhibit the proliferation of CD4, CD8, and NK cells. They induce expansion of Tregs and also interfere with the maturation of dendritic cells (DCs), enabling Mtb to evade adaptive immunity. Naïve MSCs show very low levels of surface MHC-II (HLA-DR in humans) and dysfunctional MHC-I (HLA-ABC) which reduce or nullify antigen presentation, enabling Mtb to evade immune surveillance. Anti-tuberculosis drugs may not penetrate well into MSCs localized within bone marrow, and if they do, they may be removed through ABCG2 efflux pumps

They are CD271$^+$, CD105$^+$, CD73$^+$, CD166, and CD90$^+$; and ≤2% of the population may express CD45, CD34, CD14 or CD11b, CD79a or CD19, and HLA-DR [24, 25]. MSCs are capable of differentiating into macrophage-like cells, fibroblasts in skin, astrocytes in central nervous system, stromal cells in bone marrow, adipocytes in fat tissue, osteocytes in bone, chondrocytes in cartilage, and myocytes in muscles [20, 26, 27]. Interestingly, a subset of CD14$^+$ monocytes can differentiate into MSCs [28]. The specific anatomical function and biological properties of MSCs in adult and fetal tissues continue to be a major focus of research. However, the key physiological role of MSCs is to participate in tissue repair and homeostatic maintenance of organs. Thus, MSCs have regenerative properties, and assist in replacing dead or dysfunctional cells, and maintain tissue and organ homeostasis [29, 30]. They mediate their regenerative properties through the secretion of specific growth factors, in concert with other chemokines that boost cell proliferation and angiogenesis within the tissue. They express several mitogenic proteins including transforming growth factor-alpha (TGF-α), epithelial growth factor (EGF), TGF-β, hepatocyte growth factor (HGF), basic fibroblast growth factor (FGF-2) and insulin-like growth factor-1 (IGF-1) to accelerate fibroblast, endothelial and epithelial cell division [31, 32]. MSCs release vascular endothelial growth factor (VEGF), IGF-1, EGF and angiopoietin, recruiting endothelial lineage cells to the site of injury or inflammation, and augment vascularization and regeneration of tissue [33]. Interestingly, despite being from a non-hematopoietic lineage, bone marrow-derived MSCs not only express a variety of hematopoietic cytokines, but also have hematopoietic supporting and immunomodulatory functions [34]. These observations support the hypothesis that transfused MSCs can repair damaged lungs during tuberculosis and may restore the function of hematopoietic cells if they are compromised. Thus, patients with MDR-tuberculosis who were infused with autologous naïve MSCs showed a significant clinical improvement as evidenced by chest radiographs and sputum conversion to negative bacterial status [35–37]. Furthermore, interstitial injection of naïve MSCs into a rabbit bladder tuberculosis model reduced the inflammation, deformation of wall, and fibrosis [38].

Mesenchymal Stem Cells Play an Immunomodulatory Role During Bacterial and Viral Infections

Since infections are also associated with immune activation, inflammation, and disease stage specific tissue damage, MSCs can play a significant role because of their known trophic and dual properties of immune-enhancement and immunosuppression. Although naïve MSCs appear to lack the array of macrophage receptors that participate in phagocytosis, they do express multiple TLRs, adenosine receptors on surface, and NOD-1/2 receptors in the cytosol [39]. We recently demonstrated that, the scavenger receptor-A (SR-A) and mannose receptors are functionally active on human MSCs, and endocytosed oxidized-low density lipoprotein (oxLDL) and mannosyl BSA, respectively [40]. Furthermore, SR-A of human MSCs mediated the phagocytosis of *M. bovis* BCG and Mtb. Therefore, MSCs are able to interact with bacterial pathogens including phagocytosis and viral uptake [40, 41]. Although their homing mechanisms remain unclear, and are likely dependent upon chemokine and cytokine signals, they have been found to migrate to inflamed tissue in vivo [42–44]. MSCs seem to exhibit different responses to microbial challenge and subsequently modulate the regulation of inflammatory cells [45–47]. Preclinical studies indicate that MSCs secrete many soluble factors, enhancing immune cell mediated antimicrobial function [48]. These include, the secretion of the anti-microbial peptide cathelicidin hCAP-18/LL-37 which also has anti-mycobacterial property, and indoleamine 2, 3-dioxygenase (IDO) which is a broad spectrum antimicrobial agent [49, 50]. Under in vitro settings, human bone marrow and peripheral glandular tissue derived MSCs were reported to resolve infection and inflammation by recruiting neutrophils to the site of infection and enhancing their anti-microbial function [51]. In addition, MSCs from healthy donors significantly inhibited apoptosis of neutrophils by dampening their respiratory burst [52]. The anti-apoptotic activity of MSC did not require cell-to-cell contact and was due to a STAT-3 dependent secretion of IL-6. Infusion of human MSCs enhanced the phagocytic activity of blood monocytes in an experimental gram-negative peritoneal sepsis model of mouse, leading to reduced mortality and bacteremia [45]. Recent studies show that, MSCs can chemotactically recruit $CCR2^{+}$ monocytes into the airways of mice [53]. Finally, mouse MSCs were found to inhibit gamma herpesviruses through a DNA sensing STING dependent pathway [41].

These observations support the emerging notion that MSCs can positively affect the outcome of selected bacterial and viral infections. In the context of tuberculosis, we propose that MSC can affect the outcome of tuberculosis by killing Mtb through a combination of antimicrobial mechanisms including antimicrobial peptides like cathelicidin, IDO and NO. These issues are further discussed below.

Paradoxically, MSCs may dysregulate the function of macrophages so that Mtb persists in a latent state. MSCs can program macrophages into M1 and M2 and therefore skew the outcome of bactericidal function of macrophages [54]. In an earlier study, MSCs reprogrammed macrophages via prostaglandin-2 (PGE2) to increase IL-10 production which in turn, led to a reduced mortality, and improved organ function in a mouse sepsis model [55]. Since pro-inflammatory M1 and anti-inflammatory M2 macrophages show a differential ability to inhibit mycobacteria, MSCs may similarly skew human or mouse macrophages to favor establishment of tuberculosis infection [56, 57]. Together, these observations suggest that MSC have the potential to exert an antimicrobial function, and at the same time modulate immune responses to facilitate persistence of pathogens like Mtb in the mammalian host. Additional investigations are required to determine whether pharmacological or genetic manipulation of MSCs can boost immune defense through transactivation.

Mesenchymal Stem Cells Play a Dual Role During Tuberculosis Through the Suppression of Immune Responses and Providing a Niche for Persistent Mtb

Multiple studies indicate that MSCs mediate immunomodulation through the secretion of multiple cytokines and chemokines in addition to IDO, NO, HGF, PGE2 and TGF-β1 [58, 59]. Through the combined action of these mediators, MSCs suppress the proliferation and functional activity of $CD4^+$ (both Th1 and Th17 cells), $CD8^+$ T cells and NK T cells to regulate inflammation at the site of infection and tissue damage [29, 60]. Notably, MSCs can expand T regulatory T cells (Tregs) [61]. Interestingly, MSCs seem to differentially modulate the function of naïve vs. activated CD8 T cells suggesting a dual property of activation vs. suppression on T cells [60, 62]. A biphasic suppression followed by activation has also been described for TH17 cells which suggests that immune modulation of MSCs may enable programming of specific populations of T cells [63, 64]. In addition to its effects on T cells and macrophages, human chorionic MSCs have been found to induce an anti-inflammatory phenotype in DCs [65]. Finally, chemokines and cytokines secreted by MSCs recruit and expand regulatory T cells (Tregs), which in turn reduce inflammation [66].

These studies indicate that overall, MSCs are likely to play a suppressive role during tuberculosis. In support of this observation, MSCs were found at the periphery of granulomas in a mouse model of tuberculosis and T cell response was suppressed through MSC mediated secretion of NO [16]. Although MSCs of granulomas also contain acid fast stainable Mtb, whether they directly phagocytose Mtb or pick up those released from macrophages remains unclear. It is relevant to note here that despite containing macrophages, DCs, neutrophils and T cells around a central zone of Mtb infected MNGCs, granulomas may actually prevent immune elimination of Mtb by sequestering them within macrophages [11]. Because of their suppressive properties, MSCs may contribute to this process by secreting cytokines like IL-4, IL-6, IL-13 and PGE2 and skewing macrophages towards the anti-inflammatory M2 phenotype. It is notable that human and mouse granulomas contain M1 and M2 macrophages, and additional investigations are required to determine whether Mtb infected MSCs affect macrophage phenotypes. It is important to note here that MSCs, depending upon the local micro-environment such as alveoli, may play an unanticipated immune-enhancing role. For example, MSCs chemotactically recruited $CCR2^+$ monocytes into airways of mice to suppress allergic inflammation [53]. $CCR2^+$ monocytes were reported essential during the initial immune response and later control of aerosolized tuberculosis in mice [67].

Bone Marrow Provides an Immune Privileged Site During Tuberculosis for Mtb Infected MSCs

It is well established that Mtb can infect macrophages from both mice and humans and can enter a dormant stage. Unless activated with IFN-γ prior to infection, Mtb grows within most macrophages over 7–14 days eventually killing them. However, activated macrophages produce NO, reactive species (ROS) and multiple antimicrobial peptides which can kill Mtb. Both phagosome-lysosome fusion, and autophagy mediated delivery of Mtb to lysosomes can kill the pathogen, although Mtb has multiple mechanisms of evasion [68]. While most replicating organisms die due to the concerted anti-microbial mechanisms, surviving Mtb bacilli enter into a dormant stage, and remain latent for prolonged periods. Interestingly, both NO and hypoxia induce expression of genes of Mtb that facilitate its survival during dormancy within macrophages [69].

It is intriguing to observe that MSCs also provide a niche for the persistence of dormant Mtb, and have similar mechanisms that drive Mtb into dormancy when compared to macrophages. Mtb can infect both mouse and human MSCs, but has a differential intracellular growth pattern. Mtb survived with a limited replication in human MSCs for as long as 14–21 days post infection [17, 40]. In contrast, mouse MSCs were unable to prevent the growth of Mtb in vitro, but killed avirulent *M. bovis* BCG and *M. smegmatis* through TLR-2/4 pathway-dependent expression of cationic antimicrobial peptide cathelicidin [70]. In addition, Mtb reduced the TLR2/4-MyD88-IRAK-4-p38-NF-κB-IL-1β dependent expression of cathelicidin. We found that the inability of Mtb to multiply in human MSCs in vitro was due to the dual action of innate immunity and secretion of NO [40]. Thus, human MSCs phagocytosed Mtb through SR-A, and inhibited the growth of Mtb through 'intrinsic' autophagy [40]. This was consistent with our previous observation that mycobacteria internalized through SR-A is associated with autophagy within mouse macrophages [71]. Additional studies showed that, rapamycin 'induced' autophagy in human MSCs led to an enhanced killing of Mtb. In addition, Mtb infected MSCs secreted NO to kill intracellular Mtb in vitro, and blockade of NO synthesis enhanced their growth. Others report that blockade of NO also enhances growth of Mtb within MSCs of mouse [72]. Thus, MSCs seem to have a robust innate ability to inhibit the growth of Mtb through intrinsic autophagy and NO although they are insufficient to eradicate the organisms. In addition, studies show that hypoxia, another critical micro-environmental factor that induces dormancy in Mtb, occurs within Mtb infected $CD271^+$ mouse and human BM-MSCs [73]. Finally, human MSCs secrete cathelicidin, which can kill Mtb either directly or through inducing autophagy [49, 70]. We and others have found that MSCs remain fully viable despite containing dormant Mtb for 14 days or longer. The longevity of MSCs can perhaps be explained by their ability to secrete anti-apoptotic factors [74, 75]. Together, these observations indicate that human MSCs use a combination of antimicrobial mechanisms to kill most of the growth competent Mtb, while some organisms enter into a dormant influenced by NO and hypoxia [73]. It is important to note here that, of the three stress inducing micro-environmental factors for dormancy of Mtb, NO is elaborated by naïve MSCs upon Mtb infection unlike the human macrophages, which need IFN-γ mediated activation.

Mtb organisms can remain dormant within macrophages among patients who have been successfully treated. In an interesting parallel, viable Mtb has been recovered from MSCs of both mice and humans treated with long term chemotherapy [76]. The failure of drugs to eradicate Mtb from MSCs could either be due to its bone marrow niche where drugs may not penetrate well, or the ability of MSCs to efflux drugs through ABCG2 pumps or both [77]. Bone marrow is therefore an immune privileged site for Mtb infected MSCs.

A second mechanism through which dormant Mtb may sequester successfully within MSCs is due to its low immunogenicity. In both humans and mice, Mtb infected macrophages are recognized by CD4 and CD8 T cells that bind respectively to peptide epitopes on MHC-II (HLA-DR in humans) and MHC-I (HLA-ABC in humans). T_H1 immunity mediated through cytokines like IFN-γ then enables activation of macrophages to kill Mtb through oxidants and PL fusion. In contrast, MSCs are unique among stem cells in expressing only low levels of MHC-II (HLA-DR) while, MHC-I (HLA-ABC) expression appears insufficient or dysfunctional [78]. Reduced immune presentation by Mtb infected MSCs may therefore enable them to avoid immune recognition and thereby prevent eradication of Mtb through T cell secreted cytokines. It is relevant to note here that IFN-γ mediated activation can enhance the ability of MSCs to express both MHC-II (HLA-DR) and MHC-I (HLA-ABC) although, their surface expression is still a slow process requiring many days [79].

It remains unclear how Mtb infected MSCs localize to bone marrows. MSCs are found in bone marrow, from where they migrate to other organs, but they also occur in multiple organs including lungs. Thus, it is appears that either the MSCs get infected with Mtb in the lungs during primary infection, and then migrate back to bone marrow or Mtb can infect the bone marrow resident MSCs trafficking from the lungs. In support of this observation, MSCs have been found to infiltrate both the lung parenchyma and lung alveoli during inflammation, where they can differentiate into type I and II epithelial cells, and in addition, immunomodulate the alveolar micro-environment [19, 80]. Furthermore, intravenous infusion of MSCs restored bone marrow immune function in animal models [81, 82].

These observations suggest that during the pathogenesis of tuberculosis, Mtb infected MSCs are likely to traffic between lungs and bone marrow helping mycobacterial dissemination, and local persistence in bone marrow. Whether MSCs seed Mtb to other organs remains an open question. Another important question is whether Mtb within MSCs can reactivate to result in active disease. A recent study showed that human and mouse HSCs containing Mtb or their DNA instilled into the trachea of immune-deficient $Rag2^{-/-}Il2rg^{-/-}$mice, led to an active disease of the lungs. We hypothesize that Mtb within MSCs may also reactivate during immunodeficiency of mice or humans. Similar to HSCs, MSCs are under the regulatory influence of IFN-γ, which induces enhanced expression of HLA-ABC, HLA-G and HLA-DR [79, 83, 84]. Although the mechanisms through which Mtb reactivates from MSCs remain unclear, it is possible that IFN-γ strengthens the ability of MSCs to inhibit Mtb, and in its absence, Mtb may resume replication. While MSCs targets Mtb to lysosomes through intrinsic autophagy, and secretes NO even without prior activation, IFN-γ can certainly enhance these processes as it does in macrophages [85, 86]. Finally, IFN-γ may also activate hitherto unknown anti-microbial pathways of MSCs that need to be explored.

Immunotherapy with Mesenchymal Stem Cells for Tuberculosis

Tuberculosis is a disease that has been difficult to control because of a lack of an efficient vaccine against adult tuberculosis, and the emergence of MDR-tuberculosis. Immunotherapy or host-directed therapy (HDT) for tuberculosis is therefore gaining more attention [1, 87]. Foregoing observations indicate that during tuberculosis, Mtb infected lungs suffer disease stage specific tissue damage, and MSCs internalize Mtb either during primary infection or during the granuloma associated immune cell recruitment. Mtb infected MSCs then localize to bone marrow where they provide a privileged niche although, they may be found in other organs. The goal of developing immunotherapy strategies with MSCs is therefore threefold; repairing and restoring lung function; restoration or strengthening of immune functions of macrophages, DCs, T cells and neutrophils; and elimination of the niche for dormant Mtb. A major advantage of immunotherapy here is that, MSCs can be grown in large numbers in vitro and because of their reduced HLA-ABC and HLA-DR expression they elicit less adverse reactions after transplantation. Furthermore, autologous MSCs replicate for several generations in vivo after transplantation. An intriguing observation relevant to tuberculosis is that, after intravenous infusion, a large proportion of MSCs are trapped in the lungs of animal models and humans due their large size. This indicates that, fortuitously, tuberculosis damaged lungs may get higher infiltration with MSCs than required.

Autologous transplantation of MSCs has indeed been shown to be safe and produce beneficial effects on the course of tuberculosis among MDR patients [35, 37, 88]. Chest radiographs and bacterial clearance were favorable after transfusion, which suggested that tissue repair occurred along with reduced inflammation; these observations are consistent with multiple other studies. Thus, MSCs have been used to treat inflammatory bowel disease, Type I Diabetes, Systemic Lupus Erythematosus, Scleroderma, Crohn's disease, Multiple Sclerosis and others [89].

Mtb targets many mammalian cells, though the macrophage continues to be the major phagocyte that can kill the bacteria through multiple mechanisms. However, it is becoming evident from recent studies that macrophages are heterogeneous, and pro-inflammatory M1 macrophages are better able to kill Mtb than anti-inflammatory M2 cells. The concept that a balance between M1 and M2 may determine the fate of tuberculosis is therefore gaining traction. In this event, MSCs can play an adversarial role by skewing M1 to M2 macrophages, and exacerbating tuberculosis. However, MSCs have also been documented to enhance antimicrobial activity through cathelicidin, IDO, NO and perhaps other unidentified mechanisms. We made a significant observation that even naïve MSCs inhibited Mtb in vitro through a combination of intrinsic autophagy and NO. Therefore, it appears feasible to augment the antimicrobial function of MSCs through various biological response modifiers.

Studies show that TLR mediated activation of MSCs increased their survival within transplanted hosts avoiding NK cell mediated killing [90]. Likewise, NOD1/2 activation led to a better differentiation and homing for MSCs [39]. MSCs were found to secrete exosomes which carry microRNAs, and various other biological response modifiers [91]. GATA-4 transgenic MSCs, which skewed immune responses towards T_H2, secreted exosomes and reduced the inflammatory responses in rat myocardium [91]. Importantly, infusion of mice with naive MSCs promoted, while, MSCs activated with the poly (A: U) TLR-3 agonist suppressed the *M. bovis* BCG infection [92]. Other studies show that it is possible alter the immunosuppressive phenotype of MSCs through genetic manipulations. Thus, siRNA knockdown of galeticn-3 in MSCs led to a loss of their immunosuppressive activity against T cells [93].

These observations suggest that it is possible to pharmacologically or genetically 'precondition' MSCs to selectively activate or suppress immune cells. We reported a significant paradigm in the conditioning of MSCs through rapamycin, which showed enhanced autophagy and better killing of Mtb [40]. This indicates that, the dormant focus of Mtb within MSCs can be eradicated using rapamycin particularly in combination with selected tuberculosis drugs. Furthermore, rapamycin is a candidate HDT drug for tuberculosis, and we propose that autologous transplantation with rapamycin preconditioned MSCs may yield a better treatment for MDR-tuberculosis patients [94, 95]. Finally, IFN-γ mediated activation enhances both HLA-ABC and HLA-DR expression in MSCs, and studies show that MSCs secreting a viral antigen stimulate antigen-specific antibody production in vivo [79, 96]. Bio-engineered MSCs can be therefore used in future for vaccination against tuberculosis.

Summary and Conclusions

MSCs are unique multipotent cells that are readily harvested from umbilical cord, placenta and bone marrow. Although they are immunosuppressive in their naive state, they can be pharmacologically or genetically manipulated to generate 'preconditioned' MSCs that are amenable for transplantation. Such MSCs can be used to reprogram other immune cells like macrophages, T cells and DCs to strengthen anti-tuberculosis immunity. Because of their self-renewal and regenerative capacity, they offer an exciting and relatively unexplored platform for designing immunotherapy against tuberculosis associated inflammation and tissue damage. MSCs have intrinsic autophagy that can be boosted to serve as a novel immunotherapy for eradication of dormant tuberculosis organisms.

References

1. Zumla A, et al. Host-directed therapies for infectious diseases: current status, recent progress, and future prospects. Lancet Infect Dis. 2016;16(4):e47–63.
2. Baek SH, Li AH, Sassetti CM. Metabolic regulation of mycobacterial growth and antibiotic sensitivity. PLoS Biol. 2011;9(5):e1001065.
3. Gengenbacher M, Kaufmann SH. *Mycobacterium tuberculosis*: success through dormancy. FEMS Microbiol Rev. 2012;36(3):514–32.
4. Gomez JE, McKinney JD. M. tuberculosis persistence, latency, and drug tolerance. Tuberculosis (Edinb). 2004;84(1–2):29–44.
5. Wakamoto Y, et al. Dynamic persistence of antibiotic-stressed mycobacteria. Science. 2013;339(6115):91–5.
6. Frieden TR, et al. Tuberculosis. Lancet. 2003;362(9387):887–99.
7. Smith I. Mycobacterium tuberculosis pathogenesis and molecular determinants of virulence. Clin Microbiol Rev. 2003;16(3):463–96.
8. van Crevel R, Ottenhoff TH, van der Meer JW. Innate immunity to *Mycobacterium tuberculosis*. Clin Microbiol Rev. 2002;15(2):294–309.
9. Saunders BM, Cooper AM. Restraining mycobacteria: role of granulomas in mycobacterial infections. Immunol Cell Biol. 2000;78(4):334–41.
10. Shaler CR, et al. Pulmonary mycobacterial granuloma increased IL-10 production contributes to establishing a symbiotic host-microbe microenvironment. Am J Pathol. 2011;178(4):1622–34.
11. Silva Miranda M, et al. The tuberculous granuloma: an unsuccessful host defence mechanism providing a safety shelter for the bacteria? Clin Dev Immunol. 2012;2012:139127.
12. Flynn JL, et al. Immunology studies in non-human primate models of tuberculosis. Immunol Rev. 2015;264(1):60–73.
13. Bold TD, Ernst JD. Who benefits from granulomas, mycobacteria or host? Cell. 2009;136(1):17–9.
14. Russell DG, et al. Foamy macrophages and the progression of the human tuberculosis granuloma. Nat Immunol. 2009;10(9):943–8.
15. Ramakrishnan L. Revisiting the role of the granuloma in tuberculosis. Nat Rev Immunol. 2012;12(5):352–66.
16. Raghuvanshi S, et al. Mycobacterium tuberculosis evades host immunity by recruiting mesenchymal stem cells. Proc Natl Acad Sci U S A. 2010;107(50):21653–8.
17. Das B, et al. CD271(+) bone marrow mesenchymal stem cells may provide a niche for dormant *Mycobacterium tuberculosis*. Sci Transl Med. 2013;5(170):170ra13.
18. Tornack J, et al. Human and mouse hematopoietic stem cells are a depot for dormant *Mycobacterium tuberculosis*. PLoS One. 2017;12(1):e0169119.
19. Lee JH, et al. Anatomically and functionally distinct lung Mesenchymal populations marked by Lgr5 and Lgr6. Cell. 2017;170(6):1149–1163.e12.
20. Pittenger MF, et al. Multilineage potential of adult human mesenchymal stem cells. Science. 1999;284(5411):143–7.
21. Uccelli A, Moretta L, Pistoia V. Mesenchymal stem cells in health and disease. Nat Rev Immunol. 2008;8(9):726–36.
22. Ma S, et al. Immunobiology of mesenchymal stem cells. Cell Death Differ. 2014;21(2):216–25.
23. Li X, et al. Comprehensive characterization of four different populations of human mesenchymal stem cells as regards their immune properties, proliferation and differentiation. Int J Mol Med. 2014;34(3):695–704.

24. Dominici M, et al. Heterogeneity of multipotent mesenchymal stromal cells: from stromal cells to stem cells and vice versa. Transplantation. 2009;87(9 Suppl):S36–42.
25. Pal B, Das B. In vitro culture of naive human bone marrow mesenchymal stem cells: a stemness based approach. Front Cell Dev Biol. 2017;5:69.
26. Park KS, et al. Trophic molecules derived from human mesenchymal stem cells enhance survival, function, and angiogenesis of isolated islets after transplantation. Transplantation. 2010;89(5):509–17.
27. Khan A, Hunter RL, Jagannath C. Emerging role of mesenchymal stem cells during tuberculosis: the fifth element in cell mediated immunity. Tuberculosis (Edinb). 2016;101S:S45–52.
28. Kuwana M, et al. Human circulating CD14+ monocytes as a source of progenitors that exhibit mesenchymal cell differentiation. J Leukoc Biol. 2003;74(5):833–45.
29. Le Blanc K. Mesenchymal stromal cells: tissue repair and immune modulation. Cytotherapy. 2006;8(6):559–61.
30. Rasmusson I. Immune modulation by mesenchymal stem cells. Exp Cell Res. 2006;312(12):2169–79.
31. Caplan AI, Bruder SP. Mesenchymal stem cells: building blocks for molecular medicine in the 21st century. Trends Mol Med. 2001;7(6):259–64.
32. Doorn J, et al. Pro-osteogenic trophic effects by PKA activation in human mesenchymal stromal cells. Biomaterials. 2011;32(26):6089–98.
33. Chen L, et al. Paracrine factors of mesenchymal stem cells recruit macrophages and endothelial lineage cells and enhance wound healing. PLoS One. 2008;3(4):e1886.
34. Huang X, et al. Three-dimensional co-culture of mesenchymal stromal cells and differentiated osteoblasts on human bio-derived bone scaffolds supports active multi-lineage hematopoiesis in vitro: functional implication of the biomimetic HSC niche. Int J Mol Med. 2016;38(4):1141–51.
35. Skrahin A, et al. Autologous mesenchymal stromal cell infusion as adjunct treatment in patients with multidrug and extensively drug-resistant tuberculosis: an open-label phase 1 safety trial. Lancet Respir Med. 2014;2(2):108–22.
36. Parida SK, et al. Cellular therapy in tuberculosis. Int J Infect Dis. 2015;32:32–8.
37. Skrahin A, et al. Effectiveness of a novel cellular therapy to treat multidrug-resistant tuberculosis. J Clin Tuberc Other Mycobact Dis. 2016;4:21–7.
38. Yudintceva NM, et al. Application of the allogenic mesenchymal stem cells in the therapy of the bladder tuberculosis. J Tissue Eng Regen Med. 2018;12(3):e1580–93.
39. Kim HS, et al. Implication of NOD1 and NOD2 for the differentiation of multipotent mesenchymal stem cells derived from human umbilical cord blood. PLoS One. 2010;5(10):e15369.
40. Khan A, et al. Mesenchymal stem cells internalize *Mycobacterium tuberculosis* through scavenger receptors and restrict bacterial growth through autophagy. Sci Rep. 2017;7(1):15010.
41. Yang K, et al. Mesenchymal stem cells detect and defend against gammaherpesvirus infection via the cGAS-STING pathway. Sci Rep. 2015;5:7820.
42. Rustad KC, Gurtner GC. Mesenchymal stem cells home to sites of injury and inflammation. Adv Wound Care (New Rochelle). 2012;1(4):147–52.
43. Li Y, et al. Staphylococcus aureus infection of intestinal epithelial cells induces human umbilical cord-derived mesenchymal stem cell migration. Int Immunopharmacol. 2013;15(1):176–81.
44. Fakhari S, et al. Effect of Helicobacter pylori infection on stromal-derived factor-1/CXCR4 axis in bone marrow-derived mesenchymal stem cells. Adv Biomed Res. 2014;3:19.
45. Krasnodembskaya A, et al. Human mesenchymal stem cells reduce mortality and bacteremia in gram-negative sepsis in mice in part by enhancing the phagocytic activity of blood monocytes. Am J Physiol Lung Cell Mol Physiol. 2012;302(10):L1003–13.
46. Lombardo E, et al. Mesenchymal stem cells as a therapeutic tool to treat sepsis. World J Stem Cells. 2015;7(2):368–79.
47. Mezey E, Nemeth K. Mesenchymal stem cells and infectious diseases: smarter than drugs. Immunol Lett. 2015;168(2):208–14.

48. Auletta JJ, Deans RJ, Bartholomew AM. Emerging roles for multipotent, bone marrow-derived stromal cells in host defense. Blood. 2012;119(8):1801–9.
49. Krasnodembskaya A, et al. Antibacterial effect of human mesenchymal stem cells is mediated in part from secretion of the antimicrobial peptide LL-37. Stem Cells. 2010;28(12):2229–38.
50. Meisel R, et al. Human but not murine multipotent mesenchymal stromal cells exhibit broad-spectrum antimicrobial effector function mediated by indoleamine 2,3-dioxygenase. Leukemia. 2011;25(4):648–54.
51. Brandau S, et al. Mesenchymal stem cells augment the anti-bacterial activity of neutrophil granulocytes. PLoS One. 2014;9(9):e106903.
52. Raffaghello L, et al. Human mesenchymal stem cells inhibit neutrophil apoptosis: a model for neutrophil preservation in the bone marrow niche. Stem Cells. 2008;26(1):151–62.
53. Takeda K, et al. Mesenchymal stem cells recruit CCR2(+) monocytes to suppress allergic airway inflammation. J Immunol. 2018;200(4):1261–9.
54. Lo Sicco C, et al. Mesenchymal stem cell-derived extracellular vesicles as mediators of anti-inflammatory effects: endorsement of macrophage polarization. Stem Cells Transl Med. 2017;6(3):1018–28.
55. Nemeth K, et al. Bone marrow stromal cells attenuate sepsis via prostaglandin E(2)-dependent reprogramming of host macrophages to increase their interleukin-10 production. Nat Med. 2009;15(1):42–9.
56. Tomioka H, et al. Characteristics of suppressor macrophages induced by mycobacterial and protozoal infections in relation to alternatively activated M2 macrophages. Clin Dev Immunol. 2012;2012:635451.
57. Abumaree MH, et al. Human placental mesenchymal stem cells (pMSCs) play a role as immune suppressive cells by shifting macrophage differentiation from inflammatory M1 to anti-inflammatory M2 macrophages. Stem Cell Rev. 2013;9(5):620–41.
58. Liu S, et al. Immune characterization of mesenchymal stem cells in human umbilical cord Wharton's jelly and derived cartilage cells. Cell Immunol. 2012;278(1–2):35–44.
59. Liu L, et al. Mesenchymal stem cells ameliorate Th1-induced pre-eclampsia-like symptoms in mice via the suppression of TNF-alpha expression. PLoS One. 2014;9(2):e88036.
60. Duffy MM, et al. Mesenchymal stem cell effects on T-cell effector pathways. Stem Cell Res Ther. 2011;2(4):34.
61. Melief SM, et al. Multipotent stromal cells induce human regulatory T cells through a novel pathway involving skewing of monocytes toward anti-inflammatory macrophages. Stem Cells. 2013;31(9):1980–91.
62. Glenn JD, et al. Mesenchymal stem cells differentially modulate effector CD8+ T cell subsets and exacerbate experimental autoimmune encephalomyelitis. Stem Cells. 2014;32(10):2744–55.
63. Carrion F, et al. Opposing effect of mesenchymal stem cells on Th1 and Th17 cell polarization according to the state of CD4+ T cell activation. Immunol Lett. 2011;135(1–2):10–6.
64. Cao W, et al. Mesenchymal stem cells and adaptive immune responses. Immunol Lett. 2015;168(2):147–53.
65. Abomaray FM, et al. Human chorionic villous mesenchymal stem cells modify the functions of human dendritic cells, and induce an anti-inflammatory phenotype in CD1+ dendritic cells. Stem Cell Rev. 2015;11(3):423–41.
66. de Oliveira Bravo M, Carvalho JL, Saldanha-Araujo F. Adenosine production: a common path for mesenchymal stem-cell and regulatory T-cell-mediated immunosuppression. Purinergic Signal. 2016;12(4):595–609.
67. Peters W, et al. Chemokine receptor 2 serves an early and essential role in resistance to *Mycobacterium tuberculosis*. Proc Natl Acad Sci U S A. 2001;98(14):7958–63.
68. Ernst JD. Mechanisms of *M. tuberculosis* immune evasion as challenges to TB vaccine design. Cell Host Microbe. 2018;24(1):34–42.
69. Voskuil MI, et al. Inhibition of respiration by nitric oxide induces a *Mycobacterium tuberculosis* dormancy program. J Exp Med. 2003;198(5):705–13.

70. Naik SK, et al. Mouse bone marrow Sca-1(+) CD44(+) mesenchymal stem cells kill avirulent mycobacteria but not *Mycobacterium tuberculosis* through modulation of cathelicidin expression via the p38 mitogen-activated protein kinase-dependent pathway. Infect Immun. 2017;85(10):e00471-17.
71. Bonilla DL, et al. Autophagy regulates phagocytosis by modulating the expression of scavenger receptors. Immunity. 2013;39(3):537–47.
72. Yang K, et al. Macrophage-mediated inflammatory response decreases mycobacterial survival in mouse MSCs by augmenting NO production. Sci Rep. 2016;6:27326.
73. Garhyan J, et al. Preclinical and clinical evidence of Mycobacterium tuberculosis persistence in the hypoxic niche of bone marrow mesenchymal stem cells after therapy. Am J Pathol. 2015;185(7):1924–34.
74. Rehman J, et al. Secretion of angiogenic and antiapoptotic factors by human adipose stromal cells. Circulation. 2004;109(10):1292–8.
75. Liu GY, et al. ROS activates JNK-mediated autophagy to counteract apoptosis in mouse mesenchymal stem cells in vitro. Acta Pharmacol Sin. 2015;36(12):1473–9.
76. Beamer G, et al. Bone marrow mesenchymal stem cells provide an antibiotic-protective niche for persistent viable Mycobacterium tuberculosis that survive antibiotic treatment. Am J Pathol. 2014;184(12):3170–5.
77. Lopes CS, et al. CD271+ Mesenchymal stem cells as a possible infectious niche for leishmania infantum. PLoS One. 2016;11(9):e0162927.
78. Jacobs SA, et al. Immunological characteristics of human mesenchymal stem cells and multipotent adult progenitor cells. Immunol Cell Biol. 2013;91(1):32–9.
79. Noone C, et al. IFN-gamma stimulated human umbilical-tissue-derived cells potently suppress NK activation and resist NK-mediated cytotoxicity in vitro. Stem Cells Dev. 2013;22(22):3003–14.
80. Sinclair KA, et al. Mesenchymal stromal cells are readily recoverable from lung tissue, but not the alveolar space, in healthy humans. Stem Cells. 2016;34(10):2548–58.
81. Lee ST, et al. Effect of mesenchymal stem cell transplantation on the engraftment of human hematopoietic stem cells and leukemic cells in mice model. Int J Hematol. 2008;87(3):327–37.
82. Bensidhoum M, et al. Homing of in vitro expanded Stro-1- or Stro-1+ human mesenchymal stem cells into the NOD/SCID mouse and their role in supporting human CD34 cell engraftment. Blood. 2004;103(9):3313–9.
83. Fu X, et al. Comparison of immunological characteristics of mesenchymal stem cells derived from human embryonic stem cells and bone marrow. Tissue Eng Part A. 2015;21(3–4):616–26.
84. Ding DC, et al. Characterization of HLA-G and related immunosuppressive effects in human umbilical cord stroma-derived stem cells. Cell Transplant. 2016;25(2):217–28.
85. Feng CG, et al. Interferon-inducible immunity-related GTPase Irgm1 regulates IFN gamma-dependent host defense, lymphocyte survival and autophagy. Autophagy. 2009;5(2):232–4.
86. Nathan C, Xie QW. Nitric oxide synthases: roles, tolls, and controls. Cell. 1994;78(6):915–8.
87. Wallis RS, et al. Tuberculosis--advances in development of new drugs, treatment regimens, host-directed therapies, and biomarkers. Lancet Infect Dis. 2016;16(4):e34–46.
88. Erokhin VV, et al. Systemic transplantation of autologous mesenchymal stem cells of the bone marrow in the treatment of patients with multidrug-resistant pulmonary tuberculosis. Probl Tuberk Bolezn Legk. 2008;(10):3–6.
89. Trounson A, McDonald C. Stem cell therapies in clinical trials: progress and challenges. Cell Stem Cell. 2015;17(1):11–22.
90. Giuliani M, et al. TLR ligands stimulation protects MSC from NK killing. Stem Cells. 2014;32(1):290–300.
91. Yu B, et al. Exosomes secreted from GATA-4 overexpressing mesenchymal stem cells serve as a reservoir of anti-apoptotic microRNAs for cardioprotection. Int J Cardiol. 2015;182:349–60.
92. Schwartz YS, et al. BCG infection in mice is promoted by naive mesenchymal stromal cells (MSC) and suppressed by poly(A:U)-conditioned MSC. Tuberculosis (Edinb). 2016;101:130–6.

93. Sioud M, et al. Evidence for the involvement of galectin-3 in mesenchymal stem cell suppression of allogeneic T-cell proliferation. Scand J Immunol. 2010;71(4):267–74.
94. Mahon RN, Hafner R. Immune cell regulatory pathways unexplored as host-directed therapeutic targets for *Mycobacterium tuberculosis*: an opportunity to apply precision medicine innovations to infectious diseases. Clin Infect Dis. 2015;61Suppl 3:S200–16.
95. Singh P, Subbian S. Harnessing the mTOR pathway for tuberculosis treatment. Front Microbiol. 2018;9:70.
96. Tomchuck SL, et al. Mesenchymal stem cells as a novel vaccine platform. Front Cell Infect Microbiol. 2012;2:140.

Role of *Mycobacterium tuberculosis* PE and PPE Proteins in Pathogen-Host Interactions

Govardhan Rathnaiah, Denise K. Zinniel, and Raul G. Barletta

Abstract This article reviews the discovery, structure, secretion, and role in microbial evolution and immuno-pathogenesis of a group of *Mycobacterium tuberculosis* acidic glycine rich proteins containing multiple copies of repetitive sequences. The classification of these into PE and PPE proteins is based on the presence of proline-glutamic acid (PE) or proline-proline-glutamic acid (PPE) residues at their N-terminal domains. The structural basis for their interactions in PE-PPE pairs and with mycobacterial protein family secretion systems (ESX or Type VII) is described. We also illustrate the role of these proteins in mycobacterial evolution and immuno-pathogenesis. The emergence of the various lineages and subfamilies of PE and PPE proteins and their ancestral counterparts are described in the context of the interactions of the pathogen with host cells and the elicitation of humoral and cellular immune responses.

Keywords Glycine rich proteins · Repetitive sequences · Proline · Glutamic acid · Sublineage V expansion · Type VII secretion system · ESAT-6 · PE-PPE complex · Gene clusters · Immuno-pathogenesis · Virulence determinants · Vaccine development

Introduction

The sequencing project for *Mycobacterium tuberculosis* (MTB) led to the discovery that approximately 10% of the MTB genome coding capacity is dedicated to encoding two novel protein families [1]. These families have been denominated PE (proline-glutamic acid) and PPE (proline-proline-glutamic acid) proteins for their characteristic

G. Rathnaiah · D. K. Zinniel · R. G. Barletta (✉)
School of Veterinary Medicine and Biomedical Sciences, University of Nebraska, Lincoln, NE, USA
e-mail: rbarletta@unl.edu

J. D. Cirillo, Y. Kong (eds.), *Tuberculosis Host-Pathogen Interactions*,
https://doi.org/10.1007/978-3-030-25381-3_6

amino acid residues in defined positions of their conserved N-terminal domains. The genome sequences of 205,006 bacteria covering a wide range of taxonomic groups including most mycobacterial species representing 7,311 mycobacterial sequences are available as of July 22, 2019 (https://www.ncbi.nlm.nih.gov/genome/browse#!/prokaryotes/). The application of bioinformatic analysis to these sequencing data demonstrated that PE-PPE proteins are unique to microorganisms of the taxonomical family *Mycobacteriaceae* [2] and the closely related actinobacteria (https://pfam.xfam.org). Moreover, these sequences are highly expanded in the microorganisms of the MTB complex and taxonomically related slow-growing mycobacteria such as *M. marinum*, as compared to those of the *M. avium* complex [2, 3] and fast-growing mycobacteria. In the latter group, only about 1% of their genomes encode PE or PPE proteins (Table 1). Thus, the expansion in PE and PPE coding sequences is indicative of the point of evolutionary departure for microorganisms of the MTB complex from other mycobacterial species.

Most PE and PPE gene sequences are linked to the five ESAT-6 gene clusters identified in slow-growing mycobacteria. The ESAT-6 gene clusters encode highly immunogenic low molecular weight proteins and the components of their secretion apparatus. This finding led to the hypothesis that PE-PPE/ESAT-6 regions constitute a genomic "immunogenicity island" [2]. These genes are in some cases organized in operons encompassing several PE and/or PPE members [4]. Moreover, biochemical evidence suggests that PE and PPE function in pair-wise combinations of interacting proteins exposed to the cell surface [5–7] with larger size PPE proteins providing a pocket for the PE partner [7].

Microorganisms of the *M. avium* complex carry a duplication of the ESAT-6 Region V. Further expansion of this region gave rise to the PE-polymorphic

Table 1 The number of mycobacterial PE and PPE proteins is indicated for various species

Species	PE proteins accession PF00934	PPE proteins accession PF00823	Comments[a,b]
Fast-growing species:			
M. abscessus	3	8	No PE-PGRS/PPE-MPTR No ESAT-6 region V
M. smegmatis	2	2	No PE-PGRS/PPE-MPTR No ESAT-6 region V
M. vaccae	3	4	No PE-PGRS/PPE-MPTR No ESAT-6 region V
Slow-growing species:			
M. avium paratuberculosis	9	37	No PE-PGRS/PPE-MPTR Ancestral ESAT-6 region V
M. marinum	162	106	Multiple PE-PGRS/PPE-MPTR (sublineage V)
M. tuberculosis	89	65	Multiple PE-PGRS/PPE-MPTR (sublineage V)

[a]Data collected from: https://pfam.xfam.org; Pfam 31.0; numbers may differ slightly from strain to strain and to reports in other databases

[b]See section on structure for description of protein motifs and sublineages

GC-rich sequences (PGRS) and PPE-major polymorphic tandem repeat (MPTR) sublineage V PE-PPE proteins in the MTB complex (Table 1). These subfamilies seem to play a fundamental role in MTB and *M. bovis* (MBO), the highly pathogenic slow-growing mycobacteria. Moreover, their highly polymorphic C-terminal regions led to the hypothesis of their potential roles in antigenic variation, modulation of the immune response, and protein-protein interactions that may determine tissue tropism and host range for different mycobacterial species [1, 2, 8–11].

Structure of PE and PPE Proteins

PE genes are classified in two subgroups based on the presence or absence of PGRS [2]. Those PE proteins that do not have repeats possess a unique C-terminal sequence of up to 500 amino acids (Fig. 1). Likewise, the PPE proteins have about a 180 amino acid N-terminal domain and are divided in three subgroups based on the presence of C-terminal MPTR with multiple copies of Asn-X-Gly-X-Gly-X-Gly-Asn-X-Gly repeats, the presence of a conserved Gly-X-X-Ser-Val-Pro-X-X-Trp motif around amino acid 350, or the presence of a unique C-terminal sequence of up to 400 amino acids (Fig. 1). These motifs are important because of their role as strong B and T-cell antigens, and their potential application as subunit vaccine candidates to protect against mycobacterial diseases [12].

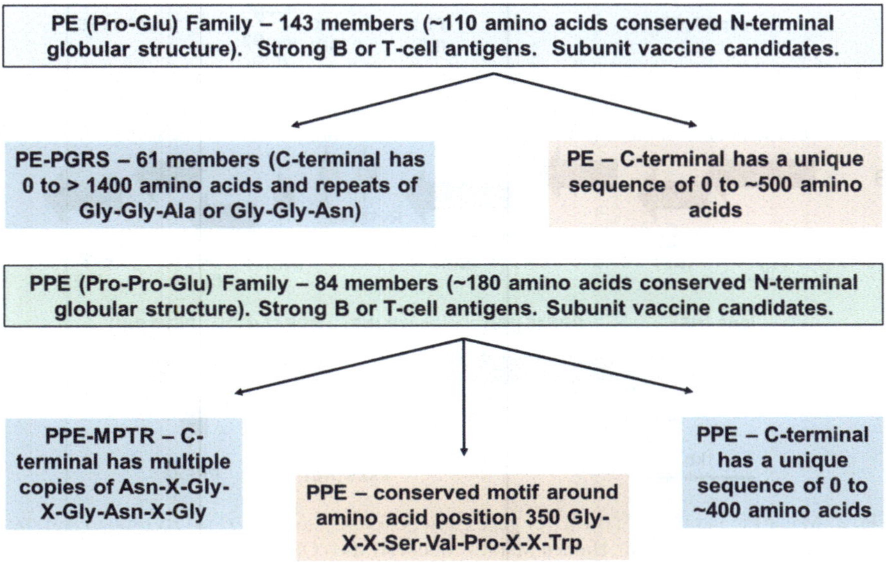

Fig. 1 PE and PPE protein classification based on the presence or absence of characteristic motifs and repeats

Interactions Between PE and PPE Proteins Themselves and the ESX Secretion Systems

PE and PPE proteins are secreted through a specialized protein export pathway called the 6-kDa early secreted antigenic target (ESAT-6) secretion system (ESX). ESX is a Type VII secretion system in mycobacteria and there are five ESX secretion systems in MTB (ESX-1 to ESX-5) [13]. Genes that encode components of each ESX secretion system are present in clusters. Except ESX-4, other ESX clusters also contains *pe* and *ppe* genes within the locus next to *esx* genes (Fig. 2). In addition, a large number of *pe* and *ppe* genes are present throughout the genome. The structural motifs of PE-PPE proteins are very similar to ESX proteins and both belong to the EsxAB protein superfamily. PPE proteins have N-termini domains that interact with PE proteins to form PPE-PE heterodimers [7]. PE proteins are composed of two antiparallel α helices connected by a loop whereas PPE proteins contain five α helices. The PE loop is stabilized by interactions with two of the helices of the PPE protein. This interaction is highly hydrophobic further suggesting that these proteins are stable only when present in a protein pair complex [7]. Bioinformatic analysis (operon/gene cluster method) also reveals that one PE gene

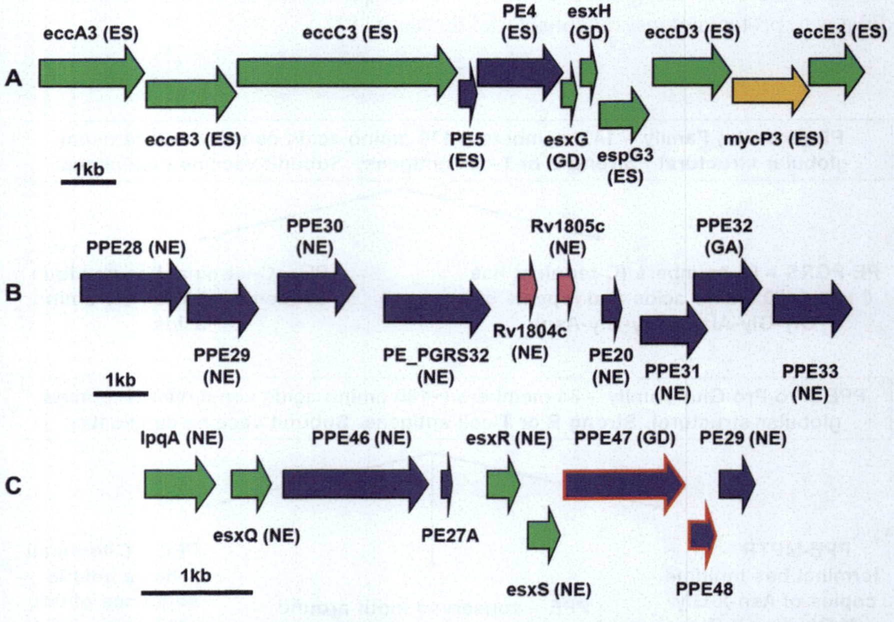

Fig. 2 Major PE and PPE MTB H37Rv gene clusters: Rv0282 to Rv0292 (**a**) Rv1800 to Rv1809 (**b**) and Rv3016 to Rv3022 (**c**). Hidden Markov Model (HMM) ORF classifications (essential, ES; growth defect, GD; growth advantage, GA; and non-essential, NE) were taken from https://mycobrowser.epfl.ch/. ORFs involved in cell wall and cell processes (■), conserved hypothetical (■), PE/PPE (■), intermediary metabolism and respiration (■), and pseudogenes (■) are depicted

is often functionally paired with one PPE gene. PPE proteins also have adaptor protein surfaces through which they interact with the ESX secretion-associated protein G (EspG) and form the PE-PPE/EspG complex [13]. EspG functions as an adaptor protein that delivers this complex to the ESX secretion system. EspG interacts with PE-PPE proteins of the same cluster as well as those involved in cross talk between different ESX systems. Each ESX cluster encodes its own EspG that determines the secretion of specific PE-PPE pairs through the cognate ESX system [14, 15]. $EspG_1$ is an ESX-1 encoded adaptor that is responsible for the secretion of its cognate PE25-PPE68 heterodimer. Similarly, $EspG_5$ is the ESX-5 encoded adaptor that forms a heterotrimeric structure through hydrophobic interactions with ESX-5 specific secretory proteins PE25-PPE41. At the molecular level, $EspG_5$ solely forms hydrophobic interactions (using the hydrophobic motif) with PPE41 and hence provides stability to PE-PPE protein pairs. Therefore, each ESX specific PPE protein has binding sites for a cognate chaperone and these sites are conformational rather than linear motifs formed because of PE-PPE pair interaction. These structures further strengthen the stringency of PE-PPE and ESX protein interactions.

Expansion of PE and PPE Proteins in Mycobacterial Evolution

PE and PPE gene families are present mostly in *Mycobacteriaceae* [2]. Moreover, these proteins co-evolve with the MTB Type VII secretion system components, the WXG100 (PF06013) protein families (e.g., ESAT-6 is a member). As indicated above, many PE-PPE proteins in the MTB complex are the result of repeated duplication events in the ESAT-6 gene cluster. Different subsets of PE-PPE proteins have originated from different ESAT-6 gene clusters. For example, the two largest subfamilies of PE-PPE proteins, PE-PGRS, and PPE-MPTR may have originated from ESAT-6 gene cluster Region V, as there are enhanced chances of duplication of PE-PPE genes in this region. Therefore, this combination of ESAT-6 locus and cognate PE-PPE proteins may be responsible for antigenic diversity.

Role of PE and PPE Proteins in Immuno-Pathogenesis

It has been hypothesized that the PE and PPE families may have immunological importance, since they are one of the main sources of antigenic variation in MTB [1]. Experimental evidence on PE-PPE proteins in MTB and other mycobacterial species is consistent with this original hypothesis. For example, the MTB protein Rv2430c (PE25) was identified as a strong B-cell antigen [16], and the seroreactivity of the *M. avium* subsp. *paratuberculosis* MAP_3420c was demonstrated in cattle [17]. In contrast, MAP_3184 (Map 39; ortholog of Rv3135 [PPE50]), the *M. avium* strain 104 MaaPE7 protein (MAV_2923), and the cell wall-associated MTB protein Rv3873 (PPE68) serve as T-cell antigens [18–21]. The PPE60 protein has been shown to potentiate Th1/Th17 responses via interactions with Toll-like receptors [22]. Interestingly, PPE37 is cleaved by a protease under low iron conditions [23] with the iron-binding N-terminal domain promoting phagocytic cell proliferation, while the C-terminal region enters the cell nucleus and induces apoptosis. Thus, these two antagonistic activities exerted extracellularly (N-domain) and intracellular (C-domain) cooperate to enhance MTB pathogenesis.

PE and PPE proteins have also been implicated in virulence. The application of the HMM to MTB saturated transposon libraries in vitro resulted in a gene classification into four categories [24]: ES (genes physiologically essential; e.g., genes do not tolerate insertions in essential domains), GD (genes whose inactivation leads to growth defects), NE (genes that tolerate inactivation without an effect on growth and are therefore non-essential), and GA (genes whose inactivation leads to a growth advantage). In this context, most PE, PPE, and PE-PGRS genes fall into the NE or GA category. Notable exceptions are Rv0285 (PE5) and the adjacent gene Rv0286 (PPE4) that are essential genes encoding a core mycobacterial component [25]. Another interesting example is Rv3021c (PPE47) that has a GD domain by HMM analysis and classified as essential by standard analysis of transposon mutagenesis data [26]. Moreover, this gene has been classified as a pseudogene due to a frameshift. Thus, its essential character for in vitro growth may be due to a possibly essential regulatory function, an explanation that has been proposed for the function of some pseudogenes [27]. Regarding genomic organization, there are several examples of PE and PPE genes that cluster together, possibly in operons. In contrast, there are very few examples of this organization for PE-PGRS genes (Fig. 2). In general, these genes can be encoded by either the positive or the negative strand of the genome. Though NE and GA genes are dispensable in vitro, some are likely to play important functions in vivo during infection [28]. For example, Rv1807 (PPE31) classifies as NE in vitro, but is required for infection in mice. Likewise, Rv3872 (PE35) and Rv3873 (PPE68) classified as NE in vitro, are required in vivo. Interestingly, the latter two ORFs are encoded by the MTB RD1 region, a 9.5 kb segment between Rv3871 and Rv3879c that is also present in virulent MBO but deleted from the vaccine strain MBO BCG. This region also encodes the immunodominant antigens Rv3874 (EsxB, Cfp10) and Rv3875 (EsxA, ESAT-6), and conserved components of the corresponding secretion system [29, 30]. Thus, these PE-PPE proteins have been proposed as targets for the construction of attenuated candidate vaccine mutant strains [12].

Recent findings, however, question whether secretion of PE-PGRS and PPE-MPTR proteins are necessary or detrimental for vaccine efficacy [31]. Indeed, secretion of these proteins requires a functional Rv2352c (PPE38) protein whose gene is in the RD5 region [32]. The vaccine strain MBO BCG, other animal host-adapted virulent strains, and highly virulent human strains of the Beijing lineage lack PPE38 and do not secrete PE-PGRS or PPE-MPTR proteins making them inaccessible to the immune system. Likewise, the deletion of *ppe38* in strains with lower virulence increased their pathogenicity. Certainly, introduction of a functional *ppe38* gene into recombinant BCG restored secretion, but it had no major effect on protection in tuberculosis mouse models [31]. These findings suggest that some of the secreted PPE proteins may inhibit antigen presentation. The authors of this study also suggest that it is possible that the role of PE-PGRS and PPE-MPTR protein in virulence may not be directly related to secretion.

Concluding Remarks

PE-PPE proteins are encoded by mycobacterial genomes. They are especially abundant in microorganisms of the MTB complex. In general, these proteins are non-essential for mycobacterial physiology but may play important roles in infection and immuno-pathogenesis. Mutants may serve as candidate live-attenuated-vaccine strains or the proteins incorporated into subunit vaccines. However, these hypotheses may need re-evaluation based on recent findings underscoring the complex interrelationship between virulence and secretion.

Acknowledgements We thank Neha Chaudhary for constructive input into this manuscript.

References

1. Cole ST, Brosch R, Parkhill J, Garnier T, Churcher C, Harris D, Gordon SV, Eiglmeier K, Gas S, Barry CE 3rd, Tekaia F, Badcock K, Basham D, Brown D, Chillingworth T, Connor R, Davies R, Devlin K, Feltwell T, Gentles S, Hamlin N, Holroyd S, Hornsby T, Jagels K, Krogh A, McLean J, Moule S, Murphy L, Oliver K, Osborne J, Quail MA, Rajandream MA, Rogers J, Rutter S, Seeger K, Skelton J, Squares R, Squares S, Sulston JE, Taylor K, Whitehead S, Barrell BG. Deciphering the biology of *Mycobacterium tuberculosis* from the complete genome sequence. Nature. 1998;393(6685):537–44. https://doi.org/10.1038/31159.
2. Gey van Pittius NC, Sampson SL, Lee H, Kim Y, van Helden PD, Warren RM. Evolution and expansion of the *Mycobacterium tuberculosis* PE and PPE multigene families and their association with the duplication of the ESAT-6 (*esx*) gene cluster regions. BMC Evol Biol. 2006;6:95. https://doi.org/10.1186/1471-2148-6-95.
3. Li L, Bannantine JP, Zhang Q, Amonsin A, May BJ, Alt D, Banerji N, Kanjilal S, Kapur V. The complete genome sequence of *Mycobacterium avium* subspecies *paratuberculosis*. Proc Natl Acad Sci U S A. 2005;102(35):12344–9. https://doi.org/10.1073/pnas.0505662102.
4. Tundup S, Akhter Y, Thiagarajan D, Hasnain SE. Clusters of PE and PPE genes of *Mycobacterium tuberculosis* are organized in operons: evidence that PE Rv2431c is co-transcribed with PPE Rv2430c and their gene products interact with each other. FEBS Lett. 2006;580(5):1285–93. https://doi.org/10.1016/j.febslet.2006.01.042.
5. Delogu G, Pusceddu C, Bua A, Fadda G, Brennan MJ, Zanetti S. Rv1818c-encoded PE_PGRS protein of *Mycobacterium tuberculosis* is surface exposed and influences bacterial cell structure. Mol Microbiol. 2004;52(3):725–33. https://doi.org/10.1111/j.1365-2958.2004.04007.x.
6. Riley R, Pellegrini M, Eisenberg D. Identifying cognate binding pairs among a large set of paralogs: the case of PE/PPE proteins of *Mycobacterium tuberculosis*. PLoS Comput Biol. 2008;4(9):e1000174. https://doi.org/10.1371/journal.pcbi.1000174.

7. Strong M, Sawaya MR, Wang S, Phillips M, Cascio D, Eisenberg D. Toward the structural genomics of complexes: crystal structure of a PE/PPE protein complex from *Mycobacterium tuberculosis*. Proc Natl Acad Sci U S A. 2006;103(21):8060–5. https://doi.org/10.1073/pnas.0602606103.
8. Banu S, Honore N, Saint-Joanis B, Philpott D, Prevost MC, Cole ST. Are the PE-PGRS proteins of *Mycobacterium tuberculosis* variable surface antigens? Mol Microbiol. 2002;44(1):9–19.
9. Brennan MJ, Delogu G, Chen Y, Bardarov S, Kriakov J, Alavi M, Jacobs WR Jr. Evidence that mycobacterial PE_PGRS proteins are cell surface constituents that influence interactions with other cells. Infect Immun. 2001;69(12):7326–33. https://doi.org/10.1128/IAI.69.12.7326-7333.2001.
10. Delogu G, Brennan MJ. Comparative immune response to PE and PE_PGRS antigens of *Mycobacterium tuberculosis*. Infect Immun. 2001;69(9):5606–11.
11. Delogu G, Sanguinetti M, Pusceddu C, Bua A, Brennan MJ, Zanetti S, Fadda G. PE_PGRS proteins are differentially expressed by *Mycobacterium tuberculosis* in host tissues. Microbes Infect. 2006;8(8):2061–7. https://doi.org/10.1016/j.micinf.2006.03.015.
12. Brennan MJ. The enigmatic PE/PPE multigene family of mycobacteria and tuberculosis vaccination. Infect Immun. 2017;85(6):e00969-16. https://doi.org/10.1128/IAI.00969-16.
13. Ekiert DC, Cox JS. Structure of a PE-PPE-EspG complex from *Mycobacterium tuberculosis* reveals molecular specificity of ESX protein secretion. Proc Natl Acad Sci U S A. 2014;111(41):14758–63. https://doi.org/10.1073/pnas.1409345111.
14. Korotkova N, Freire D, Phan TH, Ummels R, Creekmore CC, Evans TJ, Wilmanns M, Bitter W, Parret AH, Houben EN, Korotkov KV. Structure of the *Mycobacterium tuberculosis* type VII secretion system chaperone $EspG_5$ in complex with PE25-PPE41 dimer. Mol Microbiol. 2014;94(2):367–82. https://doi.org/10.1111/mmi.12770.
15. Korotkova N, Piton J, Wagner JM, Boy-Rottger S, Japaridze A, Evans TJ, Cole ST, Pojer F, Korotkov KV. Structure of EspB, a secreted substrate of the ESX-1 secretion system of *Mycobacterium tuberculosis*. J Struct Biol. 2015;191(2):236–44. https://doi.org/10.1016/j.jsb.2015.06.003.
16. Choudhary RK, Mukhopadhyay S, Chakhaiyar P, Sharma N, Murthy KJ, Katoch VM, Hasnain SE. PPE antigen Rv2430c of *Mycobacterium tuberculosis* induces a strong B-cell response. Infect Immun. 2003;71(11):6338–43.
17. Newton V, McKenna SL, De Buck J. Presence of PPE proteins in *Mycobacterium avium* subsp. *paratuberculosis* isolates and their immunogenicity in cattle. Vet Microbiol. 2009;135(3–4):394–400. https://doi.org/10.1016/j.vetmic.2008.09.066.
18. Mackenzie N, Alexander DC, Turenne CY, Behr MA, De Buck JM. Genomic comparison of PE and PPE genes in the *Mycobacterium avium* complex. J Clin Microbiol. 2009;47(4):1002–11. https://doi.org/10.1128/JCM.01313-08.
19. Nagata R, Muneta Y, Yoshihara K, Yokomizo Y, Mori Y. Expression cloning of gamma interferon-inducing antigens of *Mycobacterium avium* subsp. *paratuberculosis*. Infect Immun. 2005;73(6):3778–82. https://doi.org/10.1128/IAI.73.6.3778-3782.2005.
20. Okkels LM, Brock I, Follmann F, Agger EM, Arend SM, Ottenhoff TH, Oftung F, Rosenkrands I, Andersen P. PPE protein (Rv3873) from DNA segment RD1 of *Mycobacterium tuberculosis*: strong recognition of both specific T-cell epitopes and epitopes conserved within the PPE family. Infect Immun. 2003;71(11):6116–23.
21. Parra M, Cadieux N, Pickett T, Dheenadhayalan V, Brennan MJ. A PE protein expressed by *Mycobacterium avium* is an effective T-cell immunogen. Infect Immun. 2006;74(1):786–9. https://doi.org/10.1128/IAI.74.1.786-789.2006.
22. Su H, Zhang Z, Liu Z, Peng B, Kong C, Wang H, Zhang Z, Xu Y. *Mycobacterium tuberculosis* PPE60 antigen drives Th1/Th17 responses via toll-like receptor 2-dependent maturation of dendritic cells. J Biol Chem. 2018;293(26):10287–302. https://doi.org/10.1074/jbc.RA118.001696.

23. Ahmad J, Farhana A, Pancsa R, Arora SK, Srinivasan A, Tyagi AK, Babu MM, Ehtesham NZ, Hasnain SE. Contrasting function of structured N-terminal and unstructured C-terminal segments of *Mycobacterium tuberculosis* PPE37 protein. mBio. 2018;9(1):e01712-17. https://doi.org/10.1128/mBio.01712-17.
24. DeJesus MA, Gerrick ER, Xu W, Park SW, Long JE, Boutte CC, Rubin EJ, Schnappinger D, Ehrt S, Fortune SM, Sassetti CM, Ioerger TR. Comprehensive essentiality analysis of the *Mycobacterium tuberculosis* genome via saturating transposon mutagenesis. mBio. 2017;8(1):e02133-16. https://doi.org/10.1128/mBio.02133-16.
25. Marmiesse M, Brodin P, Buchrieser C, Gutierrez C, Simoes N, Vincent V, Glaser P, Cole ST, Brosch R. Macro-array and bioinformatic analyses reveal mycobacterial 'core' genes, variation in the ESAT-6 gene family and new phylogenetic markers for the *Mycobacterium tuberculosis* complex. Microbiology. 2004;150. (Pt 2:483–96. https://doi.org/10.1099/mic.0.26662-0.
26. Griffin JE, Gawronski JD, Dejesus MA, Ioerger TR, Akerley BJ, Sassetti CM. High-resolution phenotypic profiling defines genes essential for mycobacterial growth and cholesterol catabolism. PLoS Pathog. 2011;7(9):e1002251. https://doi.org/10.1371/journal.ppat.1002251.
27. Lerat E, Ochman H. Recognizing the pseudogenes in bacterial genomes. Nucleic Acids Res. 2005;33(10):3125–32. https://doi.org/10.1093/nar/gki631.
28. Sassetti CM, Rubin EJ. Genetic requirements for mycobacterial survival during infection. Proc Natl Acad Sci U S A. 2003;100(22):12989–94. https://doi.org/10.1073/pnas.2134250100.
29. Flint JL, Kowalski JC, Karnati PK, Derbyshire KM. The RD1 virulence locus of *Mycobacterium tuberculosis* regulates DNA transfer in *Mycobacterium smegmatis*. Proc Natl Acad Sci U S A. 2004;101(34):12598–603. https://doi.org/10.1073/pnas.0404892101.
30. Guinn KM, Hickey MJ, Mathur SK, Zakel KL, Grotzke JE, Lewinsohn DM, Smith S, Sherman DR. Individual RD1-region genes are required for export of ESAT-6/CFP-10 and for virulence of *Mycobacterium tuberculosis*. Mol Microbiol. 2004;51(2):359–70. https://doi.org/10.1046/j.1365-2958.2003.03844.x.
31. Ates LS, Sayes F, Frigui W, Ummels R, Damen MPM, Bottai D, Behr MA, van Heijst JWJ, Bitter W, Majlessi L, Brosch R. RD5-mediated lack of PE_PGRS and PPE-MPTR export in BCG vaccine strains results in strong reduction of antigenic repertoire but little impact on protection. PLoS Pathog. 2018;14(6):e1007139. https://doi.org/10.1371/journal.ppat.1007139.
32. Ates LS, Dippenaar A, Ummels R, Piersma SR, van der Woude AD, van der Kuij K, Le Chevalier F, Mata-Espinosa D, Barrios-Payan J, Marquina-Castillo B, Guapillo C, Jimenez CR, Pain A, Houben ENG, Warren RM, Brosch R, Hernandez-Pando R, Bitter W. Mutations in ppe38 block PE_PGRS secretion and increase virulence of *Mycobacterium tuberculosis*. Nat Microbiol. 2018;3(2):181–8. https://doi.org/10.1038/s41564-017-0090-6.

Co-Infection with TB and HIV: Converging Epidemics, Clinical Challenges, and Microbial Synergy

Matthew B. Huante, Rebecca J. Nusbaum, and Janice J. Endsley

Abstract Human immunodeficiency virus (HIV) and *Mycobacterium tuberculosis* (*Mtb*) are the two leading causes of infectious disease-related death today. An estimated 2.6 million people die as a result of infection with one or both of these pathogens annually, while a range of morbidities afflict tens of millions more. The resurgence of TB in the years following the start of the HIV/AIDS pandemic revealed a close relationship of these two infectious diseases. TB and HIV are now viewed as a syndemic that impedes efforts to reduce incidence of infection, complicates treatment, and promotes development of drug resistance. This chapter summarizes the complex factors whereby TB and HIV converge to drive a global health emergency and discusses ongoing research and clinical efforts to reduce dual disease.

Keywords Tuberculosis · HIV/AIDS · TB and HIV co-infection · Microbial synergy · Pathogenesis · Cellular immunity · Immune dysfunction · Innate immunity · Clinical challenges · Drug resistance

Introduction

Tuberculosis (TB) and human immunodeficiency virus (HIV) are considered a co-pandemic due to complex socio-economic, epidemiological, and biological, factors whereby these pathogens converge to cause death and disease. Following the peak of "white plague" in the fifteenth to seventeenth centuries, TB rates were at a historical low when the human immunodeficiency virus (HIV) pandemic began in the

M. B. Huante · J. J. Endsley (✉)
Department of Microbiology and Immunology, University of Texas Medical Branch at Galveston, Galveston, TX, USA
e-mail: jjendsle@utmb.edu

R. J. Nusbaum
University of Pennsylvania, Philadelphia, PA, USA

J. D. Cirillo, Y. Kong (eds.), *Tuberculosis Host-Pathogen Interactions*,
https://doi.org/10.1007/978-3-030-25381-3_7

1980s. The association of HIV with TB risk was recognized early in those with acquired immune deficiency syndrome (AIDS), though the mechanistic bases continue to be defined. By the 1990s, HIV was understood to be the main factor driving TB resurgence as a global health emergency. The tide has been turning due to access to anti-retroviral therapy (ART), the development of molecular point of care diagnostics, and implementation of integrated public health and clinical approaches to TB/HIV treatment. Despite these successes, HIV remains the most important risk factor for TB disease, and TB is the primary cause of death in those with HIV. The key factors that have driven the TB and HIV co-pandemic over the last three decades will be discussed along with new and on-going challenges to disease elimination efforts.

Tuberculosis: An Ancient Disease in Modern Man

Mycobacterium tuberculosis (*Mtb*), the etiological agent of TB, has killed more people than any other infectious disease in human history [1]. Molecular evidence from Neolithic burial remains on the Atlic peninsula definitively date *Mtb* to at least 9,000 years ago [2], while genetic mapping suggest an age of at least 70,000 years [2–12]. The spread of TB across civilizations, including pre-Columbian people of the Americas and the most famous of Egyptian pharaohs, Tutankhamun [13], is evident from molecular and skeletal analysis of mummies [3, 5, 14, 15]. The sparse population density and nomadic nature of communities likely limited TB incidence until the Neolithic era, when agricultural advances led to increasingly stationary human lifestyles [3, 4] that are more supportive of TB transmission. TB rates escalated during the fifteen to seventeenth centuries, especially in densely populated and squalid housing conditions [3, 16–21]. TB accounted for 25% of deaths during this period, which at the peak in the late 1700s comprised an incidence rate of 700–1,120 deaths per 100,000 persons [16–18, 20–22].

At the turn of the twentieth century, rates of TB were in decline due to many factors including improved living conditions, nutrition, reductions in bovine TB, and public health efforts to isolate afflicted populations [23–25]. Nonetheless, TB remained the second leading cause of infectious disease death in 1900, only surpassed by pneumonia [26]. The introduction of the TB vaccine BCG in 1921, and especially the availability and implementation of combination drug therapy in the 1950s further reduced global TB mortality and morbidity rates to historical lows by the 1970s [27]. A decade after the discovery of HIV as the cause of AIDS in 1983, the alarming resurgence in TB led to an unprecedented declaration by the WHO of TB as a global health emergency [28].

The peak of TB infection in the post HIV/AIDS era occurred in 1995 and rates of new infections and relapse are declining. Despite the decline, TB is once again the leading cause of infectious disease-related death globally and the incidence of drug resistance is increasing at a rapid pace [29]. As of the 2017 WHO report, there were 10.4 million confirmed infections and ~1.7 million deaths due to TB annually [29]. Multi-drug resistant (MDR) strains were identified in 490,000 people in 2016, among which 10% of the isolates were found to be extensively drug resistant (XDR) [29]. Importantly, roughly one-third of the world population is currently estimated to harbor latent TB and serve as a reservoir for new infections [29].

HIV/AIDS: A Pandemic Threat of the Modern Age

Infectious disease due to HIV is relatively recent in human history, having emerged late in the twentieth century. In contrast to *Mtb*, HIV did not originate as a human pathogen but rather one of non-human primates in the form of Simian Immunodeficiency Virus (SIV). The most prevalent strain of HIV today likely originated in Kinshasa, in the Democratic Republic of Congo in the 1920s [30, 31]. Estimates put the common HIV-1 ancestor as arising in the first half of the twentieth century [32], in agreement with the earliest human evidence of infection from a blood sample collected in 1959 from west-central Africa [33]. Over 90% of human disease is caused by infection with HIV-1, while cases of infection with HIV-2 occur in West Africa and more rarely in other regions [34].

It is important to note that HIV/AIDS was first identified due to the cluster of symptoms and clinical signs that developed associated with opportunistic infections (OI). In 1981 the CDC released reports of the opportunistic disease *Pneumocystis carinii* pneumonia (PCP) in previously healthy homosexual men with no known risk factors [35]. Additional cases of PCP and Kaposi's sarcoma (KS) in men who have sex with men, individuals with a history of injection drug usage, and hemophiliacs [35–38], were soon reported. The term acquired immune deficiency syndrome (AIDS) began to be used in late 1982 to define cases of "a disease, at least moderately predictive of a defect in cell-mediated immunity, occurring in a person with no known cause for diminished resistance to that disease. Such diseases include KS, PCP, and serious OIs" [39]. The viral etiology of the disease was discovered by two different research groups in 1983 and 1984 and named Lymphadenopathy-Associated Virus (LAV) or HTLV-III [40]. Subsequently, these identical viruses that caused AIDS were renamed HIV.

Although HIV-associated disease was initially observed in the United States, these cases represented the tip of the iceberg of a pandemic already underway globally and especially in Africa. By 1999, HIV was the fourth most common cause of death worldwide and the most common in Africa [41]. HIV mortality peaked in 2005, killing 1.9 million people as the leading cause of infectious disease-related death from a single pathogen [42]. The HIV pandemic is in decline due to public health education initiatives, and especially the access to ART therapy, in many endemic regions [43]. Despite this progress, HIV remains the second leading cause of infectious disease-related death; 37 million people are living with HIV worldwide and 1.1 million people still die annually from AIDS-related causes [29].

TB and HIV Converge to Drive a Deadly Syndemic

Epidemiological Overlap

Today, TB is the leading cause of death among people living with HIV (PLWH). In newly diagnosed cases of TB, 12% occur in PLWH globally, while rates exceed 50% in South Africa and other southern African countries [29]. An estimated one third of PLWH have latent TB infection and have greatly increased risk of TB reactivation compared to HIV-individuals [44]. One important factor for the dual burden of TB and HIV is the overlap of regions of endemicity. The greatest case burdens of both occur in sub-Saharan Africa and Asia [29]. TB impacts these regions disproportionally due to multiple risk factors of poverty that have been extensively reviewed [45] including malnutrition, dense populations, and poor housing conditions that facilitate greater person to person spread. The spread and persistence of HIV in these same areas is further driven by cultural barriers and educational gaps that limit implementation of practices needed to prevent spread of sexually transmitted diseases [46]. Both diseases are associated with stigma, an important social barrier that prevents people from seeking testing and treatment at clinics [47, 48].

The HIV crisis was economically devastating in many regions due to the loss and illness among those in the most productive part of their working life [49]. The fallout included the collapse of healthcare infrastructure supporting TB control in many countries including through loss or shifts in funding to HIV, and due to death and disability of healthcare workers. Treatment for TB is an intensive process that takes from six to greater than 24 months depending on the drug susceptibility of the isolate and treatment history of the subject [50]. ART is very effective against HIV, but is also a combination therapy and once initiated must be continued throughout the patient's life to maintain viral suppression [51]. These lengthy treatment periods with combination drug therapy as well as the pill burden in those with co-infection increase the likelihood of patient non-compliance [52]. Not surprisingly, then, the incidence of MDR- and XDR-TB is higher in PLWH [53] and the risk for mortality due to drug resistance forms despite treatment is also increased [54]. ART reduces the risk for TB, though a significant number of the 476,774 new cases of TB reported in HIV+ people in 2016 occurred among those on ART [29].

Today, the majority of TB and HIV medication costs, as well as some implementation support are sponsored by international aide programs supplemented to varying proportions by local governments [29]. The remaining costs to access healthcare, which may include transportation, childcare, and lost wages, are often still beyond the reach of the individual. These geographical, political, and economic barriers to consistent healthcare present especially important challenges for chronic diseases such as TB and HIV that require lengthy treatment regimens. The current delivery of ART to an estimated 15 million HIV+ people represents a major milestone that has already had a profound impact on global HIV-related deaths [55]. This milestone still falls well short of the 90% ART coverage estimated to be needed to eliminate population transmissions as part of the 90-90-90 challenge of the Stop TB partnership [55]. An important challenge in this regard is the estimated 30-50% of those with HIV infection that, unaware of their status, perpetuate cycles of virus transmission [43]. Increasing diagnostic coverage to identify HIV-infected persons in endemic regions is thus a critical component of public health efforts to reduce TB.

Clinical Challenges to Treating Co-Infection

Diagnostics

Diagnosing TB in individuals living with HIV is more challenging despite the increased risk of dual disease. Commonly used TB diagnostic depend on the activation of $CD4^{+}$T cells in order to generate the positive readout diagnostic of TB exposure. Loss and dysfunction of $CD4^{+}$T cell due to HIV compromises the delayed-type hypersensitivity reaction generated by the tuberculin skin test (TST) and the IFN-γ release assays (IGRA) used to detect exposure and exclude vaccine reactivity, respectively [56–58]. Sputum of HIV+ individuals with TB frequently contains fewer bacilli, and can lead to higher rates of false negatives [59]. Overall, this means that those who are at elevated risk for acquiring TB include the population in which TB is most challenging to diagnose.

Current efforts that demonstrate promise to overcome TB diagnostic challenges include implementation of molecular approaches with increased sensitivity to detect drug susceptible and resistant TB (e.g. GeneXPERT MTB-RIF) and identification of bacterial products (e.g. lipoarabinomannan) in blood, urine, or other samples that can serve as protein or lipid-based biomarkers [60–62]. These newer diagnostics have been frequently shown to increase case detection in those with immune compromise due to HIV, though conflicting results of sensitivity suggests subject population or other factors may reduce clinical value in some settings [63, 64]. The most important diagnostic challenges, however, are those of access and application. The estimates for TB and HIV mono-infections that remain undiagnosed due to lack of testing are estimated at 37% and 40% for TB and HIV, respectively [43, 65]. Importantly, the HIV status of an estimated 45% of TB patients is unknown due to lack of testing [66]. Increasing diagnostic coverage of populations in high burden HIV and TB regions is an important component of the WHO END TB Strategy for the year 2035 [65].

IRIS

The development of Immune Reconstitution Inflammatory Syndrome (IRIS) is another important challenge for treating co-infected subjects [67]. IRIS most often develops in HIV+ subjects with an underlying OI, following initiation of ART [67–69]. *Mtb* infection is an important OI associated with IRIS; paradoxically

Mtb-specific $CD4^+T$ cells restored by ART can drive life-threatening inflammation and neurological complications [70–73]. Treatment alternatives to broadly active corticosteroids are limited and the benefits of ART cessation to reduce inflammation do not outweigh the consequences of $CD4^+T$ cell loss and viremia [74, 75]. Despite available treatments for IRIS and positive outcomes of ART for TB disease, fear of IRIS among other reasons is a factor for HIV+ subjects to delay ART treatment [69]. Strategies to limit development of IRIS by optimizing corticosteroid implementation or testing of new interventions (e.g. COX-2 inhibitors) are currently being explored through clinical trials and may lessen the ART-related occurrence or severity of IRIS for those with TB (clinicaltrials.gov, NCT01924286 and NCT02060006).

Drug Resistance

An alarming rate of development of TB drug resistance is occurring in areas endemic for HIV [29]. The rising incidence of TB drug resistance is multifactorial, but is primarily due to clinical case management and treatment adherence issues. HIV infection does play an important indirect role, however, as a strong risk factor that increases rates of new and reactivated latent TB infections [76]. The poorer post-chemotherapy TB outcomes in HIV+ individuals, including greater rates of: treatment failure, TB relapse, and development of drug resistance also suggests a direct role for HIV to contribute to development of TB drug resistance. These poorer clinical outcomes are likely attributable to reduced complementation of the *in vivo* drug response by the host immune system. Epidemiological evidence demonstrates that TB drug resistance and association with HIV differs significantly by region and does not follow a general pattern of dual disease incidence. In several regions, over 40% of the new cases of TB diagnosed annually occur among those with HIV [29] and yet the rates of MDR- or XDR-TB have remained fairly low. In contrast, alarming rates of drug resistance are developing in some regions with low HIV co-infection rates [66]. These outcomes suggest that HIV infection provides opportunities for development of TB drug resistance; however, the occurrence can be greatly reduced with proper case management and patient adherence.

Drug Efficacy

Treatment for both TB and HIV can be complicated. Rifampin, a critical first line drug against TB, and other drugs of its class are strong inducers of cytochrome p450 [77]. This results in reduced efficacy due to p450-mediated metabolism of anti-retrovirals and increased toxicity when using these classes of drugs with some HIV medications [78]. Current clinical guidelines advise against simultaneous initiation of TB and HIV drug therapy [79, 80]. Several studies, however, demonstrate that the benefits of earlier ART outweigh the costs to the patient with regard to TB outcomes [74, 81, 82]. Other trials have demonstrated lack of clinical benefit to earlier initiation of ART in those with CD4 counts greater than 50 [83], while an increased incidence of IRIS in someone with active TB is a known risk [84]. Alternatives to rifampin have been used to further reduce the toxicity and decreased efficacy associated with simultaneous treatment [78, 85]. In patients who have previously been diagnosed with HIV and are currently tolerating ART, continuation of their therapy while initiating TB treatment is recommended [80]. Some ART can be used with rifampin, for example, patients already tolerating the combinatorial drug efavirenz. Other ART can be combined with rifabutin while drug concentrations may require alteration to ensure efficacy [80].

With the growing prevalence of dual disease, assessments of clinical interventions are increasingly designed to include, or specifically target, co-infected populations. The impact of TB drugs on bioavailability of alternative ART are also more frequently included in anti-viral assessments. As an example, the use of Efavirenz (EFV) or Lopinarvir/Ritonavir (LPV/r) with the new TB drug PA-824 was shown to support combined use of LPV/r with PA-824, but demonstrated that EFV as well as rifampicin could reduce availability of PA-824 [86]. Host directed therapies that complement TB drug activity are currently an area of intensified research including efforts to modulate innate immunity (see reviews [87, 88]) or target anti-oxidant pathways (clinicaltrials.gov, NCT03281226). These new approaches may be particularly important for use in patients with HIV where immune defects that persist even after ART can extend the treatment period, increase the rates of TB relapse, and promote development of drug resistance when *Mtb* infection fails to clear [89, 90].

Integrated TB/HIV Services

Traditionally, clinical services for TB and HIV were most often independent; occurring at distinct clinical sites, funded through separate donor or government programs, and carried out by independent health care services. The recognition of TB/HIV as linked diseases requiring coordinated health care approaches has led the WHO and many other global health organizations to strongly advocate for integration of clinical services [65, 91]. The logistical advantages include ease of tracking and communication for follow up treatment, as well as greatly increased linkage of care services. The integrated approach for this high risk population is expected to increase the overall diagnosis of dual infections and as a result, support timely implementation of ART along with TB preventive or prophylactic chemotherapy, and facilitate earlier detection of drug resistance development [29]. These efforts may further alleviate the dual stigma of HIV and TB and make access to care easier and more efficient as a "one stop shop" experience that increase the likelihood for subjects to seek care and adhere to treatment regimes. To date, implementation of integrated services has been slow though early reports advocate for this approach and demonstrate better patient outcomes without significantly increased costs [90, 92, 93].

Co-Infection Pathobiology

As discussed above, several non-biological factors have converged to promote dual disease with *Mtb* and HIV. A complementary, and sometimes synergistic pathophysiology also occurs, despite the very different routes of infection, transmission, and mechanisms of pathogenesis. Co-infection scenarios are numerous and occur in different orders or stages of infection as well as different phases of treatment or recovery. These scenarios include: new *Mtb* infection or reactivated TB in those living with HIV and/or AIDS, new HIV infection in someone with active or latent TB, and unmasked TB in HIV+ persons beginning ART, among others. Clinical presentation of TB differs in HIV+ subjects with low CD4$^+$T cell counts (≤100 cells/mm^3) with extra-pulmonary disease such as lymphadenitis, pleural effusions, and meningitis commonly observed [94]. The basis for the strong association between TB and HIV are the multi-faceted mechanisms of pathogenesis used to exploit and disrupt the immune response in a manner that is mutually beneficial to the pathogens and devastating to the human host.

Mtb: Host Response and Pathogenesis

Mtb is an intracellular, facultative, bacterial pathogen that primarily infects professional antigen-presenting cells, especially macrophages (Mϕ), of the immune system. The lung is the primary route of entry that results from *Mtb* successfully circumventing the multiple protective barriers of the respiratory tract, as recently reviewed [95]. Transmission occurs through inhalation of aerosols generated by the productive cough of someone suffering from TB disease. The majority of exposed persons (~90%) develop latent TB; a state of containment that is associated with development of a strong cell-mediated immune (CMI) response [96]. Approximately 5–10% of those exposed to *Mtb* develop an active infection that is fatal in the absence of treatment [96]. Some individuals clear infection through what increasingly appears to occur through strong innate immune responses [96].

Innate Immunity to Mtb

Alveolar Mϕ are considered the primary port of entry for *Mtb* in the lung. Mycobacteria exploit the function of cellular receptors of the immune complement and pathogen pattern recognition systems (e.g. CR3) to bind bacterial ligands as a means to gain access to the intracellular Mϕ compartment, see reviews [96–98]. Following entry, infected Mϕ use a wide repertoire of innate mechanisms intended to degrade or damage the bacterium including: phagolysosome fusion-dependent digestion, oxidative and nitrositive stress due to reactive oxygen species (ROS) and nitric oxide (NO), cell apoptosis or death, and autophagy-driven degradation [96, 97]. In addition to direct antibacterial activity via *Mtb* degradation, autophagy further directs host immune responses via delivery of antigen into antigen presentation pathways and regulation of inflammatory responses [99, 100]. To evade these protective host Mϕ responses, *Mtb* employs an array of bacterial effector molecules or stress response programs in order to proliferate, or persist in a dormant state, despite immune pressure [101, 102].

The innate immune response dominates during the first two weeks following pulmonary *Mtb* infection, due to slow activation kinetics of the acquired immune system [103]. The strong inflammatory responses to mycobacterial products can contribute to pathogenesis, through recruitment of myeloid cells that serve as new hosts for infection [104]. Inflammation networks regulated by the arachidonic acid pathway metabolites are determinants of protective or pathogenic TB outcomes. Increased LTA4H levels correlate with inflammatory responses that increase mycobacterial proliferation [105] while prostaglandin E2 serves a protective function associated with reduced bacterial burden [106]. The type I IFN pathways that are activated by *Mtb* infection were described as a signature associated with worsened clinical outcomes in human subjects [107], despite previous evidence suggesting that IFNα therapy may be beneficial in some subjects who failed to respond to conventional TB chemotherapy [108]. Investigations of susceptible mouse strains lacking type I IFN receptors demonstrate that type I IFN signaling contributes to *Mtb* virulence [108], a concept further supported by recent findings that mutation of the human IFNAR1 gene is associated with decreased susceptibility to tuberculosis [109].

Despite the varied mechanisms used by *Mtb* to exploit and evade innate immunity, a growing body of evidence suggests that innate mechanisms can provide protection in many individuals [97]. The lack of TST conversion in a subset of individuals with a high risk for repeated exposures, strongly suggests the potential of innate immunity to clear infection prior to onset of the CMI response [110]. In addition to the antibacterial role of Mϕ, other leukocytes such as neutrophils, natural killer (NK) cells, and mucosal associated invariant T-like (MAIT) cells have important roles in the innate immune response to *Mtb*. Neutrophils are recruited to sites of *Mtb* replication and play an active role in bacterial containment through phagocytic uptake, release of granules and oxygen radicals that damage mycobacteria, release of extracellular traps or nets, and production of soluble mediators that contribute to granuloma formation [111, 112]. Despite protective roles during early stages of infection, persistence of neutrophils in the lung is an important mechanism for immune-mediated pathology and pulmonary damage [113, 114]. Similarly, neutrophils contribute to immunopathology in TB of the central nervous system via the action of matrix metalloproteases [115]. Neutrophils are an important source of arachidonic acid pathway metabolites such as LTH4, an excess of which is linked to hyper-inflammatory responses and increased mycobacterial proliferation in TB disease models [105].

Natural killer cells are likely one of the earliest source of IFN-γ and other important cytokines prior to development of CMI responses to intracellular pathogens including *Mtb* [116]. Mϕ infected with *Mtb* are lysed by NK cells through interactions between the NK receptors NKG2D and NKp46 with ligands on the target cell surface [117, 118]. Human NK cells are also important sources of granulysin, a cytotoxic lymphocyte (CTL) granule protein with potent anti-mycobactericidal activity [119–121]. Thus, NK cells can mediate both the death of the infected host cell and the mycobacterial cargo. Despite the important effector function of NK, the low prevalence in the lung prior to infection suggest a requirement for recruitment from the blood where NK cells are more prevalent. In contrast, the natural killer T (NKT) cells and MAIT cells are ubiquitous in tissues and could potentially respond more rapidly to localized threats [122]. NKT cells expand after recognition of mycobacterial lipid molecules presented by CD1d while MAIT cells recognize riboflavin precursor metabolites presented by MR1 molecules [122].

Both NKT and MAIT cells mount cytolytic and cytokine helper responses similar to NK cells. NKT cells play an important role to restrict *Mtb* proliferation as part of the early granulomatous response to infection [123]. Reduced numbers of NKT are seen in human subjects with progressive disease while cellular anergy of NKT is associated with lack of *Mtb* growth restriction in mouse models [123]. The protective function of MAIT cells in immunity to *Mtb* is not yet established, though reduced activation of effector molecules (e.g. IFN-γ and granulysin) is observed in MAIT cells of those with active as compared to latent TB [124]. Poor TB outcomes are further correlated with reduced numbers of MAIT cells and expression of the exhaustion marker PD-1 [125].

Cellular Immunity to Mtb

The important role of $CD4^{+}T$ cells in the protective host response to *Mtb* is well established, in no small part due to the increased susceptibility and accelerated disease outcomes observed in those with HIV/AIDS. Development of a CMI response, including both $CD4^{+}$ and $CD8^{+}T$ cells, is associated with protective immunity and establishment of the latent TB state in approximately 90% of exposed individuals (see reviews [103, 126]). A strong Th1 response by $CD4^{+}T$ cells activates Mϕ antibacterial activity against *Mtb* via IFN-γ-dependent and independent mechanisms. In murine models, activation of Mϕ by IFN-γ promotes phagosome maturation and activates NO, resulting in the killing of *Mtb* [127, 128]. The increased risk of TB in people with heritable defects in IFN-γ activation pathways (e.g. IL-12 and STAT1), and the aggressive TB observed in mice deficient for IFN-γ, further support the central role of IFN-γ [129, 130]. TB outcomes in people living with HIV, however, correlate less strictly with $CD4^{+}T$ cell count than for other OIs [131, 132]. The role of IFN-γ, and especially of NO activation by IFN-γ, as the primary mechanism whereby $CD4^{+}T$ cells restrain *Mtb* in human Mϕ is controversial, and arguably less dominant than in mouse models. A memory Th17 cell response also develops following *Mtb* exposure and is associated with both protective and pathogenic responses through production of different cytokines such as IL-17 and IL-22 and regulation of neutrophil influx [133].

The role of $CD8^{+}T$ cells in host defense to TB is complementary to that of $CD4^{+}T$ cells. In animal models, $CD8^{+}T$ cell depletion or MHC class I pathway deficiency is associated with greater mycobacterial proliferation and pulmonary necrosis [134–136]. The $CD8^{+}T$ cell subset has been shown to mediate cytolytic, anti-bacterial, and cytokine effector function as part of the CMI response to *Mtb*. Similar to CD4$^+$T cells, *Mtb*-specific CD8$^+$T cells produce IFN-γ upon antigenic stimuli and activate downstream IFN-γ-dependent immune networks [137]. Cytolytic activity against *Mtb*-infected cells is an important function of CD8$^+$T cells that are carried out through perforin and granzyme-dependent mechanisms [138]. Direct antibacterial activity against intracellular mycobacteria is also an important function carried out by CD8$^+$T cells. In contrast to cellular cytotoxicity, the direct mycobactericidal activity of CD8$^+$T cells from mouse and human has been shown to be independent of perforin and granzyme B [139, 140]. In humans, and non-rodent TB models, the granulysin molecule stored in the cytotoxic granules of CTLs is known to mediate direct killing of mycobacteria following perforin-mediated entry into the intracellular compartment [121, 141]. Granulysin can also be produced by antigen-specific CD4$^+$ CTLs that mediate similar antibacterial activity against Mϕ infected with mycobacteria [142]. In rodent models, the granule-dependent mechanism for direct microbidical activity by CD8$^+$T cells has not yet been defined.

A role for humoral immunity against *Mtb* is controversial due to differences between human and animal model immune responses. In contrast to CMI-related defects, subjects with immunoglobulin-related deficiencies do not have higher TB risk [143]. Mice deficient for humoral immune function, and B cell depleted NHP, however, are more susceptible to *Mtb* [144–146]. TB granulomas contain frequent B cells, and development of bronchus associated lymphoid tissue (BALT) aggregates of B cells have been associated with protective responses and vaccine efficacy in an NHP model [146–148]. Human antibodies specific to *Mtb* develop following exposure and display distinct glycosylation patterns that are associated with protective interactions with innate immune cells [149]. Recently, the antibody profile was found to be strongly correlated with protective immunity in healthcare workers at high risk for TB exposure [150]. The role of B cells and immunoglobulin in TB immunity is currently an intense area of research given the implications for vaccine and diagnostic advances.

The combined effects of innate and CMI immunity successfully restrain active TB in an estimated 90% of those that are exposed. As a result, approximately one-third of the world's population, or 2.5 billion people, are estimated to harbor latent TB [65]. Skin testing results in diagnostic settings support this estimate, based on rates of detection of immune memory responses in the absence of clinical disease [66]. The risk of reactivation is low in most individuals and is estimated to be between 5 and 10% during the person's lifetime. Several risk factors are known to increase the chances of reactivation including smoking, metabolic disorders, alcohol use, immune-suppressive therapy, and especially, co-infection with HIV [151].

HIV/AIDS: Host Response and Pathogenesis

HIV is a retrovirus that primarily infects CD4$^+$T cells or monocyte/Mϕ cell populations of the human immune system [34]. Infection begins following attachment of HIV to the CD4 molecule as the primary receptor and gains entry by further binding to co-receptors such as CXCR4 and CCR5 [34]. Attachment allows fusion of the virus with the host cell membrane followed by entry and uncoating in the host cell cytoplasm. Reverse transcription to DNA in the cytosol is followed by integration into the host cell genome. The viral DNA is subsequently transcribed and translated via host enzyme-mediated events to continue the full viral life cycle. The virus is spread from person to person through biological fluids including blood, semen, vaginal fluid, and breast milk [152]. In contrast to TB, most individuals exposed to an infectious dose of HIV will fail to clear or contain infection long term. The virus initially replicates in mucosal tissues and then rapidly infects organs of the lymph system during the acute stage of disease in the weeks following infection [34, 49, 153]. A stage of clinical latency subsequently develops for several years as the host immune response restrains viral replication. Over time, a progressive depletion and dysfunction of immune cells, especially of $CD4^{+}T$ cells, leads to the severe immune compromise that is characteristic of AIDS [154, 155]. Mϕ also serve as a site of replication and are an important reservoir for latent virus that persists despite ART [156].

Innate Immunity to HIV

Several innate mechanisms slow viral replication and dissemination early in the disease process, as recently reviewed [157]. The type I IFN system plays an important role in acute HIV infection by activating host restriction factors such as SAMHD1 and APOBEC3G that mutate viral genomes and limit the nucleoside triphosphate pool needed for replication [158]. Long term, however, the type I IFN response that activates these and other host restriction factors, is suboptimal for viral clearance while viral proteins such as vpx and vpr further inhibit the anti-viral activity of host restriction factors [159]. A close association of the viral genome with the pre-integration complex limits recognition through various cytosolic pathogen pattern sensors (e.g. TLRs) and as a result, reduces the innate anti-viral response including through the type I IFN and other pathogen recognition pathways [160]. The host tetherin molecule further functions to limit viral budding at the cell surface, an important innate function that is impaired by interference from the HIV vpu protein [161].

Similar to the type I IFN pathways, autophagy drives both pro- and anti-viral innate immune responses following HIV infection. Activation of autophagy can promote apoptosis of HIV-infected cells, or restrict HIV replication via degradation of the viral transactivator tat and disruption of the HIV capsid protein via interactions with TRIM5α [162–164]. During initiation of the autophagic process, however, autophagosomes support both viral particle production and viral protein processing [165]. Viral proteins (e.g. nef) can further limit the anti-viral role of autophagy by blocking degradation of accumulated autophagosomes through interactions with autophagy pathway intermediates such as Beclin 1 [165].

Despite the multitude of innate immune evasion mechanisms employed by HIV, a lack of detectable immune memory in apparently non-infected persons at high risk for exposures (e.g. sex workers) indicate that innate immunity may be sufficient for viral clearance in a small percent of populations [166]. NK cells are able to lyse HIV-infected host cells through an NKG2D-dependent mechanism and are likely to play an important cytotoxic role that complements that of the acquired immune response [167, 168]. Recent studies suggest that NK cell-mediated antibody-dependent cellular cytotoxicity (ADCC) may be an important outcome associated with protection [167, 168]. As chronic HIV develops, NK cells are found to become increasingly dysfunctional, potentially due to reduced production of cytokines that regulated homeostasis and effector function [169]. Release of soluble NKG2D by HIV-infected $CD4^{+}T$ cells has also been described as potential immune escape mechanism [170].

MAIT cells play an important role in protection of mucosal tissues, though a specific role in innate immunity to HIV has not been characterized [171]. The progressive loss of MAIT cells that occurs in those with HIV infection, and is not recovered following ART [172], is currently postulated to contribute to susceptibility to opportunistic infections [171]. Neutrophil influx to tissues is also a common finding in HIV+ subjects that is associated with immune activation [173, 174], though a definitive anti-viral role for neutrophils specific to HIV is not well established. Neutrophils may be a factor contributing to T cell exhaustion through high expression of PD-L1, the ligand for the PD-1 marker expressed on exhausted T cells [175].

Adaptive Immunity to HIV

Adaptive immunity develops in the first few weeks following infection and determines the viral set point at the onset of the chronic stage of disease, as reviewed [34]. The HIV-specific antibodies that are generated form the basis for accurate diagnostics including point of care tests employed in resource limited settings. Humoral immunity fails to provide long term protection, however, due to the rapid development of viral escape mutants [176]. The B cells that produce antibody are found to be increasingly dysfunctional over time in people living with HIV, due to exhaustion from chronic activation and loss of Th1-derived cytokines and co-stimulatory signals [177]. Depletion of $CD4^{+}T$ cells is a hallmark feature of HIV, that along with increasing viral load, signals development of AIDS. The Th17 population of $CD4^{+}T$ cells are also highly susceptible to HIV infection and become significantly depleted in PLWH [178–180]. The role of Th17 in immunity to HIV is not well described to date, though regulation of gut mucosa barrier recovery and suppression of microbial translocation are suggested functions [181].

$CD8^{+}T$ cells play an important antiviral role in HIV infection, primarily through CTL activity against infected cells [182]. This antiviral CTL response is the key mechanism that restrains viral replication during the lengthy chronic stage that can last for many years. HIV-specific $CD8^{+}T$ cells control the viral set point and delay disease progression in animal models. The effect of $CD4^{+}T$ cell depletion on viremia is in part attributed to the loss of Th1 help needed to maintain antiviral CTL activity of the memory $CD8^{+}T$ cell pool [182]. Over time, chronic inflammation, progressive depletion of CD4⁺T cells that provide helper function to CTLs, and development of CTL escape mutants facilitates progression to the AIDS stage. In general, the protective function of antibody and T cells only slows the viral replication and delays progression to the severe immune suppression stage. The exception is a rare population (<1%) of infected persons described as elite controllers with unique HLA alleles (e.g. HLA-B∗5701) that have undetectable viral loads despite known exposure and seroconversion [183, 184].

Co-Infection Pathogenesis: Immune Disturbances that Promote Microbial Synergy and Aggressive Disease

A positive HIV status significantly shifts the paradigm for clinical TB outcomes through effects on both the innate and CMI responses. Those with HIV are more likely to develop active infection upon new *Mtb* exposure and less likely to develop latent TB or clear *Mtb* infection through innate immune mechanisms [89, 151]. The risk of re-activation of latent infection in someone who becomes HIV+ increases substantially [151]. The clinical course of TB in PLWH is also accelerated and more severe compared to HIV- individuals [45, 76, 185]. Similarly, pulmonary HIV replication is increased in those with TB and an accelerated course of HIV has been described in co-infected persons [186, 187]. At different stages of each disease, defects and dysregulations of innate and acquired immune defenses contribute to complementary and/or synergistic mechanisms that promote HIV and *Mtb* proliferation and exacerbate disease.

Innate Immune Disturbances Provide Unique Opportunities for Growth

Due to the role of the innate immune system in the first 2 weeks of a new *Mtb* infection, defects in innate immunity of those living with HIV infection are presumably an important factor for increased susceptibility to *Mtb*. Infection of lung resident CD4⁺T cells and alveolar Mϕ occurs in the acute stage of HIV infection, an association that was determined early in the HIV/AIDS epidemic as a factor likely to increase susceptibility to opportunistic pulmonary infections including *Mtb* [188]. HIV has well-described effects on pulmonary epithelial barrier integrity and endothelium function that are likely to disrupt innate immunity to *Mtb* [189], though experimental evidence in co-infected animals is limited to date. Phagocytes, including neutrophils, monocytes, and Mϕ from the blood and alveolar lavage of those with HIV have reduced phagocytic activity compared to healthy controls [173].

Several anti-microbial functions of phagocytic cells are also perturbed due to HIV infection, including reduced microbicidal activity, disturbances in cell death and autophagy pathways, and decreased production of cytokine mediators [131, 190]. The effects of co-infection on autophagy are increasingly understood to play an important role in microbial synergy due to the additive effects observed in Mϕ [190]. As a result of these various mechanisms whereby HIV infection compromises Mϕ function, *Mtb* is presumed to be able to more easily resist damage from microbicidal molecules, evade degradation in endosomal or autophagic vesicles, and complete more cycles of replication in the host cell. Host directed therapies such as Vitamin D that promote autophagy hold potential for boosting immunity [191], though activation of authophagy via mTOR inhibition suggest a paradoxical and detrimental outcome in co-infected Mϕ [192].

The pro-inflammatory anti-viral responses that are observed in many stages of HIV disease, and can persist after ART [193–195], are also a factor for co-infection. Pro-inflammatory responses that augment microbicidal and antigen-presenting function of APC are protective against *Mtb* [196–198], while other inflammatory processes driven by HIV (e.g. type I IFN) may actually promote *Mtb* proliferation [106, 107]. The type I IFN pathways activated by HIV infection are generally not protective in chronic stages of HIV/AIDS, and in the setting of co-infection could further exacerbate type I IFN driven responses linked to worsened TB outcomes [108]. The strong innate immune response to *Mtb* products that agonize pathogen pattern recognition systems such as Toll like receptors can also promote HIV replication. Mϕ infection with *Mtb* activates a strong chemokine transcriptional response, including upregulation of the CXCR4 and CCR5 chemokine receptors [199, 200] that function as important co-receptors for HIV viral entry. The innate cytokines IL-1β, IL-6, TNF-α, and GM-CSF are activated early in the immune response to *Mtb* and have been shown in animal models to be essential TB protective mechanisms. These same cytokines, however, activate HIV transcription through direct effects on the viral LTR and indirect mechanisms [201, 202]. Inflammatory responses can also drive recruitment and activate receptor and co-receptor expression by potential new hosts for both pathogens. HIV infection additionally impacts cellular trafficking through changes in surface receptors such as CD62L [174] that regulate tissue recruitment and entry.

Increased NK cells are found in lavage of those with HIV or TB, while co-infection does not significantly shift this pulmonary influx [173]. Increasing dysfunction of NK cells is observed in those with HIV, however, including reduced proliferative responses, cytokine production, and cytotoxic functions. Impairments in STAT5 signaling due to HIV infection have been described as a basis for reduced NK cell activation in response to survival and activation signals through IL-7 and IL-15 receptors [203, 204]. In vitro studies further suggest that the glutathione-dependent activation of Mϕ bactericidal activity by NK cells is also disrupted by HIV infection [205] while defects in NK cell expression of granulysin due to HIV may limit direct microbicidal activity of NK cells [203]. In contrast to NK cells, MAIT cells are found to be depleted in those with HIV or HIV/TB co-infection [172, 206]. Importantly, these mucosal resident cells do not appear to fully recover following initiation of ART [172] and could reflect a residual defect in pulmonary surveillance needed to protect against *Mtb*. HIV infection has also been described to increase expression of the PD-1 marker on MAIT cells [206], suggesting functional exhaustion of this cell type.

The inflammatory processes that converge in TB/HIV co-infection promote increased neutrophil influx and are associated with exacerbated lung damage.

Neutrophil influx has an established protective role in early stages of pulmonary TB [207], while persistent neutrophilia at later stages of infection appear to mediate lung tissue pathology [208]. In those with HIV, blood neutrophil counts have been found to be predictive of increased sputum *Mtb* load [209]. Co-infected human subjects [210–212] as well as humanized mice experimentally challenged with *Mtb* and HIV [213] display a marked increase in lung neutrophils and exacerbated pulmonary pathology. Investigations of lung lavage and tissue supernatants suggest that HIV modulates the *Mtb*-infected lung microenvironment to increase chemokines such as IL-8 and MCP-1 with roles in neutrophil and inflammatory monocyte/Mϕ recruitment [213, 214]. The increased expression of PD-L1 by neutrophils in those with HIV [175] could also function to subdue activation of *Mtb*-specific T cells that are recruited to sites of co-infection in the lung (Table 1).

Acquired Immune System Activation and Dysfunction Further Facilitate Microbial Synergy

The predilection of HIV for activated immune cells, especially CD4⁺T cells, provides continual opportunities for infection and viral replication in the lymphoid cells and system of the *Mtb*-infected host. The strongly activated memory CD4⁺T cells and Th17 T cells that are important for host immunity to TB are especially susceptible to HIV infection [178, 215]. Due to the increased susceptibility of activated and memory T cells to HIV infection, *Mtb*-specific T cell populations are disproportionally disrupted and depleted in those with HIV [216]. These losses due to HIV result in reduced production of IFN-γ and other important cytokines and chemokines that function to activate bactericidal activity of infected Mϕ, orchestrate protective functions of multiple immune cells, and maintain the organization of TB granulomas. The antibacterial activity of CD4⁺T cells mediated via granule proteins may also be impaired following HIV infection [217].

CD8⁺T cells play an important cytotoxic and antibacterial role in the immune response to both HIV and *Mtb*, and further provide redundant helper function through production of IFN-γ and other cytokines. In contrast to CD4⁺T cells, the CD8⁺T cell populations are not directly infected or depleted as a result of HIV infection. These attributes make CD8⁺T cells an attractive target for TB vaccine development and host directed therapies for those at risk for HIV [218]. Similar to innate lymphocytes such as NK and MAIT cells, however, the function of CD8⁺T cells is also impaired in those with HIV. Activation of *Mtb*-specific CD8⁺T cell polyfunctional cytokine and cytotoxic/anti-bacterial function is suppressed due to HIV across the spectrum of TB disease stages [219, 220].

An important defect of lymphocytes in PLWH that could suppress the function of multiple T cell subsets, and innate lymphocytes such as NK cells, is reduced signaling through the common γ chain (γ_c) cytokine networks. The γ_c cytokines include IL-2, IL-4, IL-7, IL-9, IL-15, and IL-21 and regulate survival, proliferation, and activation of effector function by lymphocytes [221]. Suppression of γ_c networks likely serves an important anti-viral role, by limiting activation events that

Table 1 Roles and dysfunction of important immune cell populations in TB/HIV co-infection

		Mycobacterium tuberculosis (Mtb)	Human immunodeficiency virus (HIV)	Co-infection pathogenesis
Macrophages	Infectability	*Yes* • Exploits pathogen recognition systems to gain entry, reside, and replicate in AMϕ [97, 98, 101] • Evades degradation in vacuoles by inhibiting phagosome/lysosome fusion [97, 98, 227]	*Yes* • CD4 receptor and CCR5 co-receptor mediate Mϕ entry [34, 228] • Small AMϕ preferentially infected [229] • Mϕ are infected early and are viral reservoir [156]	• *Mtb* increases expression of HIV co-receptors CCR5 and CXCR4 [230, 231] • Increased HIV replication and *Mtb* proliferation in co-infected Mϕ [232–234]
	Immune role	• Produce cytokines/chemokines that orchestrate inflammation, activate microbicidal activity, and direct acquired immunity [104, 235] • Bactericidal activity via phagocytosis, proteases, ROS, NO, autophagy, and apoptosis [100, 236]	• Express host restriction factors (e.g. SamHD1), that limit viral replication [158] • Produce cytokines/chemokines that direct inflammation and antiviral programs [237]	• Activation of SOCS1 by *Mtb* and HIV supports viral replication and suppresses bactericidal activity in Mϕ [238, 239] • Increased pro-inflammatory cytokines recruit new hosts and promote pathogen proliferation [132]
Neutrophils	Infectability	*Not definitive*: contribute to dissemination? [240]	*No* [241]	–
	Immune role	• *Early*: phagocytic and bactericidal activity via granules, O_2 radicals, and traps/nets [112, 242] • *Early*: produce cytokines/chemokines that drive Mϕ and DC differentiation, and granuloma formation [112] • *Late*: excessive influx causes lung pathology and promotes *Mtb* proliferation [240, 243]	• Anti-viral role via ROS, MPO, α-defensins and traps/NETs [241] • Production of cytokines/chemokines (e.g. IL-8, TNF-α) that promote inflammation [241] • Expression of PD-L1 may promote T cell exhaustion [175]	• HIV infection reduces phagocytosis, respiratory burst, and NET activity relevant to *Mtb* control [241] • Excessive neutrophils associated with pulmonary damage in co-infected lung [211, 213] • Blood neutrophil counts predict sputum *Mtb* load in HIV+ subjects [209]

(continued)

Table 1 (continued)

		Mycobacterium tuberculosis (Mtb)	Human immunodeficiency virus (HIV)	Co-infection pathogenesis
Natural killer (NK) cells	Infectability	*No*	*No*	–
	Immune role	• Cytotoxic role via CTL granules and NK receptor (NKG2D, NKp46)-mediated lysis [116–118] • *Mtb* growth inhibition via Glutathione (GSH) and granulysin [205, 244, 245] • Produce cytokines/chemokines (e.g. IFN-γ, TNF-α, IL-22) [246]	• Cytolysis of infected cells via NKG2D [167, 168] • Production of cytokines/chemokines (MIP1β, IFN-γ) to activate antiviral response [247]	• Reduced production of granulysin and GSH [203, 205] • Decreased cytokines (e.g. IFN-γ) [248] • Reduced NK cell numbers and cytotoxic function [169, 249]
MAIT cells	Infectability	*No*	*Yes*: infects and depletes MAIT cells [172]	–
	Immune role	• Recognize riboflavin precursors presented via MR1 [122] • Cytotoxic/antimicrobial granule repertoire differs between latent and active TB [124] • Produce helper cytokines: IFN-γ, TNF-α, and IL-17 [250, 251] • Exhaustion correlates with severe TB [125]	• General role in mucosal immunity known [171], but no HIV-specific role defined yet • Produce cytokines/chemokines: IL-17, IFN-γ, TNF-α [171] • Progressive depletion due to HIV is not restored by ART [172]	• HIV-mediated MAIT exhaustion and depletion in mucosa and periphery is potential mechanism for susceptibility to OIs [171] • MAIT cells from TB/HIV co-infected subjects display exhausted (PD-1) phenotype [206]

CD4+ T cells	Infectability	*No*	*Yes* • Primary host for infection and replication [34] • Memory $CD4^+$ T cells preferentially infected and depleted from gut mucosa and other sites [34] • Th17 cells highly susceptible to infection [178, 180]	• *Mtb* increases HIV co-receptors CCR5 and CXCR4 [200, 231] • Inflammatory cytokines/chemokines recruit new cell hosts and promote HIV replication [132] • Activation by specific antigen promotes infection of *Mtb* and HIV memory T cell pools [131, 132]
	Immune role	• Th1 cells have key immune role and are important component of granulomas [252] • Effector function via production of cytokines/chemokines (e.g. IFN-γ, TNF-α) and CTL activity [142, 252] • Th17 cytokines (e.g. IL-17, IL22) drive both protective and pathogenic inflammation [133]	• Critical T helper role for activation of B cell antibody production and antiviral $CD8^+$T cell activity [34, 182] • Th17 cells may regulate gut mucosa recovery and reduce microbial translocation [181]	• HIV-mediated infection and depletion of memory $CD4^+$T cell pools compromises immunity to both pathogens [131, 132] • Loss of Th1 and Th17 helper cytokines could compromise function of multiple immune cells of the innate and acquired immune system [132, 133, 181]
CD8+ T cells	Infectability	*No*	*No*	–
	Immune role	• Deficiency increases TB susceptibility in animal models [134–136] • Mediate cytolytic and antibacterial activity against infected cells [121, 139] • Important source of cytokines/chemokines: IFN-γ, IL-2, TNF-α [246]	• CTL activity against HIV-infected cells, strongly correlates with elite control [182] • Immune surveillance at HIV infection sites [182] • Important target for vaccine development [218]	• Loss of *Mtb* and HIV antigen-specific $CD8^+$ T cell cytolytic/antibacterial, and polyfunctional cytokine function due to HIV infection [219, 220] • HIV-mediated defects in cytotoxic/antibacterial molecule signaling pathways compromises CTL function against both pathogens [223, 253]

increase cellular susceptibility to HIV infection and reducing signaling intermediates such as STAT5 that bind the viral promoter [222]. An important consequence to the host with regards to TB, however, is reduced production of cytokines and granule proteins such as IFN-γ, perforin, and granulysin, due to HIV-dependent decreases in STAT3 and STAT5 phosphorylation events that regulate gene expression of these effector molecules [223].

The effects of HIV on innate immune function of professional antigen-presenting cells also disrupts activation of *Mtb*-specific T cell populations. Mϕ exposed to HIV have reduced MHC class I and II expression [173], as well as defects in phagosome maturation that initiate degradation of pathogen epitopes for MHC II presentation. The sum of these effects is reduced APC function and as a result, less efficient activation of *Mtb*-specific $CD4^+$ and $CD8^+$T cell populations. High levels of IL-10 are found in serum and BAL of HIV+ subjects, an effect that is exacerbated by *Mtb* co-infection in humans and animal models [213, 214]. Though IL-10 plays an important role in limiting HIV replication, the downstream immune-regulatory activity of IL-10 suppresses the activation of T cells as well innate immune cells such as Mϕ and NK cells [202, 214].

A loss of TB granuloma organization is a consistent feature observed in co-infected human lung and in tissue from animal models of HIV or SIV co-infection with *Mtb* [211, 213, 224]. A multitude of HIV-driven events may prevent protective development, or break down the protective structure, of TB granulomas in the lung, as has been thoroughly reviewed [225]. A recent development is the observation that SIV infection greatly reduces BALT in NHP with latent TB, an effect that was strongly associated with TB reactivation [226]. HIV infection compromises B cell function and has been shown to alter the overall production and glycosylation patterns of immunoglobulins that determine interactions with Fc-bearing phagocytic cells [149, 177]. To date, the effects of HIV to disrupt humoral immunity to *Mtb* are poorly understood with regard to co-infection pathobiology.

Summary

The TB/HIV syndemic arose over the last three decades from multiple factors that converged due to overlapping epidemiology, inadequate availability or access to diagnostics and drugs, unique clinical challenges, and a synergistic pathogenesis. The global response to HIV and continually expanding coverage of ART has contributed to significantly reduced rates of death due to HIV as well as TB. More recent efforts such as: point of care TB diagnostics with increased sensitivity; earlier introduction of ART in those with TB; new drugs that are more effective against drug resistant TB forms; and implementation of integrated clinical services for TB and HIV, are further expected to improve disease outcomes.

The fact that HIV and TB infections and deaths are in decline, however, is overshadowed by the combined annual death of approximately 2.6 million people today. Despite the positive trends for infection and mortality, HIV remains the largest risk factor for TB; likewise, TB is the leading cause of death in people living with HIV. The development of drug resistant forms of TB associated with the HIV pandemic, is a rapidly emerging threat to the world population. Addressing this co-pandemic threat requires a global investment in the development of vaccines, host directed therapies, novel point of care diagnostics, and new drugs. Phase I-III clinical trials are currently underway to test seventeen TB drugs and twelve TB vaccine candidates and include several trials that are aimed at, or include, HIV+ populations [29]. Along with these potential new clinical interventions, new approaches that improve access to care and implementation of best clinical practices are similarly critical to efforts to limit TB, HIV, and especially dual infection. An aggressive pace on these multiple fronts is essential to ending the deadly syndemic of TB and HIV co-infection.

References

1. Paulson T. Epidemiology: a mortal foe. Nature. 2013;502(7470):S2–3.
2. Hershkovitz I, et al. Detection and molecular characterization of 9,000-year-old *Mycobacterium tuberculosis* from a Neolithic settlement in the Eastern Mediterranean. PLoS One. 2008;3(10):e3426.
3. Rom WN, Garay SM, editors. Tuberculosis. 1st ed. Boston: Little, Brown; 1996. xxv, 1002 p.
4. Brothwell DR, Sandison AT. Diseases in antiquity; a survey of the diseases, injuries, and surgery of early populations. Springfield, IL: C. C. Thomas; 1967. xix, 766 p.
5. Donoghue HD. Insights gained from palaeomicrobiology into ancient and modern tuberculosis. Clin Microbiol Infect. 2011;17(6):821–9.
6. Rothschild BM, et al. *Mycobacterium tuberculosis* complex DNA from an extinct bison dated 17,000 years before the present. Clin Infect Dis. 2001;33(3):305–11.
7. Wirth T, et al. Origin, spread and demography of the *Mycobacterium tuberculosis* complex. PLoS Pathog. 2008;4(9):e1000160.
8. Bos KI, et al. Pre-columbian mycobacterial genomes reveal seals as a source of New World human tuberculosis. Nature. 2014;514(7523):494–7.
9. Formicola V, Milanesi Q, Scarsini C. Evidence of spinal tuberculosis at the beginning of the fourth millennium BC from Arene Candide cave (Liguria, Italy). Am J Phys Anthropol. 1987;72(1):1–6.
10. Zink A, et al. Molecular analysis of skeletal tuberculosis in an ancient Egyptian population. J Med Microbiol. 2001;50(4):355–66.
11. Morse D, Brothwell DR, Ucko PJ. Tuberculosis in ancient Egypt. Am Rev Respir Dis. 1964;90:524–41.
12. Faerman M, Jankauskas R. Paleopathological and molecular evidence of human bone tuberculosis in Iron Age Lithuania. Anthropol Anz. 2000;58(1):57–62.
13. Nicholas A, Boire VAAR, Parrish NM, Riedel S. Tuberculosis: from an untreatable disease in antiquity to an untreatable disease in modern times? J Anc Dis Prev Rem. 2013;1(2):1.
14. Verano JW, Ubelaker DH, National Museum of Natural History (U.S.). Disease and demography in the Americas. Washington, DC: Smithsonian Institution Press; 1992.. x, 294 p.
15. Allison MJ, Mendoza D, Pezzia A. Documentation of a case of tuberculosis in Pre-Columbian America. Am Rev Respir Dis. 1973;107(6):985–91.
16. Bloom BR. Tuberculosis: pathogenesis, protection, and control. Washigngton, DC: ASM Press; 1994.
17. Webb GB. Tuberculosis. New York: P. B. Hoeber, Inc; 1936. xv, 205 p.

18. Waksman SA. The conquest of tuberculosis. Berkeley: University of California Press; 1964. xiv, 241 p.
19. Porter JDH, Grange JM. Tuberculosis: an interdisciplinary perspective. London: Imperial College Press; 1999.
20. Dubos RJ, Dubos J. The white plague; tuberculosis, man and society. 1st ed. Boston: Little; 1952. viii, 277 p.
21. Daniel TM. The history of tuberculosis. Respir Med. 2006;100(11):1862–70.
22. Krause AK. Tuberculosis and public health. Am Rev Tuberc. 1928;28(3):271–322.
23. Fairchild AL, Oppenheimer GM. Public health nihilism vs pragmatism: history, politics, and the control of tuberculosis. Am J Public Health. 1998;88(7):1105–17.
24. Newsholme A. Poverty and Disease, as illustrated by the Course of Typhus Fever and Phthisis in Ireland: (Presidential Address). Proc R Soc Med. 1908;1(Sect Epidemiol State Med):1–44.
25. Wilson LG. The historical decline of tuberculosis in Europe and America: its causes and significance. J Hist Med Allied Sci. 1990;45(3):366–96.
26. Jones DS, Podolsky SH, Greene JA. The burden of disease and the changing task of medicine. N Engl J Med. 2012;366(25):2333–8.
27. Warner DF, Mizrahi V. Complex genetics of drug resistance in *Mycobacterium tuberculosis*. Nat Genet. 2013;45(10):1107–8.
28. World Health Organization. Global tuberculosis programme. Framework for effective tuberculosis control. Geneva, Switzerland. WHO/TB/94.179, 1994.
29. WHO. Global tuberculosis report. Geneva: World Health Organization; 2017.
30. Sharp PM, Hahn BH. Origins of HIV and the AIDS pandemic. Cold Spring Harb Perspect Med. 2011;1(1):a006841.
31. Vidal N, et al. Unprecedented degree of human immunodeficiency virus type 1 (HIV-1) group M genetic diversity in the Democratic Republic of Congo suggests that the HIV-1 pandemic originated in Central Africa. J Virol. 2000;74(22):10498–507.
32. Faria NR, et al. HIV epidemiology. The early spread and epidemic ignition of HIV-1 in human populations. Science. 2014;346(6205):56–61.
33. Gao F, et al. Origin of HIV-1 in the chimpanzee Pan troglodytes troglodytes. Nature. 1999;397(6718):436–41.
34. Deeks SG, et al. HIV infection. Nat Rev Dis Primers. 2015;1:15035.
35. CDC. Pneumocystis pneumonia—Los Angeles. In: MMWR. Morbidity and Mortality Weekly Report. Atlanta, GA: CDC; 1981. p. 1–3.
36. CDC. A cluster of Kaposi's sarcoma and *Pneumocystis carinii* pneumonia among homosexual male residents of Los Angeles and range Counties, California. In: MMWR. Morbidity and Mortality Weekly Report. Atlanta, GA: CDC; 1982. p. 305–7.
37. CDC. Opportunistic infections and Kaposi's sarcoma among Haitians in the United States. In: MMWR. Morbidity and Mortality Weekly Reports. Atlanta, GA: CDC; 1982. p. 353–4.
38. CDC. Epidemiologic notes and reports pneumocystis carinii pneumonia among persons with Hemophilia A. In: MMWR. Morbidity and Mortality Weekly Reports. Altanta, GA: CDC; 1982. p. 365–7.
39. CDC. Current trends update on acquired immune deficiency syndrome (AIDS)—United States. In: MMWR. Morbidity and Mortality Weekly Reports. Atlanta, GA: CDC; 1982. p. 513–4.
40. Popovic M, et al. Detection, isolation, and continuous production of cytopathic retroviruses (HTLV-III) from patients with AIDS and pre-AIDS. Science. 1984;224(4648):497–500.
41. WHO. The world health report 1999. Geneva: World Health Organization; 1999.
42. UNAIDS. Global report: UNAIDS report on the global AIDS epidemic 2013. Geneva: UNAIDS; 2013.
43. UNAIDS. UNAIDS Global AIDS update 2016. Geneva: UNAIDS; 2016.
44. Ai JW, et al. Updates on the risk factors for latent tuberculosis reactivation and their managements. Emerg Microbes Infect. 2016;5:e10.
45. Corbett EL, et al. The growing burden of tuberculosis: global trends and interactions with the HIV epidemic. Arch Intern Med. 2003;163(9):1009–21.

46. Laga M, Piot P. Prevention of sexual transmission of HIV: real results, science progressing, societies remaining behind. AIDS. 2012;26(10):1223–9.
47. Craig GM, et al. Tuberculosis stigma as a social determinant of health: a systematic mapping review of research in low incidence countries. Int J Infect Dis. 2017;56:90–100.
48. Rueda S, et al. Examining the associations between HIV-related stigma and health outcomes in people living with HIV/AIDS: a series of meta-analyses. BMJ Open. 2016;6(7):e011453.
49. Levy JA. HIV pathogenesis: 25 years of progress and persistent challenges. AIDS. 2009;23(2):147–60.
50. World Health Organization. WHO treatment guidelines for drug resistant tuberculosis: World Health Organization; 2016.
51. World Health Organization. Consolidated guidelines on the use of antiretroviral drugs for treating and preventing HIV Infection. Recommendations for a public health approach: World Health Organization; 2016.
52. Gebremariam MK, Bjune GA, Frich JC. Barriers and facilitators of adherence to TB treatment in patients on concomitant TB and HIV treatment: a qualitative study. BMC Public Health. 2010;10:651.
53. Mesfin YM, et al. Association between HIV/AIDS and multi-drug resistance tuberculosis: a systematic review and meta-analysis. PLoS One. 2014;9(1):e82235.
54. Chung-Delgado K, et al. Mortality among MDR-TB cases: comparison with drug-susceptible tuberculosis and associated factors. PLoS One. 2015;10(3):e0119332.
55. (UNAIDS), J.U.N.P.o.H.A. 90-90-90 An ambitious treatment target to help end the AIDS epidemic. 2014.
56. Cattamanchi A, et al. Interferon-gamma release assays for the diagnosis of latent tuberculosis infection in HIV-infected individuals: a systematic review and meta-analysis. J Acquir Immune Defic Syndr. 2011;56(3):230–8.
57. Cheallaigh CN, et al. Interferon gamma release assays for the diagnosis of latent TB infection in HIV-infected individuals in a low TB burden country. PLoS One. 2013;8(1):e53330.
58. Mandalakas AM, et al. High level of discordant IGRA results in HIV-infected adults and children. Int J Tuberc Lung Dis. 2008;12(4):417–23.
59. Montales MT, et al. HIV-associated TB syndemic: a growing clinical challenge worldwide. Front Public Health. 2015;3:281.
60. Kerkhoff AD, et al. Disseminated tuberculosis among hospitalised HIV patients in South Africa: a common condition that can be rapidly diagnosed using urine-based assays. Sci Rep. 2017;7(1):10931.
61. LaCourse SM, et al. Urine TB lipoarabinomannan (LAM) predicts mortality in hospitalized HIV-infected children. Clin Infect Dis. 2018;66:1798.
62. Kaur R, et al. Diagnostic accuracy of xpert test in tuberculosis detection: a systematic review and meta-analysis. J Glob Infect Dis. 2016;8(1):32–40.
63. Thit SS, et al. The clinical utility of the urine-based lateral flow lipoarabinomannan assay in HIV-infected adults in Myanmar: an observational study. BMC Med. 2017;15(1):145.
64. Li S, et al. Diagnostic accuracy of Xpert MTB/RIF for tuberculosis detection in different regions with different endemic burden: a systematic review and meta-analysis. PLoS One. 2017;12(7):e0180725.
65. World Health Organization. The end TB strategy: global strategy and targets for tuberculosis prevention, care and control after 2015: World Health Organization; 2015.
66. WHO. 2015 global tuberculosis report. Geneva: World Health Organization; 2015.
67. Lai RP, Meintjes G, Wilkinson RJ. HIV-1 tuberculosis-associated immune reconstitution inflammatory syndrome. Semin Immunopathol. 2016;38(2):185–98.
68. Manabe YC, et al. Immune reconstitution inflammatory syndrome: risk factors and treatment implications. J Acquir Immune Defic Syndr. 2007;46(4):456–62.
69. Marais S, et al. Management of patients with the immune reconstitution inflammatory syndrome. Curr HIV/AIDS Rep. 2009;6(3):162–71.
70. Bahr N, et al. Central nervous system immune reconstitution inflammatory syndrome. Curr Infect Dis Rep. 2013;15(6):583–93.

71. Johnson T, Nath A. Neurological complications of immune reconstitution in HIV-infected populations. Ann N Y Acad Sci. 2010;1184:106–20.
72. Nath A, Berger JR. Complications of immunosuppressive/immunomodulatory therapy in neurological diseases. Curr Treat Options Neurol. 2012;14(3):241–55.
73. Mahnke YD, et al. Selective expansion of polyfunctional pathogen-specific CD4(+) T cells in HIV-1-infected patients with immune reconstitution inflammatory syndrome. Blood. 2012;119(13):3105–12.
74. Blanc FX, et al. Earlier versus later start of antiretroviral therapy in HIV-infected adults with tuberculosis. N Engl J Med. 2011;365(16):1471–81.
75. Meintjes G, et al. Corticosteroid-modulated immune activation in the tuberculosis immune reconstitution inflammatory syndrome. Am J Respir Crit Care Med. 2012;186(4):369–77.
76. Moreno S, et al. Risk for developing tuberculosis among anergic patients infected with HIV. Ann Intern Med. 1993;119(3):194–8.
77. Zilly W, Breimer DD, Richter E. Pharmacokinetic interactions with rifampicin. Clin Pharmacokinet. 1977;2(1):61–70.
78. Sterling TR. Treatment of pulmonary tuberculosis in HIV-infected adults. In UpToDate. Reyn CFv, Baron EL, editors. 2016.
79. Erratum: New Guidelines for the Treatment of Drug-Susceptible Tuberculosis from the American Thoracic Society, Centers for Disease Control and Prevention, and the Infectious Diseases Society of America: Now Comes the Hard Part. Am J Respir Crit Care Med. 2017;195(11):1540.
80. Nahid P, et al. Official American Thoracic Society/Centers for Disease Control and Prevention/Infectious Diseases Society of America Clinical Practice Guidelines: treatment of Drug-Susceptible Tuberculosis. Clin Infect Dis. 2016;63(7):e147–95.
81. Abdool Karim SS, et al. Timing of initiation of antiretroviral drugs during tuberculosis therapy. N Engl J Med. 2010;362(8):697–706.
82. Velasco M, et al. Effect of simultaneous use of highly active antiretroviral therapy on survival of HIV patients with tuberculosis. J Acquir Immune Defic Syndr. 2009;50(2):148–52.
83. Havlir DV, et al. Timing of antiretroviral therapy for HIV-1 infection and tuberculosis. N Engl J Med. 2011;365(16):1482–91.
84. Naidoo K, et al. The immune reconstitution inflammatory syndrome after antiretroviral therapy initiation in patients with tuberculosis: findings from the SAPiT trial. Ann Intern Med. 2012;157(5):313–24.
85. Bartlett JG, Sax PE. Selecting antiretroviral regimens for the treatment-naïve HIV-infected patient. In UpToDate. Hirsch MS, Mitty J, editors. 2016.
86. Dooley KE, Chaisson RE. Tuberculosis and diabetes mellitus: convergence of two epidemics. Lancet Infect Dis. 2009;9(12):737–46.
87. Kroesen VM, et al. Non-steroidal anti-inflammatory drugs as host-directed therapy for tuberculosis: a systematic review. Front Immunol. 2017;8:772.
88. Zumla A, et al. Towards host-directed therapies for tuberculosis. Nat Rev Drug Discov. 2015;14(8):511–2.
89. Getahun H, et al. HIV infection-associated tuberculosis: the epidemiology and the response. Clin Infect Dis. 2010;50(Suppl 3):S201–7.
90. Mudzengi D, et al. The patient costs of care for those with TB and HIV: a cross-sectional study from South Africa. Health Policy Plan. 2017;32:iv48.
91. World Health Organization. WHO policy on collaborative TB/HIV activities. Guidelines for national programmes and other stakeholders: World Health Organization; 2012.
92. Gilbert JA, et al. Integrating community-based interventions to reverse the convergent TB/HIV epidemics in rural South Africa. PLoS One. 2015;10(5):e0126267.
93. Owiti P, et al. Integrating tuberculosis and HIV services in rural Kenya: uptake and outcomes. Public Health Action. 2015;5(1):36–44.
94. Tornheim JA, Dooley KE. Tuberculosis associated with HIV infection. Microbiol Spectr. 2017;5(1). https://doi.org/10.1128/microbiolspec.TNMI7-0028-2016.

95. Torrelles JB, Schlesinger LS. Integrating lung physiology, immunology, and tuberculosis. Trends Microbiol. 2017;25(8):688–97.
96. Philips JA, Ernst JD. Tuberculosis pathogenesis and immunity. Annu Rev Pathol. 2012;7:353–84.
97. Liu CH, Liu H, Ge B. Innate immunity in tuberculosis: host defense vs pathogen evasion. Cell Mol Immunol. 2017;14:963.
98. Queval CJ, Brosch R, Simeone R. The macrophage: a disputed fortress in the battle against *Mycobacterium tuberculosis*. Front Microbiol. 2017;8:2284.
99. Jagannath C, et al. Autophagy enhances the efficacy of BCG vaccine by increasing peptide presentation in mouse dendritic cells. Nat Med. 2009;15(3):267–76.
100. Castillo EF, et al. Autophagy protects against active tuberculosis by suppressing bacterial burden and inflammation. Proc Natl Acad Sci U S A. 2012;109(46):E3168–76.
101. Awuh JA, Flo TH. Molecular basis of mycobacterial survival in macrophages. Cell Mol Life Sci. 2017;74(9):1625–48.
102. Dutta NK, Karakousis PC. Latent tuberculosis infection: myths, models, and molecular mechanisms. Microbiol Mol Biol Rev. 2014;78(3):343–71.
103. Orme IM, Robinson RT, Cooper AM. The balance between protective and pathogenic immune responses in the TB-infected lung. Nat Immunol. 2015;16(1):57–63.
104. McClean CM, Tobin DM. Macrophage form, function, and phenotype in mycobacterial infection: lessons from tuberculosis and other diseases. Pathog Dis. 2016;74(7):ftw068.
105. Tobin DM, et al. An enzyme that inactivates the inflammatory mediator leukotriene b4 restricts mycobacterial infection. PLoS One. 2013;8(7):e67828.
106. Mayer-Barber KD, et al. Host-directed therapy of tuberculosis based on interleukin-1 and type I interferon crosstalk. Nature. 2014;511(7507):99–103.
107. Berry MP, et al. An interferon-inducible neutrophil-driven blood transcriptional signature in human tuberculosis. Nature. 2010;466(7309):973–7.
108. Donovan ML, et al. Type I interferons in the pathogenesis of tuberculosis: molecular drivers and immunological consequences. Front Immunol. 2017;8:1633.
109. Zhang G, et al. A proline deletion in IFNAR1 impairs IFN-signaling and underlies increased resistance to tuberculosis in humans. Nat Commun. 2018;9(1):85.
110. Hall NB, et al. Polymorphisms in TICAM2 and IL1B are associated with TB. Genes Immun. 2015;16(2):127–33.
111. Sia JK, Georgieva M, Rengarajan J. Innate immune defenses in human tuberculosis: an overview of the interactions between mycobacterium tuberculosis and innate immune cells. J Immunol Res. 2015;2015:747543.
112. Warren E, Teskey G, Venketaraman V. Effector mechanisms of neutrophils within the innate immune system in response to Mycobacterium tuberculosis infection. J Clin Med. 2017;6(2):E15.
113. Mishra BB, et al. Nitric oxide prevents a pathogen-permissive granulocytic inflammation during tuberculosis. Nat Microbiol. 2017;2:17072.
114. Dallenga T, Schaible UE. Neutrophils in tuberculosis—first line of defence or booster of disease and targets for host-directed therapy? Pathog Dis. 2016;74(3):ftw012.
115. Ong CW, et al. Complex regulation of neutrophil-derived MMP-9 secretion in central nervous system tuberculosis. J Neuroinflammation. 2017;14(1):31.
116. Esin S, Batoni G. Natural killer cells: a coherent model for their functional role in *Mycobacterium tuberculosis* infection. J Innate Immun. 2015;7(1):11–24.
117. Vankayalapati R, et al. Role of NK cell-activating receptors and their ligands in the lysis of mononuclear phagocytes infected with an intracellular bacterium. J Immunol. 2005;175(7):4611–7.
118. Vankayalapati R, et al. The NKp46 receptor contributes to NK cell lysis of mononuclear phagocytes infected with an intracellular bacterium. J Immunol. 2002;168(7):3451–7.
119. Hanson DA, et al. Biosynthesis of granulysin, a novel cytolytic molecule. Mol Immunol. 1999;36(7):413–22.

120. Houchins JP, et al. Genomic structure of NKG5, a human NK and T cell-specific activation gene. Immunogenetics. 1993;37(2):102–7.
121. Stenger S, et al. An antimicrobial activity of cytolytic T cells mediated by granulysin. Science. 1998;282(5386):121–5.
122. Chandra S, Kronenberg M. Activation and Function of iNKT and MAIT Cells. Adv Immunol. 2015;127:145–201.
123. Arora P, Foster EL, Porcelli SA. CD1d and natural killer T cells in immunity to Mycobacterium tuberculosis. Adv Exp Med Biol. 2013;783:199–223.
124. Jiang J, et al. Mucosal-associated invariant T cells from patients with tuberculosis exhibit impaired immune response. J Infect. 2016;72(3):338–52.
125. Jiang J, et al. Mucosal-associated invariant T-cell function is modulated by programmed death-1 signaling in patients with active tuberculosis. Am J Respir Crit Care Med. 2014;190(3):329–39.
126. Huang L, Russell DG. Protective immunity against tuberculosis: what does it look like and how do we find it? Curr Opin Immunol. 2017;48:44–50.
127. Schaible UE, et al. Cytokine activation leads to acidification and increases maturation of *Mycobacterium avium*-containing phagosomes in murine macrophages. J Immunol. 1998;160(3):1290–6.
128. Herbst S, Schaible UE, Schneider BE. Interferon gamma activated macrophages kill mycobacteria by nitric oxide induced apoptosis. PLoS One. 2011;6(5):e19105.
129. Bustamante J, et al. Mendelian susceptibility to mycobacterial disease: genetic, immunological, and clinical features of inborn errors of IFN-gamma immunity. Semin Immunol. 2014;26(6):454–70.
130. Cooper AM, et al. Disseminated tuberculosis in interferon gamma gene-disrupted mice. J Exp Med. 1993;178(6):2243–7.
131. Pawlowski A, et al. Tuberculosis and HIV co-infection. PLoS Pathog. 2012;8(2):e1002464.
132. Shankar EM, et al. HIV-Mycobacterium tuberculosis co-infection: a 'danger-couple model' of disease pathogenesis. Pathog Dis. 2014;70(2):110–8.
133. Shen H, Chen ZW. The crucial roles of Th17-related cytokines/signal pathways in *M. tuberculosis* infection. Cell Mol Immunol. 2018;15(3):216–25.
134. Flynn JL, et al. Major histocompatibility complex class I-restricted T cells are required for resistance to Mycobacterium tuberculosis infection. Proc Natl Acad Sci U S A. 1992;89(24):12013–7.
135. Villarreal-Ramos B, et al. Investigation of the role of CD8+ T cells in bovine tuberculosis in vivo. Infect Immun. 2003;71(8):4297–303.
136. Chen CY, et al. A critical role for CD8 T cells in a nonhuman primate model of tuberculosis. PLoS Pathog. 2009;5(4):e1000392.
137. Prezzemolo T, et al. Functional signatures of human CD4 and CD8 T cell responses to *Mycobacterium tuberculosis*. Front Immunol. 2014;5:180.
138. Walch M, et al. Cytotoxic cells kill intracellular bacteria through granulysin-mediated delivery of granzymes. Cell. 2014;157(6):1309–23.
139. Canaday DH, et al. CD4(+) and CD8(+) T cells kill intracellular *Mycobacterium tuberculosis* by a perforin and Fas/Fas ligand-independent mechanism. J Immunol. 2001;167(5):2734–42.
140. Cooper AM, et al. The course of *Mycobacterium tuberculosis* infection in the lungs of mice lacking expression of either perforin- or granzyme-mediated cytolytic mechanisms. Infect Immun. 1997;65(4):1317–20.
141. Endsley JJ, et al. Characterization of bovine homologues of granulysin and NK-lysin. J Immunol. 2004;173(4):2607–14.
142. Endsley JJ, et al. *Mycobacterium bovis* BCG vaccination induces memory CD4+ T cells characterized by effector biomarker expression and anti-mycobacterial activity. Vaccine. 2007;25(50):8384–94.
143. Glatman-Freedman A, Casadevall A. Serum therapy for tuberculosis revisited: reappraisal of the role of antibody-mediated immunity against Mycobacterium tuberculosis. Clin Microbiol Rev. 1998;11(3):514–32.

144. Maglione PJ, Xu J, Chan J. B cells moderate inflammatory progression and enhance bacterial containment upon pulmonary challenge with Mycobacterium tuberculosis. J Immunol. 2007;178(11):7222–34.
145. Vordermeier HM, et al. Increase of tuberculous infection in the organs of B cell-deficient mice. Clin Exp Immunol. 1996;106(2):312–6.
146. Phuah JY, et al. Activated B cells in the granulomas of nonhuman primates infected with Mycobacterium tuberculosis. Am J Pathol. 2012;181(2):508–14.
147. Kaushal D, et al. Mucosal vaccination with attenuated *Mycobacterium tuberculosis* induces strong central memory responses and protects against tuberculosis. Nat Commun. 2015;6:8533.
148. Tsai MC, et al. Characterization of the tuberculous granuloma in murine and human lungs: cellular composition and relative tissue oxygen tension. Cell Microbiol. 2006;8(2):218–32.
149. Lu LL, et al. A functional role for antibodies in tuberculosis. Cell. 2016;167(2):433–43.. e14
150. Li H, et al. Latently and uninfected healthcare workers exposed to TB make protective antibodies against Mycobacterium tuberculosis. Proc Natl Acad Sci U S A. 2017;114(19):5023–8.
151. Narasimhan P, et al. Risk factors for tuberculosis. Pulm Med. 2013;2013:828939.
152. WHO. W.H.O., HIV/AIDS fact sheet: WHO; 2016.
153. Hileman CO, Funderburg NT. Inflammation, immune activation, and antiretroviral therapy in HIV. Curr HIV/AIDS Rep. 2017;14(3):93–100.
154. Sheppard HW, Ascher MS. The natural history and pathogenesis of HIV infection. Annu Rev Microbiol. 1992;46:533–64.
155. Naif HM. Pathogenesis of HIV infection. Infect Dis Rep. 2013;5(Suppl 1):e6.
156. Abbas W, et al. Eradication of HIV-1 from the macrophage reservoir: an uncertain goal? Viruses. 2015;7(4):1578–98.
157. Schott K, Riess M, Konig R. Role of innate genes in HIV replication. Curr Top Microbiol Immunol. 2018;419:69.
158. Bosinger SE, Utay NS. Type I interferon: understanding its role in HIV pathogenesis and therapy. Curr HIV/AIDS Rep. 2015;12(1):41–53.
159. Bosinger SE, et al. Gene expression profiling of host response in models of acute HIV infection. J Immunol. 2004;173(11):6858–63.
160. Sandstrom TS, Ranganath N, Angel JB. Impairment of the type I interferon response by HIV-1: potential targets for HIV eradication. Cytokine Growth Factor Rev. 2017;37:1–16.
161. Neil SJ, Zang T, Bieniasz PD. Tetherin inhibits retrovirus release and is antagonized by HIV-1 Vpu. Nature. 2008;451(7177):425–30.
162. Mandell MA, et al. TRIM proteins regulate autophagy: TRIM5 is a selective autophagy receptor mediating HIV-1 restriction. Autophagy. 2014;10(12):2387–8.
163. Sagnier S, et al. Autophagy restricts HIV-1 infection by selectively degrading Tat in CD4+ T lymphocytes. J Virol. 2015;89(1):615–25.
164. Espert L, et al. Autophagy is involved in T cell death after binding of HIV-1 envelope proteins to CXCR4. J Clin Invest. 2006;116(8):2161–72.
165. Kyei GB, et al. Autophagy pathway intersects with HIV-1 biosynthesis and regulates viral yields in macrophages. J Cell Biol. 2009;186(2):255–68.
166. Kulkarni PS, Butera ST, Duerr AC. Resistance to HIV-1 infection: lessons learned from studies of highly exposed persistently seronegative (HEPS) individuals. AIDS Rev. 2003;5(2):87–103.
167. Alsahafi N, et al. Impaired downregulation of NKG2D ligands by Nef proteins from elite controllers sensitizes HIV-1-infected cells to antibody-dependent cellular cytotoxicity. J Virol. 2017;91(16):e00109.
168. Madhavi V, et al. HIV-1 Env- and Vpu-specific antibody-dependent cellular cytotoxicity responses associated with elite control of HIV. J Virol. 2017;91(18):e00700.
169. Ansari AW, et al. Natural killer cell heterogeneity: cellular dysfunction and significance in HIV-1 immuno-pathogenesis. Cell Mol Life Sci. 2015;72(16):3037–49.
170. Matusali G, et al. Soluble ligands for the NKG2D receptor are released during HIV-1 infection and impair NKG2D expression and cytotoxicity of NK cells. FASEB J. 2013;27(6):2440–50.

171. Saeidi A, et al. Functional role of mucosal-associated invariant T cells in HIV infection. J Leukoc Biol. 2016;100(2):305–14.
172. Cosgrove C, et al. Early and nonreversible decrease of CD161++ /MAIT cells in HIV infection. Blood. 2013;121(6):951–61.
173. Bonecini-Almeida Mda G, et al. Functional activity of alveolar and peripheral cells in patients with human acquired immunodeficiency syndrome and pulmonary tuberculosis. Cell Immunol. 1998;190(2):112–20.
174. Hayes PJ, et al. Alterations in blood leucocyte adhesion molecule profiles in HIV-1 infection. Clin Exp Immunol. 1999;117(2):331–4.
175. Bowers NL, et al. Immune suppression by neutrophils in HIV-1 infection: role of PD-L1/PD-1 pathway. PLoS Pathog. 2014;10(3):e1003993.
176. Bonsignori M, et al. Antibody-virus co-evolution in HIV infection: paths for HIV vaccine development. Immunol Rev. 2017;275(1):145–60.
177. Ruffin N, Hani L, Seddiki N. From dendritic cells to B cells dysfunctions during HIV-1 infection: T follicular helper cells at the crossroads. Immunology. 2017;151(2):137–45.
178. Christensen-Quick A, et al. Human Th17 cells lack HIV-inhibitory RNases and are highly permissive to productive HIV infection. J Virol. 2016;90(17):7833–47.
179. Prendergast A, et al. HIV-1 infection is characterized by profound depletion of CD161+ Th17 cells and gradual decline in regulatory T cells. AIDS. 2010;24(4):491–502.
180. El Hed A, et al. Susceptibility of human Th17 cells to human immunodeficiency virus and their perturbation during infection. J Infect Dis. 2010;201(6):843–54.
181. Valverde-Villegas JM, et al. New insights about Treg and Th17 cells in HIV infection and disease progression. J Immunol Res. 2015;2015:647916.
182. Munier CM, et al. The role of T cell immunity in HIV-1 infection. Curr Opin Virol. 2013;3(4):438–46.
183. Fellay J, et al. A whole-genome association study of major determinants for host control of HIV-1. Science. 2007;317(5840):944–7.
184. International, H.I.V.C.S, et al. The major genetic determinants of HIV-1 control affect HLA class I peptide presentation. Science. 2010;330(6010):1551–7.
185. Selwyn PA, et al. A prospective study of the risk of tuberculosis among intravenous drug users with human immunodeficiency virus infection. N Engl J Med. 1989;320(9):545–50.
186. Collins KR, et al. Impact of tuberculosis on HIV-1 replication, diversity, and disease progression. AIDS Rev. 2002;4(3):165–76.
187. Whalen C, et al. Accelerated course of human immunodeficiency virus infection after tuberculosis. Am J Respir Crit Care Med. 1995;151(1):129–35.
188. Meltzer MS, et al. Role of mononuclear phagocytes in the pathogenesis of human immunodeficiency virus infection. Annu Rev Immunol. 1990;8:169–94.
189. Brune KA, et al. HIV impairs lung epithelial integrity and enters the epithelium to promote chronic lung inflammation. PLoS One. 2016;11(3):e0149679.
190. Espert L, Beaumelle B, Vergne I. Autophagy in *Mycobacterium tuberculosis* and HIV infections. Front Cell Infect Microbiol. 2015;5:49.
191. Campbell GR, Spector SA. Vitamin D inhibits human immunodeficiency virus type 1 and Mycobacterium tuberculosis infection in macrophages through the induction of autophagy. PLoS Pathog. 2012;8(5):e1002689.
192. Andersson AM, et al. Autophagy induction targeting mTORC1 enhances Mycobacterium tuberculosis replication in HIV co-infected human macrophages. Sci Rep. 2016;6:28171.
193. Duprez DA, et al. Inflammation, coagulation and cardiovascular disease in HIV-infected individuals. PLoS One. 2012;7(9):e44454.
194. Graziosi C, et al. Kinetics of cytokine expression during primary human immunodeficiency virus type 1 infection. Proc Natl Acad Sci U S A. 1996;93(9):4386–91.
195. Sinicco A, et al. Cytokine network and acute primary HIV-1 infection. AIDS. 1993;7(9):1167–72.
196. Cooper AM, Torrado E. Protection versus pathology in tuberculosis: recent insights. Curr Opin Immunol. 2012;24(4):431–7.

197. Ernst JD. The immunological life cycle of tuberculosis. Nat Rev Immunol. 2012;12(8):581–91.
198. Huynh KK, Joshi SA, Brown EJ. A delicate dance: host response to mycobacteria. Curr Opin Immunol. 2011;23(4):464–72.
199. Juffermans NP, et al. Up-regulation of HIV coreceptors CXCR4 and CCR5 on CD4(+) T cells during human endotoxemia and after stimulation with (myco)bacterial antigens: the role of cytokines. Blood. 2000;96(8):2649–54.
200. Juffermans NP, et al. Patients with active tuberculosis have increased expression of HIV coreceptors CXCR4 and CCR5 on CD4(+) T cells. Clin Infect Dis. 2001;32(4):650–2.
201. Briken V, et al. Mycobacterial lipoarabinomannan and related lipoglycans: from biogenesis to modulation of the immune response. Mol Microbiol. 2004;53(2):391–403.
202. Kedzierska K, et al. The influence of cytokines, chemokines and their receptors on HIV-1 replication in monocytes and macrophages. Rev Med Virol. 2003;13(1):39–56.
203. Hogg A, et al. Activation of NK cell granulysin by mycobacteria and IL-15 is differentially affected by HIV. Tuberculosis (Edinb). 2011;91(Suppl 1):S75–81.
204. Judge CJ, et al. CD56bright NK IL-7Ralpha expression negatively associates with HCV level, and IL-7-induced NK function is impaired during HCV and HIV infections. J Leukoc Biol. 2017;102(1):171–84.
205. Guerra C, et al. Control of Mycobacterium tuberculosis growth by activated natural killer cells. Clin Exp Immunol. 2012;168(1):142–52.
206. Saeidi A, et al. Attrition of TCR Valpha7.2+ CD161++ MAIT cells in HIV-tuberculosis co-infection is associated with elevated levels of PD-1 expression. PLoS One. 2015;10(4):e0124659.
207. Pedrosa J, et al. Neutrophils play a protective nonphagocytic role in systemic *Mycobacterium tuberculosis* infection of mice. Infect Immun. 2000;68(2):577–83.
208. Keller C, et al. Genetically determined susceptibility to tuberculosis in mice causally involves accelerated and enhanced recruitment of granulocytes. Infect Immun. 2006;74(7):4295–309.
209. Kerkhoff AD, et al. Blood neutrophil counts in HIV-infected patients with pulmonary tuberculosis: association with sputum mycobacterial load. PLoS One. 2013;8(7):e67956.
210. Bezuidenhout J, et al. Pleural tuberculosis in patients with early HIV infection is associated with increased TNF-alpha expression and necrosis in granulomas. PLoS One. 2009;4(1):e4228.
211. de Noronha AL, et al. Lung granulomas from *Mycobacterium tuberculosis*/HIV-1 co-infected patients display decreased in situ TNF production. Pathol Res Pract. 2008;204(3):155–61.
212. Plaza V, et al. Bronchoalveolar lavage cell analysis in patients with human immunodeficiency virus related diseases. Thorax. 1989;44(4):289–91.
213. Nusbaum RJ, et al. Pulmonary tuberculosis in humanized mice infected with HIV-1. Sci Rep. 2016;6:21522.
214. Vanham G, et al. Examining a paradox in the pathogenesis of human pulmonary tuberculosis: immune activation and suppression/anergy. Tuber Lung Dis. 1997;78(3-4):145–58.
215. Massanella M, et al. CD4 T-cell hyperactivation and susceptibility to cell death determine poor CD4 T-cell recovery during suppressive HAART. AIDS. 2010;24(7):959–68.
216. Geldmacher C, et al. Preferential infection and depletion of *Mycobacterium tuberculosis*-specific CD4 T cells after HIV-1 infection. J Exp Med. 2010;207(13):2869–81.
217. Zheng CF, et al. Late expression of granulysin by microbicidal CD4+ T cells requires PI3K- and STAT5-dependent expression of IL-2Rbeta that is defective in HIV-infected patients. J Immunol. 2008;180(11):7221–9.
218. Wijesundara DK, et al. Emerging targets for developing T cell-mediated vaccines for human immunodeficiency virus (HIV)-1. Front Microbiol. 2017;8:2091.
219. Ongaya A, et al. Mycobacterium tuberculosis-specific CD8+ T cell recall in convalescing TB subjects with HIV co-infection. Tuberculosis (Edinb). 2013;93(Suppl):S60–5.
220. Day CL, et al. Detection of polyfunctional *Mycobacterium tuberculosis*-specific T cells and association with viral load in HIV-1-infected persons. J Infect Dis. 2008;197(7):990–9.

221. Sirskyj D, et al. Disruption of the gamma c cytokine network in T cells during HIV infection. Cytokine. 2008;43(1):1–14.
222. Crotti A, et al. Naturally occurring C-terminally truncated STAT5 is a negative regulator of HIV-1 expression. Blood. 2007;109(12):5380–9.
223. Hogg AE, et al. Induction of granulysin in CD8+ T cells by IL-21 and IL-15 is suppressed by human immunodeficiency virus-1. J Leukoc Biol. 2009;86(5):1191–203.
224. Kaushal D, et al. The non-human primate model of tuberculosis. J Med Primatol. 2012;41(3):191–201.
225. Diedrich CR, O'Hern J, Wilkinson RJ. HIV-1 and the *Mycobacterium tuberculosis* granuloma: a systematic review and meta-analysis. Tuberculosis (Edinb). 2016;98:62–76.
226. Foreman TW, et al. CD4+ T-cell-independent mechanisms suppress reactivation of latent tuberculosis in a macaque model of HIV coinfection. Proc Natl Acad Sci U S A. 2016;113(38):E5636–44.
227. Mwandumba HC, et al. Mycobacterium tuberculosis resides in nonacidified vacuoles in endocytically competent alveolar macrophages from patients with tuberculosis and HIV infection. J Immunol. 2004;172(7):4592–8.
228. Koppensteiner H, Brack-Werner R, Schindler M. Macrophages and their relevance in Human Immunodeficiency Virus Type I infection. Retrovirology. 2012;9:82.
229. Jambo KC, et al. Small alveolar macrophages are infected preferentially by HIV and exhibit impaired phagocytic function. Mucosal Immunol. 2014;7(5):1116–26.
230. Mancino G, et al. Infection of human monocytes with *Mycobacterium tuberculosis* enhances human immunodeficiency virus type 1 replication and transmission to T cells. J Infect Dis. 1997;175(6):1531–5.
231. Rosas-Taraco AG, et al. Mycobacterium tuberculosis upregulates coreceptors CCR5 and CXCR4 while HIV modulates CD14 favoring concurrent infection. AIDS Res Hum Retrovir. 2006;22(1):45–51.
232. Hoshino Y, et al. Maximal HIV-1 replication in alveolar macrophages during tuberculosis requires both lymphocyte contact and cytokines. J Exp Med. 2002;195(4):495–505.
233. Nakata K, et al. Mycobacterium tuberculosis enhances human immunodeficiency virus-1 replication in the lung. Am J Respir Crit Care Med. 1997;155(3):996–1003.
234. Pathak S, Wentzel-Larsen T, Asjo B. Effects of in vitro HIV-1 infection on mycobacterial growth in peripheral blood monocyte-derived macrophages. Infect Immun. 2010;78(9):4022–32.
235. Hossain MM, Norazmi MN. Pattern recognition receptors and cytokines in *Mycobacterium tuberculosis* infection—the double-edged sword? Biomed Res Int. 2013;2013:179174.
236. Pahari S, et al. Reinforcing the functionality of mononuclear phagocyte system to control tuberculosis. Front Immunol. 2018;9:193.
237. Rodrigues V, et al. Myeloid cell interaction with HIV: a complex relationship. Front Immunol. 2017;8:1698.
238. Carow B, et al. Silencing suppressor of cytokine signaling-1 (SOCS1) in macrophages improves Mycobacterium tuberculosis control in an interferon-gamma (IFN-gamma)-dependent manner. J Biol Chem. 2011;286(30):26873–87.
239. Ryo A, et al. SOCS1 is an inducible host factor during HIV-1 infection and regulates the intracellular trafficking and stability of HIV-1 Gag. Proc Natl Acad Sci U S A. 2008;105(1):294–9.
240. Lowe DM, et al. Neutrophils in tuberculosis: friend or foe? Trends Immunol. 2012;33(1):14–25.
241. Yaseen MM, et al. The role of polymorphonuclear neutrophils during HIV-1 infection. Arch Virol. 2018;163(1):1–21.
242. Eruslanov EB, et al. Neutrophil responses to *Mycobacterium tuberculosis* infection in genetically susceptible and resistant mice. Infect Immun. 2005;73(3):1744–53.
243. Dallenga T, et al. M. tuberculosis-induced necrosis of infected neutrophils promotes bacterial growth following phagocytosis by macrophages. Cell Host Microbe. 2017;22(4):519–30. e3.
244. Allen M, et al. Mechanisms of control of *Mycobacterium tuberculosis* by NK cells: role of glutathione. Front Immunol. 2015;6:508.
245. Lu CC, et al. NK cells kill mycobacteria directly by releasing perforin and granulysin. J Leukoc Biol. 2014;96(6):1119–29.

246. Domingo-Gonzalez R, et al. Cytokines and chemokines in Mycobacterium tuberculosis infection. Microbiol Spectr. 2016;4(5). https://doi.org/10.1128/microbiolspec.TBTB2-0018-2016.
247. Scully E, Alter G. NK cells in HIV disease. Curr HIV/AIDS Rep. 2016;13(2):85–94.
248. Azzoni L, et al. Sustained impairment of IFN-gamma secretion in suppressed HIV-infected patients despite mature NK cell recovery: evidence for a defective reconstitution of innate immunity. J Immunol. 2002;168(11):5764–70.
249. Alter G, et al. Sequential deregulation of NK cell subset distribution and function starting in acute HIV-1 infection. Blood. 2005;106(10):3366–9.
250. Gold MC, Napier RJ, Lewinsohn DM. MR1-restricted mucosal associated invariant T (MAIT) cells in the immune response to *Mycobacterium tuberculosis*. Immunol Rev. 2015;264(1):154–66.
251. Jiang J, et al. Enhanced immune response of MAIT cells in tuberculous pleural effusions depends on cytokine signaling. Sci Rep. 2016;6:32320.
252. Jasenosky LD, et al. T cells and adaptive immunity to *Mycobacterium tuberculosis* in humans. Immunol Rev. 2015;264(1):74–87.
253. White L, et al. Differential effects of IL-21 and IL-15 on perforin expression, lysosomal degranulation, and proliferation in CD8 T cells of patients with human immunodeficiency virus-1 (HIV). Blood. 2007;109(9):3873–80.

Optical In Vivo Imaging in Tuberculosis Research

Riti Sharan, Thushara Galbadage, Panatda Saenkham, Madeleine Moule, Preeti Sule, Ying Kong, and Jeffrey D. Cirillo

Abstract Tuberculosis remains one of the greatest challenges to global health, making the development of novel diagnostics and therapeutics for tuberculosis a high priority. However, the unique cause, *Mycobacterium tuberculosis*, demonstrates a number of characteristics that have hindered progress in tuberculosis research. These challenges include an unusually slow growth rate that makes traditional microbiological methods time consuming, a unique glycolipid-rich cell wall that causes bacterial aggregation and complicates enumeration of bacterial loads, and a highly variable disease progression including both acute and chronic stages of infection that can complicate in vivo studies due to variation between infected animals. One strategy that has proven to be remarkably successful in overcoming these challenges is the application of in vivo optical imaging to the study of *M. tuberculosis*. This approach allows the progress of an infection to be followed in individual animals over time, enabling researchers to better understand this important pathogen and assay new vaccines, treatments, and diagnostic tests more accurately. In this chapter, we discuss the techniques and tools that have been developed to facilitate application of bioluminescent and fluorescent in vivo imaging to tuberculosis research. We also summarize the progress and potential contributions of real-time imaging to the tuberculosis field. Based on recent progress, optical imaging has the potential to transform the field, leading to more rapid discovery of therapeutics, vaccines and mechanisms of pathogenesis.

R. Sharan · T. Galbadage · M. Moule · P. Sule
Department of Microbial Pathogenesis and Immunology, Medical Research and Education Building, Texas A&M Health Science Center, Bryan, TX, USA

P. Saenkham
Molecular and Human Genetics Department, Baylor College of Medicine, Houston, TX, USA

Y. Kong (✉)
The University of Tennessee Health Science Center, Memphis, TN, USA
e-mail: ykong3@uthsc.edu

J. D. Cirillo (✉)
Department of Microbial Pathogenesis and Immunology, Texas A&M University College of Medicine, Bryan, TX, USA
e-mail: jdcirillo@tamu.edu

J. D. Cirillo, Y. Kong (eds.), *Tuberculosis Host-Pathogen Interactions*,
https://doi.org/10.1007/978-3-030-25381-3_8

Keywords Fluorescent proteins · Bacterial bioluminescence · Eukaryotic bioluminescence · Reporter enzyme fluorescence · Animal models · Bioluminescence substrates · Codon-optimization · Optical imaging · Tuberculosis

Introduction

Non-invasive optical imaging has emerged as an important tool to monitor a growing number of diseases in real-time [1–8]. Bioluminescence and fluorescence are key optical imaging techniques used to visualize progress of infectious diseases and study therapeutic efficacy in small animals [9–15]. Bioluminescent or fluorescent signal is measured by imaging to quantify the bacteria within the site of infection in real-time. This approach avoids sacrificing a group of animals at each time-point to determine colony forming units (CFU) and allows for the same group of animals to be imaged over many time points; thereby, reducing costs for maintaining animals and reducing the number of animals overall for an experiment. Bioluminescent and fluorescent imaging techniques are rapid and relatively easy to use, allow imaging of whole animals, necropsied tissues, tissue homogenates, infections in cell lines and pure bacterial cultures, making them useful in both drug and vaccine development as well as virulence studies [16, 17].

There are two principle strategies of bioluminescent imaging in living cells. One strategy utilizes an ATP and O_2 dependent reactions wherein, an exogenous substrate, D-luciferin, is converted into oxy-luciferin by the enzyme luciferase. Pathogens or mammalian cells engineered to express luciferase gene(s) under the control of promoter(s) of interest are used to generate light by administering the substrate and measuring the signal output via a highly-sensitive charge coupled–device (CCD) camera [4, 18]. The other strategy is to stably transfer the complete bacterial lux operon containing genes that express both the bacterial luciferase and produce the substrate, as is found naturally in *Photorhabdus luminescens* and several other bacterial species, producing continuous bioluminescent signal without the need of substrate administration [19, 20]. Thus, bioluminescent imaging uses photon emission in a naturally evolved biological context and is broadly compatible with biological systems. Fluorescence imaging is based on the excitation of fluorophores using illumination at certain wavelengths and detecting fluorescence emission using a CCD camera. Absorption of photons at a certain wavelength range by the fluorescent molecule causes its electrons to get excited to a higher energy state. The loss of this energy when the electrons relax back into the ground state releases photons in an emission spectrum that has lower energy than the initial photons absorbed producing longer wavelengths than the absorption spectrum [21, 22]. The increased stability of fluorescently labelled molecules [17], low hazard quotient in a clinical setting [23] and commercial availability of substrates has allowed successful implementation of fluorescent imaging in a wide array of applications including cancer typing, tracking drug metabolism and monitoring response to treatment [24, 25].

Both bioluminescent and fluorescent imaging probes have been developed for tuberculosis research [1, 3, 26–33]. A number of these probes have been applied to in vivo imaging of *Mycobacterium tuberculosis* infections [1, 27, 28, 32, 33] and we will discuss these further.

Fluorescent Proteins

Tremendous effort has been made to develop fluorescent proteins (FPs) with novel characteristics and enhanced fluorescence to improve visualization of dynamic processes within living cells. FPs have been widely used in cellular and whole animal imaging to track cellular movement in embryogenesis and inflammatory processes [34, 35], to monitor pathogen migration within the host [36–38], and to study cancer processes in live animals [8, 39–42]. Creation of red-shifted FPs [43] has allowed an increased fluorescent intensity within the key spectral window of 650–1100 nm favorable for tissue-penetration and most suitable for whole body imaging. Several factors contribute to the choice of the optimal FP for imaging. The FP should be non-toxic to the host, efficiently expressed and good signal-to-noise ratios resulting from an appropriate Stokes shift and desirable wavelength range [44]. The excitation and emission wavelengths of FP for whole animal imaging should be between 650 and 900 nm [22], because hemoglobin and water have their lowest absorption coefficients in this region of the spectrum [17], often called the near infrared (NIR) window. FPs that have emission wavelengths within the NIR window can penetrate through animal body with minimal absorbance by hemoglobin and water. The brightness of the mature protein and photostability of the FP also impact in vivo fluorescence imaging. TdTomato and mCherry demonstrate high photostability, and tdTomato is among the brightest FP among the variants of DsRFP [44]. Thus, these two FPs are often chosen for in vivo fluorescent imaging of *M. tuberculosis* infections [32, 45].

Research on tuberculosis (TB) has been impeded by the slow growth rate of *M. tuberculosis*, the bacteria responsible for the disease. *M. tuberculosis* divides once every 15–20 h. Quantification of *M. tuberculosis* normally relies on counting bacterial CFU on agar plates. It takes at least 4 weeks for *M. tuberculosis* to form visible colonies on agar plates [46–48]. Non-invasive optical imaging technologies have facilitated both in vitro and in vivo studies greatly accelerating TB research by allowing nearly instantaneous quantification of *M. tuberculosis*. The tdTomato and mCherry FPs have been selected for in vivo fluorescent imaging of *M. tuberculosis* infection based on their photostability and brightness [32, 45]. Kong et al. constructed FP expressing *Mycobacterium bovis* BCG strains for in vivo imaging to track bacterial location and quantify bacterial load in live animals [45]. tdTomato, mCherry, mPlum, mKate, Katushka and mKeima were cloned into mycobacteria and their fluorescent signals were compared both in vitro and in vivo. The tdTomato expressing strain was found to have the brightest fluorescent signal in vivo, and was used to study efficacy of rifampicin and isoniazid in vitro and in vivo [45]. Zelmer et al. has used H37Rv strains expressing tdTomato and mCherry to study efficacy of moxifloxacin treatment in live mice [32]. In addition, mCherry labelled *M. smegmatis* has been used to visualize pulmonary infections in living mice by Kong et al. [49]. Thus, mCherry and tdTomato display great promise for facilitating tuberculosis research.

Bioluminescence

Luciferases commonly used for bioluminescence imaging can be divided into three groups based on substrate and chemical reaction [50]. The first group is based on the *lux* operon, *luxCDABE*, present in several bacterial strains [51]. The *luxAB* genes encode the luciferase and *luxCDE* genes encode the fatty acid reductase complex responsible for synthesizing fatty aldehydes used in the luminescence reaction. Bacterial cells expressing the *lux* operon can produce light continuously without requiring exogenous substrate, since the reaction utilizes a substrate synthesized and recycled by the products of genes present within the operon [52]. However, bacterial luciferases produce light with a short emission wavelength that is less than ideal for in vivo imaging due to absorbance of its signal by hemoglobin [17, 52]. This problem has not prevented use of this system for in vivo imaging because the absence of the need for an exogenous substrate allows long photon acquisition times, but it does limit the threshold of detection for bacteria to approximately 10^5–10^6 in those systems [53–55]. The second group of bioluminescent systems used for imaging have luciferases that utilize coelenterazine as a substrate. Coelenterazine substrate luciferases include the *Renilla* luciferase and *Gaussia* luciferase originating from the sea pansy [56]. One of the main problems with these systems is the limitation in bioavailability of coelenterazine, because of its low membrane permeability [4]. The third group of bioluminescent systems includes beetle luciferases, such as firefly luciferase (FFluc) and click-beetle red luciferase (CBRluc) that use luciferin as their substrates for light production [57, 58]. In the case of the beetle luciferases, the chemical reaction involves luciferase, oxygenation of luciferin and ATP. FFluc produces a broad spectral range of emission though it has a maximum at 560 nm [59]. The fact that the spectral properties of FFluc and CBRluc bridge the 600 nm range, which is within the NIR window, makes them valuable as reporters in live animals [60].

Bioluminescence allows investigation of molecular and cellular events in all organs of a live animal simultaneously [4]. One advantage of bioluminescence imaging is that it is not restricted by delivery of an excitation wavelength, that can heat and/or damage tissue due to prolonged exposure or high intensity. Luciferases are routinely used for antimicrobial studies, possibly because they display a rapid loss of signal due to the requirement for ATP in light production. However, the temporal kinetics of substrate distribution must be determined prior to use of bioluminescent substrates to ensure that consistent levels of substrate and, thereby, signal are obtained, so that signal correlations with infectious agent are quantitatively accurate [61]. Chang et al. developed optimized bioluminescence systems using

CBRluc and FFluc to study mycobacterial infection kinetics in real-time. The different spectral maxima of the two luciferases allows unmixing of mixed cultures and hence, simultaneous detection of multiple mycobacterial strains in vivo [62]. In addition, Andreu et al. [27] have optimized the use of firefly, Gaussia and bacterial luciferases in mycobacteria as well as developing auto-luminescent *M. tuberculosis* and *M. smegmatis* to allow non-invasive detection of TB in living mice. Together, these bioluminescent systems allow a great deal of flexibility and offer the potential to spectrally unmix and quantify as many as three different strains of bacteria within a single animal using imaging.

Reporter Enzyme Fluorescence

Reporter enzyme fluorescence (REF), a newly developed enzymatic imaging system, utilizes fluorescent or bioluminescent substrates that are specific for enzymes expressed by target organisms. The most common REF probes are fluorescence-generating substrates for β-lactamase (BlaC), a constitutively expressed *M. tuberculosis* enzyme. All tuberculosis-complex bacteria, including *M. bovis* BCG, the vaccine strain, carry the *blaC* gene, encoding BlaC that belongs to the class A β-lactamase family [63, 64]. BlaC is highly conserved in clinical isolates, which is the central biochemical mechanism responsible for β-lactam-antibiotic resistance in *M. tuberculosis* [63, 65, 66]. When β-lactamase is expressed in mammalian cells it is quite stable, with a half-life of 206 min [67]. A portion of the *M. tuberculosis* BlaC is secreted and released from the bacteria, but it is mostly surface-localized, which allows the REF probes to label *M. tuberculosis* without the need to cross the bacterial membrane. Quenched REF probes carry a near infrared fluorescent dye connected to a quencher through the β-lactam ring, and generate fluorescence when BlaC hydrolyzes the β-lactam ring to release the quencher. Most optical imaging technologies require high pathogen numbers, usually in the range of 10^6 bacteria, to produce detectable signals in deeper tissues of mice. One of the first-generation REF probes, CNIR5, was able to lower the detection threshold to 10^4 bacteria in the lungs of mice [28, 68]. The second-generation REF probe, CNIR800, has higher sensitivity, detecting as low as ~10^3 CFU of *M. tuberculosis* in mouse lungs [69]. The improved sensitivity of REF imaging is ascribed to the NIR dyes of the probes and the special designed probe structures as well as the robust catalytic nature of the BlaC enzyme. The REF probes carry an acetylated D-glucosamine connected to the carboxylate of cysteine through γ-amino-butyric acid producing a charged molecule, which facilitates uptake into eukaryotic cells [70]. After being hydrolyzed by BlaC, the fluorescent products are less membrane permeable and build up within infected cells over time, leading to very high sensitivity [28, 68]. Furthermore, REF imaging allows detection of all strains of *M. tuberculosis*, including clinical strains, in living mice and in all other conditions, for that matter, without the need to express foreign genes that might potentially impact bacterial fitness. The ability to immediately quantify M. tuberculosis under almost any condition can profoundly impact TB research as it can speed both basic and translational studies.

Optical Imaging Models

Bioluminescent and fluorescent imaging has been extensively used in imaging bacterial infections in small animals. Far-red fluorescent protein, Katushka, has been used to visualize living cells in *Xenopus laevis* [41]. Imaging has been used to understand attachment of bioluminescent *E. coli* O157:H7 to beef carcasses and to understand the interaction of food-borne pathogens to animal tissue surfaces [71]. It has been demonstrated that *luxCDABE* operon expressing bioluminescent *Citrobacter rodentium* signal accurately reflects bacterial numbers in the caecum of infected mice both in vitro and in vivo [72]. Real-time antibiotic efficacy of a bioluminescent engineered *Staphylococcus aureus* was studied in a rat model of infection [73]. The suitability of mCherry expressing *E. coli*, *Pseudomonas aeruginosa* and *Edwardsiella tarda* for visualizing microbial communities has been demonstrated [74]. The impact of indole and 7HI on *P. aeruginosa* colonization in guinea pigs can be investigated using bioluminescence [75]. A luxCDABE expressing *Brucella suis* strain has been developed to facilitate in vivo imaging in the guinea pig model of infection [76]. Adult zebrafish prove advantageous for mechanistic studies, since they are easy to raise, are small and genetically manipulatable. However, adult zebrafish lose their transparency and the use of fluorescent reporter proteins is impacted by the fact that the detection of fluorescent cells is semi-quantitative and more limited to cells closer to the body surface [77]. Reports on luciferase imaging in zebrafish have been sparse and limited to embryos [78–80]. Fluorescence- and luciferase-based detection has been compared in adult zebrafish by expressing mCherry and FFluc from a single transcript [77]. Bioluminescent imaging of ferrets infected with H1N1 virus was used to study influenza virus transmission efficiency for risk-assessment [81]. Insight into the mechanisms involved in *Mycobacterium marinum* colonization of *Caenorhabditis elegans* was gained by performing confocal microscopy on *C. elegans* infected with tdTomato (Fig. 1) expressing *M. marinum* [82]. Transgenic *C. elegans* expressing green fluorescent protein (GFP) from a heat-shock protein promoter was employed to elucidate the molecular basis for effects on life-span [83]. In addition, the safety and efficacy of fetal adeno-associated virus gene delivery in rhesus monkeys was studied using long-term monitoring of transgene expression by bioluminescence imaging [84]. The same group had earlier shown that firefly luciferase can be used to detect transgene expression at multiple time points in fetal and infant monkeys in vivo without any adverse effects [85].

Recent advances have been made in the use of near-infrared fluorescence imaging in humans. The cause of pediatric lymphedema was investigated using near-infrared fluorescence lymphatic imaging in a 21-month old boy [86]. NIR fluorescence imaging has demonstrated sensitivity for molecular imaging of cancer-positive lymph nodes using indocyanine green (ICG) in breast, skin and gastric cancers in humans [87]. Two pilot studies of human breast imaging using intravenous administration of ICG have been reported [88, 89]. Recently, whole body dynamic near-infrared fluorescence has been developed for adult human subjects to explore the possibility of dynamic whole-body fluorescence imaging and to detect

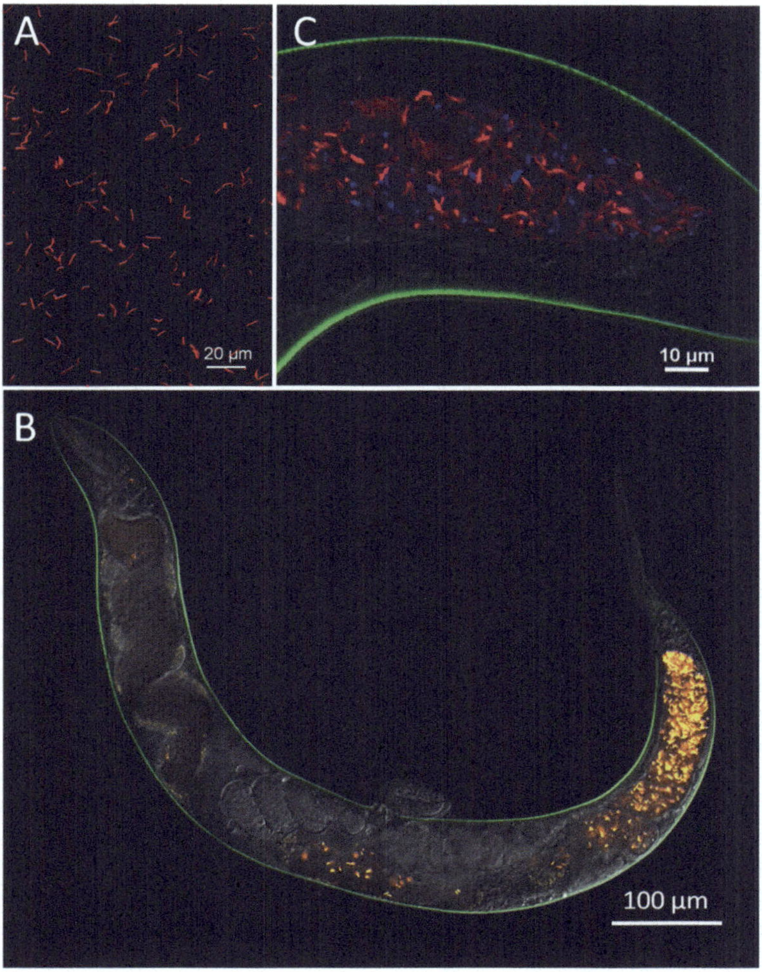

Fig. 1 Imaging fluorescently tagged mycobacteria in the *C. elegans* model. (**a**) Fluorescent confocal microscopy of *Mycobacterium smegmatis (Ms)* strain ψms23 expressing tdTomato (red) fluorescent protein. (**b**) Images showing *C. elegans* that can be used as a model system to study the innate immune response to mycobacterial infection. eGPF (green) expressing *C. elegans* (TP12) infected with *Mycobacterium marinum (Mm)* expressing tdTomato (pseudocolor gold). *Mm* is internalized by *C. elegans* and visible in the nematode gut. (**c**) *Mm* competitive infections with two bacterial strains within a single *C. elegans*. Two strains of *Mm*, one expressing tdTomato (red) and the other expressing mCherry (pseudocolor blue) in the gut, near the tail of an eGFP (green) expressing *C. elegans* (TP12)

modulations in skin perfusions using the fluorescent probe, ICG [90]. ICG-enhanced near infrared fluorescence imaging has also been used to illuminate high-risk histologic plaque features of human carotid atherosclerosis [91]. A multicolor bioluminescent imaging platform can be used to monitor the cell number and viability by genetically modifying a human breast cancer cell line to express green, red and blue light emitting luciferases [92]. Overall, these studies demonstrate the broad flexibility of optical imaging for numerous pre-clinical and clinical studies.

Optical Imaging of Tuberculosis

Factors Affecting Imaging with FP-Expressing Strains

Fluorescent Proteins

A large number of fluorescent proteins (FPs) have been engineered from *Aequorea victoria* GFP or from various Anthozoan marine organisms such as corals or anemones, providing different fluorescent colors across the entire optical spectrum (450–650 nm) [93]. FPs do not require any additional enzymes or cofactors except for molecular oxygen during the formation of the chromophore. FPs have been characterized based on their peak of excitation and emission. Violet FP has a peak of excitation and emission of 355 and 424 nm, respectively. Sireus is the violet FP that has the shortest emission wavelength, peaking at 424 nm with high photo and pH stability [94]. The blue FP, EBFP, has excitation/emission peaking at 380–400/450 nm. FPs in the cyan has excitation and emission peaking at 430–460 and 480–490 nm. FPs in this group are ECFP and its variants [95] SCFPs [96], TagCFP (Evrogen JSC), and mTurquoise [97]. FPs in the green group (excitation/emission peaked at 490/510 nm) have been extensively studied and developed, and a number of good monomeric green FP have come out of these studies, including EGFP, mEGFP, mWasabi, Emerald (EmGFP), Superfolder GFP, and TagGFP2. The yellow FPs, EYFP, (excitation/emission peaked at 515/530 nm) and enhanced versions, Citrine [98], Venus [99], Topaz [100], and TagYFP [101], have been developed including what may be the brightest one, YPet. FPs with excitation/emission peak at 550/560 nm produce an orange color of light (Orange FPs). There are several bright variants of orange FPs available, including mKO (monomeric Kusabira Orange) [102] and mOrange and their variants, mKO2 and mOrange2. A group of red FPs derived from the coral *Discosoma* sp. FP "DsRed" have been developed by introducing mutations into the original protein, including mRFP1, mHoneydew, mBanana, mOrange, dTomato, tdTomato, mTangerine, mStrawberry, mCherry, and mMars. These FPs have various excitation and emission wavelengths at 560–580 and 570–610 nm, respectively. The mRaspberry, mPlum [103], mKate2 [104], and mNeptune [105] FPs have excitation and emission peaks in the far-red wavelength (Far red FPs) at 590 and 630–650 nm, respectively. Other red FPs have been developed by multiple groups, including Katushka, mKate [41], and mKeima [106]. Katushka and mKate share the same excitation and emission wavelengths, with an emission peak at 635 nm, which is very close to the NIR window. Interestingly, mKeima has a large Stokes shift with the excitation and emission peaks far away from each other, 440 nm vs 620 nm. Different FPs also have different brightness,

Table 1 Commonly used fluorescent proteins

Fluorescent protein	Excitation coefficient of FP (M^{-1} cm^{-1})	λ of FP [35][a]	
		Excitation	Emission
GFP	21,000	395	509
mCherry	72000	587	610
mOrange	71,000	548	562
Turbo-635	65000	588	635
tdTomato	138000	554	581
mBanana	6000	540	553
mCitrine	77,000	516	529
DsRed/RFP	75,000	558	583
mPlum	41,000	590	649
mRasberry	86,000	598	625
mRuby	112,000	558	605

[a]Wavelengths (λ) are represented by maxima of excitation (ex) and emission (em) spectra

half-lives, and photo stabilities. The parameters of these FPs are summarized in the Table 1. The brightness of FPs can often be improved through mutagenesis. For example, mEGFP is a variant of EGFP with the point mutation A206K. FPs can be applied to numerous studies in living systems, including protein labelling, promoter tracking, subcellular localization and cell and tissue labelling.

One of the major advantages of the zebrafish model is that the natural optical transparency of zebrafish embryos and early swimming larvae allows lower wavelength fluorophores such as GFP, which does not penetrate mammalian tissue effectively, to be used [37, 107]. In addition to allowing imaging with GFP which is bright, stable, and readily available, the opportunity to image with a broader spectrum of fluorescent proteins allows use of multiple fluorophores in a single experiment. Examples of this include coinfections with multiple strains of mycobacteria labelled with fluorophores of different wavelengths [108–110] and infection of transgenic zebrafish expressing fluorescent labelled host proteins with bacteria labelled with fluorophores of contrasting wavelengths [111, 112]. As new FPs have been developed, the range of FPs used in the zebrafish model has expanded to include those with a wide variety of properties including mCherry, tdTomato, mWasabi, mEos, eGFP, and E2-Crimson [113–116].

GFP has been used for protein labelling to monitor localization and to visualize cellular events. Since GFP does not required a substrate or any co-factors, the proteins of interest can be monitored by measuring expression through fluorescent signals detected using fluorescence microscopy. Unlike other techniques (eg. immunocytochemistry, luminescences), GFP-fusion proteins are non-toxic to live cells since detection does not required any fixation, permeabilization, other enzymes or adding substrates. However, GFP tags may sometimes interfere with the natural functions of protein of interest. Since hemoglobin, melanin and water absorb almost all light below 600 nm [117], using the FPs in the short wavelength range can result in more interference and more background, resulting in less efficient imaging for deep tissue or whole animals. Red-shifted FPs showed reduced autofluorescence, lower light-scattering, and lower phototoxicity. These properties make red-shifted FPs excellent probes for in vivo imaging, particularly in deep tissues and for imaging approaches that require low background [118].

Variants in Fluorescent Proteins Provide New Tools

Fluorescent markers can be used as pH indicators that have the ability to measure pH at specific intracellular sites. There are several advantages of using this methods including: little background signal, absence of indicator leakage and no toxicity like that associated with chemical indicators that have invasive loading procedures. Optimal fluorescent markers for pH sensing need specific characteristics: a rapid signal response to pH changes, high pH sensitivity and specificity, and good optical properties. For quantification of its intensity, an increase in fluorescence of at least 50% for every 1 pH unit change is desirable.

Several fluorescent markers, including GFP, can respond very rapidly to pH changes. For in vivo studies, fluorescent markers are good indicators because they are nontoxic, chemically inert, and targetable to selected intracellular locations without leakage or migration. Fluorescence energy transfer between GFP mutants has been used in the design of protein sensors to measure protease activity [119] and calcium concentrations [120, 121]. This is done using florescent proteins and their mutants that have different affinities at a given pH and having distinguishable excitation and emission wavelengths.

The use of fluorescence as intracellular pH indicators permits measurements that cannot be easily accomplished using existing chemical pH indicators. Targeting of these proteins to the lumen of organelles allows direct measurement of intra-organelle pH and analysis of pH regulatory mechanisms [122]. These markers can be driven by pH inducible promoters to be differentially expressed in high or low pH conditions. These methods have been employed to help characterize the environment where mycobacteria reside intracellularly.

Fluorescent fusion proteins (FFPs) are FPs attached to either the N-terminus or C-terminus of a protein of interest. FFPs containing the full-length protein fused to a FP are valuable tools that can be used to study a protein's function, localization or Interacting partners in its native environment. The simplest FFPs are FPs fused to targeting sequences (e.g., a nuclear localization sequence or a signal sequence) to mark an organelle or cellular domain of interest. Such FFPs allow co-localization of a protein of interest with a specific organelle, protein, intracellular location or other molecule in a living cell [123]. In addition, these FFPs can be coupled with photobleaching methods to quantify the density, movement or number of units within a cellular environment [123, 124].

FFPs are useful as markers to understand protein and organelle dynamics. However, the temporal aspects of FP maturation may place constraints on the utility of FFPs. For example, FFPs can be more difficult to implement for following the behavior of nascent proteins within the first few minutes of translation. This is because most versions of EGFP take up to 30 min to fold and display strong fluoresce in solution [125]. However, EGFP may become fluorescent more rapidly in cells [126]. The Discosoma red fluorescent protein (DsRed) is thought to be slower and can take up to 48 h to allow 90% of newly synthesized proteins fluorescent [127]. However, new red FP variants are available that fold in <1 h [128]. The slow folding of one DsRed variant, DsRed-E5, has been exploited to visually distinguish proteins younger and older than 9 h [129].

Fusion of FP to another protein represents a significant addition to a protein and thus may have steric consequences for protein folding, function, or targeting. GFP variants and the coral FPs are about 27 kDa. The crystal structures of all FPs show β-barrels that are 3 nm in diameter and 4 nm in length [130]. In addition, many of the coral FPs exist as obligate tetramers of β-barrels [127], which not only increase their size but also can lead to formation of aggregates. Usually FPs are not a small percentage of the total final protein fusion product, and some proteins do not fold properly or are nonfunctional following the addition of a FP [131]. Therefore, it is always important to consider FP-related changes and their potential impact on protein function. In order to reduce transcriptional effects on gene regulation, codon-optimized variants of FPs are available for mammalian, fungal, and plant cells [130, 132, 133]. Use of codon-optimized genes represents a first step in helping to ensure that unwanted effects of making this type of fusion are observed; however, it is critical to be aware that both transcriptional and post-transcriptional events may impact how these fusions perform in biological systems.

GFP folds to form a β-barrel bearing a triplet of internal amino acids (SYG) that produce a fluorophore within the barrel [125]. Wild-type GFP does not fold efficiently, is sensitive to pH, and can undergo reversible photo-bleaching [134], as shown in FRAP (fluorescence recovery after photo-bleaching) and FLIP (fluorescence loss in photo-bleaching) experiments. To improve the utility of GFP, the codon bias has been modified to make the protein more suitable for expression in mammalian cells, and two amino acids were mutated to enhance brightness and protein folding (S65T and P64L). The resulting variant is termed EGFP (enhanced green fluorescent protein). Furthermore, EGFP and its variants have been further improved and optimized for various target organisms or model systems, making this protein very versatile and widely used in a large number of diverse studies.

Promoter-induced vector instability is a concern for fluorescent reporters in *M. tuberculosis*. The promotor Phsp60 has been linked to frameshift mutations and large deletions in either the promoter or coding region in *M. tuberculosis* at a relatively high frequency (2×10^{-3}). In plasmids containing fluorescent reporters, plasmid stability is dependent on the specific gene being expressed. In addition, increasing plasmid copy number can have a deleterious effect on the organism by having an increased number of FPs and producing fewer clones expressing FPs well. The increase in plasmid instability can result from negative selection against increased expression levels of FPs and a strong selective pressure for deletion of plasmids.

Use of FPs also has the advantage of increased sensitivity at low cell densities, where other reporters may be below the limit of detection. Fluorescent reporters offer the advantages of increased sensitivity as well as the ability to measure activity sequentially in live cells. These reporters allow detection of bacterial gene expression profiles during long-term persistence. FPs used in gene expression studies have helped identify genes up-regulated under conditions relevant to infection [135].

It has been demonstrated that fluorescent protein reporters can be very stable, even after long-term excitation, allowing the advantage of serial imaging [3]. Fitness assays have demonstrated that relatively high-levels of expression are not normally detrimental to growth of mycobacterial species. Expression of these reporters has shown not to cause any major impact on growth or virulence of *M. tuberculosis* in vitro. Optimized FPs are also instrumental in imaging of *M. tuberculosis* during infections. FP expressing mycobacterial strains can be used to track bacterial location and quantify bacterial load in animal models [45, 136]. Therefore, fluorescent reporters allow the development of tools to analyze pathogenesis of *M. tuberculosis* in real-time.

Choice of Proteins to Be Used as Markers

Both fluorescent and luciferase protein tagged strains of *M. tuberculosis* have been developed [1, 3, 27, 33, 137]. A variety of proteins have been used for different infection models, chosen for characteristics that make them more advantageous in each system (Table 1). All of the FPs are large and can cause problems in protein folding of tagged protein or even have physiological changes in the bacilli due to aggregation. Therefore, it is important to understand the characteristics of the reporter system used.

GFP was the initial fluorophore to be used. Now the color spectrum of the GFP-like fluorophores have been extended toward the red emission range of light for different advantageous reasons. Red light penetrates to deeper tissue in whole body imaging of model organisms. This makes it easy to image *M. tuberculosis* in the lungs of infected mice or even during dissemination of the bacteria to extrapulmonary sites. Fluorophores with an emission range in the red wavelengths are in a wavelenth region of the spectrum where auto-fluorescence is lower, resulting in less background signal in imaging (Table 1).

FP expressing strains do not require administration of a substrate or time for the substrate to reach peak levels in tissues. These characteristics offer the advantage that the FP reporter strains can be repeatedly imaged over very short periods of time, without having to wait for clearance of previously administered probes [45]. However, when using a FP as a reporter, a modified mycobacterial strain containing the FP needs to be used, which can limit its utility in some cases.

Effects of Molecular Constructs on Fluorescent Protein Signal

Stable expression of fluorescent markers can be achieved in mycobacteria by introducing an extrachromosomal or integrating plasmid with the gene of interest expressed from an appropriate promoter. A replicating plasmid will contain an origin of replication in mycobacteria, maintaining it separate from the genomic DNA. Several copies of the plasmid normally exist in each of the bacilli, resulting in greater fluorescent signal. Plasmids that are able to integrate into the mycobacterial genomic DNA will have one copy of the plasmid and fluorescent reporter in each bacilli. While the overall expression of fluorescence is often lower using these plasmids, the resulting strains are more likely to correlate better with the bacterial load. Therefore, depending on the purpose and function of the fluorescent markers, single-copy or multi-copy plasmids can be chosen as appropriate.

The use of different promoters for expression of a fluorescent marker can have an impact on levels of expression. When expressed from the L5 promoter, there appears to be a greater level of expression of fluorescent signal than from the Hsp60 promoter. However, in studies when the plasmid DNA copy number was compared, the L5 promoter strain had a higher copy number than in the Hsp60 promoter strain. It is possible that some fluorophores are more toxic to bacilli than others. Although the L5 promoter strain carries more copies of the plasmid than the Hsp60 promoter strain, the L5 promoter strain only expresses slightly more tdTomato transcript numbers, minimizing the toxicity of tdTomato to the bacteria [45].

Strains carrying plasmids expressing multi-copy FPs have been used to show that the plasmids are stable in mycobacterial strains over days to weeks, even in the absence of antibiotic selection [3]. Single copy constructs that are site-specifically integrated into the mycobacterial chromosome can be used to help ensure that mycobacteria express these FPs in a more stable manner. These integrating constructs usually contain a mycobacterial plasmid with the phage attachment site attP and the L5 integrase (int) gene from the mycobacteriophage L5 genome. Although the integrated strains carry a single copy of the FP gene in their chromosomal DNA, it does not necessarily result in lower fluorescent signal than strains carrying higher copy number plasmids.

Studies comparing different fluorescent and luminescent signals in *M. tuberculosis* strains carrying either high, low or single copy (chromosomal) plasmids carrying reporter genes showed that single copy reporter had the highest levels of expression [3, 27]. This could be explained by two different mechanisms. Either the increased expression of FP in multi-copy plasmids caused deleterious effects to the bacilli, leading to a decrease in the number of bacilli carrying the plasmid or a greater number of bacteria that eliminate the plasmid carrying the FP during replication. With the strains carrying FPs in chromosome, long-term animal or cell infection experiments can be conducted in the absence of plasmid selection, making these preferable in most cases.

Codon-optimization by changing amino acids in the FP sequence to optimize translation of the protein it encodes in a particular bacterial species and ensure RNA transcripts produced are translated efficiently. In mycobacteria, codon-optimization has shown to increase the fluorescent signal obtained using mCherry and tdTomato. The optimized fluorescent sequence for translation after transcription can reduce formation of secondary structures that may terminate transcription due to improved ribosomal reading of the RNA, thus, producing more fluorescent signal overall. This codon-optimization process makes each fluorophore more specific to a bacterial species, which can make them less efficient for expression in other bacterial species.

Over-expression of certain fluorophores, including tdTomato, can result in toxicity for mycobacterial species. However, when these FPs are expressed in a carefully regulated manner, they do not have any apparent impact on growth, bacterial physiology or virulence in vitro or during infections [3]. Therefore, each FP can be codon optimized to provide a stable, non-toxic yet robust reporter in mycobacteria. Successful approaches to imaging reporter gene expression require efficient production of the reporter protein. Production depends on the characteristics of the expression vector used, copy number, promotor, and transcriptional and translational signals present. It is important that the report signals correlate well with copy number of either the protein or bacteria being studied. The fluorescent signal in labeled bacteria usually correlates very well with bacterial numbers as determined by CFU [3, 32, 45]. Imaging offers a unique way to more rapidly evaluate new TB therapeutic regimens in vitro and in vivo using florescent tagged mycobacteria for detection.

Factors Affecting Bioluminescence Imaging Results

Comparison of Different Bioluminescence Systems

Bioluminescent imaging enables analysis of specific cellular and biological processes in living animals [138–140]. More than 30 different chemically unrelated bioluminescence systems exist in nature, from bacteria and fungi to fireflies and fishes, exhibiting emission ranges from blue-violet to red. While bacterial luciferase systems have been extensively used in prokaryotic and plant hosts [141], eukaryotic luciferases are extensively used in mammalian systems. The *lux* operon from *P. luminescens* contains genes for both the luciferases and for aldehyde substrate synthesis negating the need for administration of substrates [142]. This is not the case with marine luciferase or luciferase from American firefly *Photinus pyralis,* which require the exogenous substrates coelenterazine or D-luciferin. The *P. luminescens lux* operon has been successfully transfected into a plethora of microorganisms. Although this operon functions well in Gram-negative bacteria, it does not translate well in Gram-positive bacteria due to lack of appropriate ribosome-binding sites in the mRNA sequences [19]. It is imperative to produce stable integration of the luciferase operon into the bacterial chromosome to avoid loss of plasmids over time. Oxygen can be a limiting factor for optimal luciferase activity since all luciferases are inherently oxidizing and require significant oxygen to function optimally. Beetle luciferases require cellular ATP and their activity can be reduced or completely absent in the absence of sufficient ATP. Luciferases that need external administration of substrate, such as D-luciferin require the molecule to penetrate target cells, making pharmacokinetics and bio-distribution of the substrate an important factor to consider for in vivo imaging.

Dual-luciferase systems have been developed where two reporter genes are combined with one serving as the experimental reporter and the other as an internal control. Combination of *Renilla* and firefly luciferase has been successful, but both are not very stable in media. Determination of their optimal activity requires cell lysis which can be a limiting factor when continuously monitoring dynamic changes in gene expression in response to stimuli. An engineered luciferase from a subunit of *Oplophorus gracilirostris* luciferase, named NanoLuc [143] has been constructed. It is only 19kDA and uses the novel substrate furimazine. It is stable in medium and exists in a secreted form. NanoLuc has a specific activity ~150-fold greater than that of firefly or *Renilla* luciferases with a similar glow-type luminescence. NanoLuc has been shown to have a higher stability (7.7 days in HEK 293 lysates at 37 °C) than other luciferases (firefly, 7.3 min in HEK293 lysates at 37 °C; Rluc, 1.7 h in HEK293 lysates at 37 °C) [144]. Another dual reporter system combines two secreted luciferases CLuc (produced by crustacean *Cypridina*) and GLuc (by marine copepod *Gaussia*). Transfection of mammalian cells with cDNA from *Cypridina* luciferase and *Guassia* luciferase leads to its secretion into the medium via the endoplasmic reticulum and subsequent quantification of the light intensity with their respective substrates (luciferin-CLuc; coelenterazine-GLuc) [145]. Bacterial luciferase emits blue-green light at 490 nm by oxidizing flavin mononucleotide (FMNH2) and a long-chain fatty aldehyde [146]. Genes coding for bacterial luciferase subunits *luxAB* and flanking genes *luxCDE*, responsible for aldehyde substrate biosynthesis, have been cloned and sequenced from *lux* operons of luminescent bacteria: *Photobacterium, Vibrio* and *Xenorhabdus* [147]. Uninduced continuous measurement of functional luciferase in the same sample is one of the advantages of bacterial luminescence systems. Other benefits include no cost for substrates and high stability of bacterial luciferases from *Vibrio harveyi* and *Xenorhabdus luminescens* at 37 °C [141]. In vivo bioluminescent imaging using either one of the aforementioned systems has been used to effectively validate mouse studies for a number of infections. Photodynamic therapy of wound infections caused by *Pseudomonas aeruginosa* was examined using a bioluminescent strain constructed by transformation with a plasmid containing the *luxCDABE* operon from *P. luminescens* [148]. Loss of luminescence correlated well with loss of bacterial viability and demonstrated dose-response curves similar to those obtained by CFU. Luminescent measurements could be achieved within minutes as opposed to hours with conventional CFU methods. Antibiotic treatment of *S. aureus* infections of skin were evaluated using the bioluminescent strain Xen 36 in mice [149]. An immediate reduction in bioluminescence was observed when wounds were treated with nisin or mupirocin. This was attributed to the mode of action of the antibiotics, i.e., inhibition of cell wall synthesis and rapid cell lysis of *S. aureus* Xen 36. Dermal needle scratch and dermal abrasion infections have been monitored by bioluminescent imaging using bioluminescent methicillin-resistant *S. aureus* (MRSA) in BALB/c mice [150, 151]. In the study by Dai et al., bioluminescent MRSA Xen31 constructed by transforming *S. aureus* ATCC 33591 with a chromosomal copy of the modified *P. luminescens luxABCDE* operon was used to mimic abrasion wound infection of humans in mice. Bioluminescent imaging allowed real-time monitoring of the extent of chronic and persistent infections in mouse wounds, did not waste animals, was non-laborious and could be easily used to study particularly less-invasive bacteria like MRSA. Luciferase from Italian firefly *Luciola italica* has 64% amino acid identity with the luciferase from *P. pyralis*. Notably, its total bioluminescence output was found to be ~twofold greater than that of *P. pyralis* luciferase due to extended light emission decay kinetics. The other advantage of this luciferase over Fluc is thermostability and higher enzyme turnover [152]. Maguire et al. further characterized codon-optimized variants of red-emitting liFluc for in vivo bioluminescence imaging in small animals [153]. The liFluc luciferase had the advantage of much lower absorption by pigmented molecules such as melanin and hemoglobin as well as scattering by mammalian tissues since the emission wavelength of liFluc is relatively long, 610 nm.

In order to help overcome difficulties with the emergence of multi-drug resistant strains of *M. tuberculosis*, slow in vitro growth rate and highly infectious nature of the bacteria, optical reporter systems have been used as a surrogate biomarkers to replace conventional CFU methods for drug discovery, vaccine or treatment studies [154]. Demonstration of bioluminescent imaging for *Mycobacterium bovis* BCG in immunodeficient mice has been accomplished [155]. However, the disadvantage of this study was the administration of a relatively toxic aldehyde substrate, decanal, for mycobacterial visualization, since the strain carries only the *luxAB* genes, not those for substrate production. A recombinant bioluminescent *Mycobacterium ulcerans* strain expressing *luxAB* from *V. harveyi* has been used for real-time evaluation of antimicrobials [156]. Though this system enables rapid assessment of novel drugs, the requirement of repeated injections of substrate and its poor diffusion reduces sensitivity. *M. tuberculosis* expressing either FLuc or Lux for in vivo mycobacterial detection in the lungs of infected mice was accomplished in 2010 [27]. *M. tuberculosis* expressing the complete bacterial luciferase operon has also been exploited in drug and vaccine efficacy studies to measure bioluminescence in homogenates of organs from mice [33]. An apparently fully virulent and reasonably stable autoluminescent strain of *M. tuberculosis* was developed that enabled distinguishing active from inactive anti-tuberculosis drugs in <5 days. Advantages of using imaging in these studies are lower costs, reduced need for biosafety level 3 animal housing, reduced need to handle infected tissues and no requirement for exogenous substrate. Disadvantages include incomplete stability of the integrated *luxCDABE* operon as demonstrated by the presence of non-luminescent revertants, and a weaker correlation of luminescence to CFU when the organisms enter stationary phase. A major limitation of this system is the number of bacteria needed for detection with the detection threshold of 10^6 CFU. An improved FFluc reporter (FFlucRT) was developed to visualize *M. tuberculosis* in severe combined immunodeficiency (SCID) mice and to validate use in high-throughput in vivo testing of drug efficacy [1]. The improved reporter produces a thermostable red-emitting luciferase, showing an emission spectrum shift towards the red (620 nm) as compared to FFluc (560 nm). Additionally, FFlucRT displays a better correlation of luminescence with CFU during stationary phase, with thresholds of detection as low as 10^3 and 10^5 CFU ex vivo and in vivo, respectively, in the lungs of mice. Optical reporters CBRlux and FFlux, both having emissions spectra in the far-red wavelengths, have been developed by codon-optimizing the genes for mycobacteria. This system allows thresholds by subcutaneous infection of 10^3 CFU. Mixed cultures of these two markers could be spectrally unmixed to quantify the two luciferases, permitting simultaneous imaging of both strains in the same animal. This system facilitates quantitative differentiation of bacterial numbers expressing these luciferases. Detection of these strains in the lungs of mice found that the signal was sensitive to antibiotic treatment, making them appropriate for rapid evaluation of novel intervention strategies.

Recent advances in rat genetic engineering have resulted in development of luciferase-expressing transgenic rats to evaluate immunological antigenicity against the luciferase in conventional skin-grafting. Skin from luciferase tagged rats is less immunogenic than GFP tagged skin and transplantation of organs showed sustained organ viability and graft survival. These characteristics make transgenic rats an innovative tool for a better understanding of organ transplantation [157]. The ability to use luciferase tagged human cytomegalovirus to track its persistence in both adult and neonate guinea pigs has been examined [158]. Bioluminescence imaging allows rapid determination of the extent of viral dissemination into spleen, liver and lung over a 2-week period indicating that the depth of the animal tissue does not dramatically reduce the intensity of signal. Individual zebrafish cells transfected with a luciferase reporter have been developed to study circadian rhythms that drift out of phase in darkness and are resynchronized in light [159]. Based on this initial study, transgenic zebrafish expressing the firefly *luc* gene were developed to monitor the roles of environmental stimuli on circadian rhythms during development. However, this system is somewhat limited by temperature as well as the days where light-day cycles are required for robust bioluminescent rhythms [160]. Bacterial bioluminescence-based metabolic assays have been developed to assess the impact of human activities on the environment and public health. Firefly luciferase expressing *C. elegans* have been used to assess effects of sublethal chronic exposure to cadmium. This system utilizes a rapid, quantitative metabolic end-point, bioluminescence instead of energy-related end-points that are constrained by their labor-intensive nature [161]. Non-invasive bioluminescence imaging can be used to detect optimally radiolabeled human embryonic stem cells expressing firefly luciferase transplanted into fetal monkey kidneys. This system enables monitoring of transplanted cells in real-time over extended periods of time, without showing toxicity or an effect on gene expression or functionality of transplanted cells [162]. More recently, bioluminescent imaging has been used in a zebrafish model to more efficiently screen anti-mycobacterial compounds. These studies utilized *M. marinum* strains tagged with either a codon-optimized red-shifted firefly luciferase or a modified *P. luminescens* luciferase cassette to monitor bacterial infections of zebrafish via caudal vein. Infected zebrafish larvae were treated with either Rifampicin or one of four nitroimidazole-derived next-generation drugs and monitored for bioluminescence to determine drug efficacy. Both luciferase tagged strains appeared to be effective, the bacterial luciferase system was superior in terms of time and cost, and that five of the six antibacterial compounds tested were able to reduce luminescence in infected animals to background levels [163]. These studies demonstrated that while zebrafish lack some of the relevance of mammalian models, they are an effective model for quickly and easily screening therapeutic compounds that can then be confirmed in larger models [163].

Effects of Variation in Bioluminescence Genes

Bioluminescent bacteria are thought to be the most abundant bioluminescent organisms in nature. Common bacterial luciferases and other enzymes involved in luminescence (*lux*) are marine bacteria in the *Vibrio*, *Photobacterium* genera, and terrestrial bacteria in the *Xenorhabdus* genus. *Vibrio harveyi*, *Vibrio fischeri*, *Photobacterium phosphoreum, Photobacterium leiognathi*, and *Xenorhabdus luminescens* species are good examples [51, 146, 164]. A common *lux* gene organization (*LuxCDABE*) is composed of the luciferase genes (*luxAB*) and the genes involved in synthesis of its fatty aldehyde substrate (*luxCDE*). This gene organization is modulated by the presence of specific genes involved in regulation, flavin binding and metabolism (*luxFI,L,R,Y*), found to be somewhat different in different luminescent bacterial species. The *luxAB* genes encode the bacterial luciferase subunits. The bacterial luciferase is a heterodimer that is composed of two subunits, α (*luxA*) and β (*luxB*) subunits. These two subunits have approximately 30% identity in amino acid sequence and the α subunit dictates the primary kinetic properties of the enzyme. Bacterial luciferase catalyzes the oxidation of reduced flavin mononucleotide ($FMNH_2$) and a long-chain fatty aldehyde, requiring molecular oxygen and leading to emission of a blue-green light at 490 nm. Oxygen and $FMNH_2$ are naturally occurring products within the cell.

$$FMNH_2 + RCHO + O_2 \rightarrow FMN + H_2O + RCOOH + hv_{490\,nm}$$

The *luxCDE* genes encode the fatty acid reductase polypeptides that are required for conversion of fatty acids into the long chain aldehyde substrate for the luminescent reaction. The *luxD* gene encodes a transferase responsible for attachment of an endogenous myristyl group to water to form myristic acid. The *luxE* gene encodes a synthase that then activates the acid via addition of an AMP group in order to prepare the reduction of the activated acid to aldehyde through the reductase encoded by *luxC*.

The *luxF* gene encodes a flavoprotein related in sequence to the luciferase subunits. The LuxF protein is apparently not necessary for luminescence. It may play a specific role in the luminescence of *Photobacterium* species found in mid or deep water, but it is absent in a *P. leiognathi* species that is a symbiont of a shallow water fish [165]. The *luxL* and *luxY* genes are related to sequences of riboflavin synthesis genes [166, 167]. The *luxI* gene is required for synthesis of an autoinducer that controls expression of luminescence. It is located upstream and transcribed in the same direction as the *luxCDABE* operon, suggesting it is in the same operon. The autoinducers are species-specific for induction of luminescence. The β-ketocaproyl-N-homoserine and 3-hydroxybutyryl-Nhomoserine lactones are specific for *V. fischeri* and *V. harveyi* lux systems, respectively [168, 169]. The *luxR* gene product functions as a receptor for the autoinducer and activates expression of *lux* operon [170, 171]. Regulation of bacterial luminescence is dependent on cell density, resulting in autoinduction, commonly referred to as quorum sensing. *In V. fischeri*, during the initial stages of growth, the *luxICDABEG* operon is expressed at a very low level with the autoinducer concentration gradually increasing in cells and media. After reaching a critical concentration, the autoinducer causes luminescence expression by binding to the LuxR regulatory protein that interacts with the operator region between the *IuxICDABEG* and *luxR* operons [170].

Since bioluminescent bacteria expressing the *lux* operon produce light without the need for an exogenous substrate, the *luxCDABE* has been transferred a large number of bacterial species for imaging studies. There are many different publications that use bacterial bioluminescence as a reporter for imaging to study host-pathogens interaction and microbial pathogenesis. An early microbial pathogenesis study by Contag and colleagues [53], used the plasmid containing *luxCDABE* from *P. luminescens* to transform three strains of *Salmonella typhimurium*. Luminescent bacteria could be detected in the whole body of live C57BL/6 or BALB/c mice following infection and allowed localization of the bacteria to specific tissues. Oxygen plays a key role in light production by the *lux* operon. The ability to detect extracellular bacteria in anaerobic microenvironments, such as the lumen of the intestine, by bioluminescence imaging may be reduced. The ilium and colon of *Salmonella*-infected mice, where the luminescent signal was not detectable, became detectable when air was injected into the ilium and colon. Bioluminescence imaging has been applied to monitor antibiotic efficacy in vitro and in vivo, using *luxCDABE*-transformed *E. coli* to determine minimal inhibitory concentrations and minimal bactericidal concentrations (MBC) of antibiotics in broth culture and in a soft tissue model of infection. Growth curves generated by bioluminescence imaging correlate well with CFU. There were differences in the magnitude of inhibition as measured by BLI as compared to colony forming units. This result may be explained by the fact that the luminescent signal at different time points is derived from exactly the same animals, while CFU are derived from different groups of animals. These results suggest that imaging offers an advantage for quantifying responses to treatment in the same mice over time [172]. Bioluminescent *Citrobacter* was constructed by integrating *luxCDABE* operon into the *Citrobacter* genome and mice were orally inoculated to monitor bacterial colonization and clearance in the colon by bioluminescence imaging and CFU. Interestingly, it was found that *Citrobacter* colonize the caecal patch before colonizing the rest of the colon, and bacteria are cleared from the caecum before being cleared from the rest of the colon [173].

Gram-positive bacteria *Staphylococcus aureus* or *Streptococcus pneumoniae* do not translate the *luxCDABE* operon from *P. luminescens* well because of Gram-positive ribosomes do not bind and translate the mRNA well. The *luxCDABE* genes have been modified to allow expression by Gram-positive bacteria [54]. Gram-positive ribosome binding sites (RBS) were inserted upstream of each gene in the operon and the gene order was modified to increase expression of the luciferase, resulting in a cassette called *luxABCDE*. The *luxABCDE* transformed *S. aureus* produces bright light and emits optimally at 37 °C. This strain produces bioluminescence that correlates well with CFU and decreases upon antibiotic treatment using a mouse model of *S. aureus* thigh infection. A transposon was used to stably integrate *luxABCDE* into the genome of *Streptococcus pneumoniae* [55]. Clinical isolates of *S. pneumoniae* were made bioluminescent in a similar manner for study of its virulence and examination of antibiotic therapy using imaging. Another research group used the same cassette (*luxABCDE*) to generate bioluminescent *Listeria monocytogenes* carrying *luxABCDE* stably integrated in the chromosome [174]. They identified new regions of in the lumen of the mouse gall bladder where *Listeria* can replicate.

The sequence of the natural *luxCDABE* operon is AT-rich, making expression less efficient in high-GC bacteria, like *Mycobacteria* and *Streptomyces*. Translation in the high GC organisms favors G and C residues in the wobble position of amino acid codons [175]. The *luxCDABE* operon of *P. luminescens* is rich in codons having either A or T in the wobble position (69%), suggesting these genes would not be efficiently expressed in *Streptomyces*, *Mycobacterium* or other high-GC organisms. In *Streptomyces coelicolor* there is only one tRNA for the leucine codon TTA, while there are 63 TTA codons in *luxCDABE* operon. The entire *luxCDABE* gene cluster has been optimized for expression in high-GC bacteria, removing TTA codons and producing the majority of codons ending in G or C [176] The optimized synthetic *luxCDABE* genes are functional in *S. coelicolor* and luminescence appears to accurately reflect expression profiles for genes, including the housekeeping sigma factor *hrdB*, a gene involved in spore-formation, *ramC*, and a gene required for production of spore-associated pigment, *whiE*.

This *luxCDABE* cassette has been used to construct bioluminescent *Mycobacterium marinum* for use in a zebrafish model system as a tool for rapid high-throughput screening of antimicrobials. This system may reduce time and resources needed to screen compounds, though they must then be confirmed in mammalian models. Comparison of a *M. marinum* strains tagged with FFluc and those expressing *luxABCDE* suggest that the bacterial luciferase was more effective despite being less bright than FFluc, possibly because of decreased background when an exogenous substrate is not required [137]. Based on these studies, bacterial luminescent systems show promise for future studies. The bacterial *lux* operon has been further optimized for *Mycobacteria* using a combination of vectors, promoters, and codon-optimized genes [27]. Cloning the *luxABCDE* operon, modified for expression in Gram-positive bacteria by replacement of the ribosome binding sites and reorganization of the genes [177] into the three different expression vectors: (1) pSMT3, low copy number with 2–5 copies per cell [178, 179] (2) pSMT3M [3], medium copy number with 32–64 copies per cell [180] and (3) pMV306hsp, single copy by integrating into the chromosome [179]. The pMV306hsp plasmid carrying the *luxABCDE* operon (pMV306hsp + Lux) displays the greatest signal. Improved signal can be obtained by increasing the amount of substrate synthesized through insertion of a strong promoter, $P_{G13,}$ in front of *luxC* in pMV306hsp + Lux (pMVhsp + LuxAB + G13 + CDE), resulting in a sixfold increase in signal over pMV306hsp + Lux, allowing detection of bacteria in the lungs of mice infected with *M. smegmatis* pMVhsp + LuxAB + G13 + CDE [27].

Bioluminescence imaging is useful for mammalian-based whole animal imaging due to low background from endogenous structures in animals [60]. Firefly luciferase is heat labile and has a short half-life of 3 min at 37 °C [181]. Luciferase from both beetle and marine aequorin need exogenous substrates to produce signal. The *lux* operon would be useful as a mammalian bioluminescent reporter, since it does not require an exogenous substrate. A challenge of constructing a *luxCDABE* operon to work in mammalian cells is that the genes are not efficiently expressed. The *P. luminescens luxA, B, C* and *E* genes were cloned into yeast expression vectors that allow for bi-directional constitutive or inducible expression of the individual *luxA, B, C*, and *E* genes. The *luxD* gene was fused to a yeast internal ribosomal entry site (IRES) to ensure high bi-cistronic expression. A flavin oxidoreductase gene (*frp*) from *Vibrio harveyi* was co-expressed to provide sufficient concentrations of the $FMNH_2$ co-factor required for bioluminescence, which stabilizes and enhances bioluminescence of the *lux* operon [182]. A bacterial *lux* operon based-mammalian bioluminescence reporter has been constructed. The *lux* and *frp* genes were re-synthesized base on codons optimized by GENSCAN analysis (http://genes.mit.edu) and cloned as a multi-bicistronic construct, which functions well in *S. cerevisiae*. The *lux* genes are grouped into pairs and separated by encephalomyocarditis virus IRES elements to more efficiently drive translation in mammals. HEK293 cells containing codon optimized *lux* display strong bioluminescence in cell culture and in nude mice [183].

Variants in Eukaryotic Bioluminescence Genes

Insect luciferases are a single protein with a molecular weight of approximately 62 kDa and do not require the posttranslational modifications for enzymatic activity [58]. The best-known insect bioluminescence is that of beetles, from the family Lampyridae, (eg. Fireflies, *Photinus pyralis*) or the family of Elateridae (eg. click beetles *Pyrophorus plagiophtalamus*). Firefly luciferases (FFluc) are classified as *Photinus*-luciferin: oxygen 4-oxidoreductase (decarboxylating, ATP-hydrolysing) (EC 1.13. 12.7). The enzyme requires a substrate that is a heterocyclic water-soluble acid (benzothiazoyl-thiazole), luciferin, ATP, and O_2. The reactions catalyzed by firefly luciferase are:

$$\text{Mg2}+$$

1. Luciferase + luciferin + ATP $\leftrightarrow$ luciferase luciferyl − AMP + PP_i
2. Luciferase luciferyl − AMP + O_2 $\rightarrow$ luciferase + oxyluciferin + AMP + CO_2 + hv

The formation of an enzyme-bound luciferyl-adenylate occurs in the first step. During the second reaction, the luciferyl-adenylate undergoes an oxidative decarboxylation that produces CO_2, oxyluciferin, AMP, and light [184]. The reaction catalyzed by firefly luciferase emits yellow-green light at pH 7.5–8.5, with the peak emission at 560 nm. FFluc is heat labile and unstable above 30 °C and pH-sensitive.

FFluc shifts to >610 nm (612–617 nm) at below pH 7.5, temperatures above 35 °C and addition of denaturants or heavy metals [60, 185].

Click beetle luciferase (CBluc) is similar to FFluc catalyzing a two-step reaction (adenylation and oxygenation) and using the same substrate, luciferin. CBluc emits a broad wavelength from green to orange (544–593 nm). In nature, the click beetle emits green light from its dorsal organ (wavelength from 548–565 nm), and green to orange (547–594 nm) by the ventral organ. The green and orange alleles of the click beetle luciferases have been further engineered to widen the gap between their emission peaks. The resulting luciferases have an emission peak at 537 nm for the green luciferase (CBGluc) and 613 nm for the red luciferase (CBRluc). The main difference between firefly and click beetle luciferases is that click beetle luciferases are not pH-sensitive.

The coelenterazine-dependent luciferases oxidize the substrate benzylimidazopyrazinone coelenterazine (coelenterazine) independent of ATP or $FMNH_2$. The well-known coelenterazine-dependent luciferases are from the sea pansy *Renilla reniformis* (Rluc,) and the copepod *Gaussia princeps* (Gluc). Rluc is a 35 kDa monomer that emits light at 480 nm. Gluc is naturally secreted, consisting of a monomeric structure with a molecular mass of 19 kDa and emitting light at 480 nm. The intensity of light emitted by Cluc is greater than Rluc, but both produce 'flash-type' bioluminescence with peak signal 10 s after substrate addition and declining to background levels over 10 min. In animals, GLuc and RLuc produce signal 1–2 min post-intravenous administration of substrate (coelenterazine) [186]. These luciferases are relatively stable at 37 °C [187–189]. Rluc and Cluc emit blue light, compromising in vivo performance due to absorption by mammalian tissue. Blue light is absorbed by mammalian tissue, particularly highly vascularized tissues with greater hemoglobin than other tissues. Since Cluc is a secreted protein, the distribution of Gluc in the bloodstream increases background. A membrane-bound version of Gluc can be used to reduce this problem [190]. *Oplophorus gracilirostris* (deep sea shrimp) derived luciferase (NanoLuc) is a relatively small (19.1 kDa) protein that uses coelenterazine as a substrate and does not require ATP. Bioluminescence is improved when the coelenterazine analogue furimazine is used. NanoLuc has an emission peak of 460 nm, which hampers the effectiveness of obtaining signal from deep tissues [143, 191].

D-luciferin has favorable pharmacologic properties for in vivo imaging. Intraperitoneal (IP) administration is commonly used and luciferin becomes distributed throughout the animal and can penetrate blood-tissue barriers such as brain and placenta within 15 min [192, 193]. Coelenterazine (substrate of Rluc and Gluc) is commonly administered to animals intravenously. This substrate results in more background because of oxidation in serum [194]. The substrate coelenterazine is excluded from some tissues by drug transport proteins [195].

Insect luciferases are widely used in research on viruses and eukaryotes and occasionally been used in bacterial research. These luciferases are intracellular enzymes that need ATP within the cell for light emission. However, the wavelength of light produced by FFluc and CBluc is more appropriate for in vivo imaging than that of the bacterial LuxAB luciferase [59, 60]. A red-optimized click beetle luciferase (CBRluc) has been developed as a luminescent reporter for *L. monocytogenes* and compared with a previously described bacterial *lux*-luminescent *L. monocytogenes* [196]. The CBRluc begins to emit bright signal in exponential phase and maintains bright signal throughout stationary phase, while a *lux*-based system produces light signals that peak during exponential phase and significantly reduce during stationary phase. The light from CBRluc labeled bacteria showed better penetration in an in vitro tissue depth model, a cell invasion assay and a systemic murine infection model than the light from *lux* labeled bacteria. These observations suggest that CBRluc is well suited for bioluminescence imaging and may provide enhanced sensitivity relative to *lux* in *Listeria* infection models [197]. FFluc has also successfully been used to tag *M. marinum* in the zebrafish model, but was found to be less effective than bacterial luminescence in this model [163].

FFluc can be modified to improve its spectral properties and stability. The peak emission is important in the bioluminescence imaging because absorbance by host tissues is much less for red-shifted light. An improved FFluc reporter (FFlucRT) for *M. tuberculosis* to use for high-throughput in vivo testing of drug efficacy [1]. The codon-optimized FFluc from previous studied was modified by substitution of nine amino acids. Three amino acids, Ile423Leu, Asp436Gly and Leu530Arg, were mutated to enhance bioluminescence intensity [198] and six amino acids, Ser284Thr, Thr214Ala, Ala215Leu, Ile232Ala, Phe295Leu and Glu354Lys, were mutated to produce a more thermostable red-emitting luciferase. FFlucRT demonstrated an emission spectrum shifted towards the red from 560 nm for FFluc to 620 nm for FFlucRT. The detection threshold is 1.7×10^3 and 7.5×10^4 CFU of the resulting FFlucRT luminescent *Mycobacterium* in culture and in the lungs of infected mice, respectively. Furthermore, luminescence in living mice given isoniazid display markedly reduced signal [199]. FFluc and click beetle red luciferase (CBRlux) emit distinct bioluminescent spectra and use the same luciferin substrate, allowing dual bioluminescence to study mycobacterial infections in vivo. Codon-optimized FFluc and CBRluc have been constructed for mycobacteria and they have been expressed in *Mycobacterium bovis*, bacillus Calmette-Guérin (BCG) [62]. These luciferases do not appear to cause growth defects in BCG and allow localization to the site of infection with detection limits as low as 10^3 CFU during subcutaneous inoculation. These reporters can be used to evaluate therapeutic efficacy in real-time since they display a sensitive response to antibiotic treatment. The results demonstrate feasibility for simultaneous detection of multiple mycobacterial strains during infection in animal models.

In order to use FFluc in *Candida albicans*, all the CUG codons in the luciferase gene, adapted for expressed in mammalian cells, must be replaced by CUU codons. This modification allows correct translation of the gene into a functional protein because CUG codons code for leucine and are translated to serine in *C. albicans* [200]. This modified FFluc is suitable to visualize persistence of *C. albicans* within the vaginal lumen of mice during infection. The luciferin substrate can be directly applied to the vaginal lumen and light emission correlates well with *C. albicans* numbers. When this optimized FFluc is expressed from a constitutively active promoter in hyphae inducing conditions it displays lower luminescent signal than in yeast cells. This reduction in signal is most likely because the uptake of luciferin substrate is interfered with by the reorganized cell wall in hyphae. A cell-wall-anchored Gluc was generated by fusing Gluc with glycophosphoinositol linked cell wall protein PGA59 of *C. albicans.* The resulting luminescent *C. albicans* produces similar levels of signal in both yeast and hyphae. This luminescent strain is suited for examining the progression of infection after subcutaneous, cutaneous and vaginal infections where the coelenterazine is added at the site of infection. The limited distribution of coelenterazine after intraperitoneal inoculation is likely responsible for poor signal during systemic *C. albicans* infection in animal models [201]. A *C. albicans* codon-optimized firefly luciferase has been constructed to improve the detection limits for *C. albicans* in infected mice. The mutations used were S284T, causing a red-shift in light emission, and L295F, improving thermal stability [199, 202]. This modified firefly luciferase displays increased bioluminescence in *C. albicans* as shown by the sensitivity of bioluminescence imaging in systemic infections as compared to the original luciferase and the intensity of emitted light correlated well with fungal load in an oropharyngeal candidiasis animal model [203].

Genetically modified mice expressing luciferase reporters allow researchers to examine the host response to bacterial or virus infection as well as interventions. Normally, a luminescent reporter mouse strain will express a luciferase gene under the control of a promoter for the gene of interest. One system has been developed where a *S. pneumoniae* strain expresses the bacterial *lux* operon, while a transgenic mouse expresses FFluc under control of the promoter for glial fibrillary acidic protein (GFAP), an established marker for astrocyte activation. The luminescence from these two systems can be differentiated by the different wavelengths of emission at 490 nm for bacterial luciferase and 610 nm for FFluc. The valuable finding that the host pro inflammatory response is a major factor causing morbidity and mortality in this disease came out of using this system, demonstrating the importance of having host and pathogen markers for imaging infections [204].

There are several D-luciferin and coelenterazine analogs developed that have potentially advantageous properties. A 6′-aminoluciferin analog was created by substitution of the 6′-hydroxyl group of D-luciferin with a 6′-amino group producing red-shifted light emission. It shows higher affinity for luciferase, but lower maximal light emission and lower cell-permeability [205]. Several 6′-aminoluciferin analogs including long-chain 6′-alkylaminoluciferins, 5′,6′-cyclic alkylaminoluciferins and dialkylaminoluciferins were synthesized. These substrates have higher affinities for luciferase than 6′-aminoluciferin and emit light at even longer wavelengths [206–208]. Mutations in FFluc can allow discrimination between D-luciferin and aminoluciferin analogs in vitro and in live cells [209, 210]. These luciferase and substrate modifications can be useful to further development of selective luciferases to expand the power of bioluminescence and allow multiple events to be imaged in the same live animal. The main focus of development of coelenterazine is to obtain an improved luminescence output. Red- and blue-shifted analogues of coelenterazine have been developed by imidazopyrazinone C-6 extended substitution [211]. Recently, new coelenterazine analogs (6etOH-, 6etOH-, 6piOH-2H-, 6etOH- and 6piOH-2H-coelenterazine) have been synthesized to selectively allow production of light from a specific luciferase with unique luciferase selectivity. These analogs were modified by changing the functional groups at the C-2 and C-6 positions of the imidazopyridine backbone of coelenterazine which leads to the ability of the substrate to selectively target a specific luciferase. These coelenterazine analogs show potential for multiplex imaging of in vivo reporter assays [212]. The commercially available modified coelenterazine substrate, ViviRen™, is a coelenterazine where the oxidation site is protected to reduce spontaneous substrate degradation and autoluminescence. This substrate appears to produce brighter signal than natural coelenterazine [213]. Gluc has been used to examine exocytosis in synaptic regions of neurons. The coelenterazine substrate for Gluc is highly membrane permeant. This substrate can diffuse across synaptic and vesicular membranes and react with the luciferase before exocytosis, resulting in high background. A less membrane permeant coelenterazine derivative has been made by alkylation of coelenterazine with a linker containing a terminal anionic phosphonate moiety. This derivative has the potential to reduce background and improve imaging of synapses.

Substrates Improved for Bioluminescent Signal Production

FLuc emits a yellow green signal at 562 nm while GLuc emits at 485 nm and RLuc at 480 nm. Auto-oxidation of coelenterazine by serum increases background, making it less favorable for in vivo imaging. Additionally, coelenterazine is unable to cross the blood-brain barrier making it inappropriate for some studies [194, 214]. On the other hand, D-luciferin is able to diffuse throughout the animal and can cross the blood-brain [192] and placental barriers [215]. Modification of D-luciferin to produce a red-shifted emission above 650 nm would be a great advantage for in vivo imaging as this wavelength produces maximumal tissue penetration [216]. Interactions between the 6′–hydroxy group of oxyluciferin and the binding site and the polarity of the microenvironment at the binding site are known to influence the emission spectrum of luciferase. A green-yellow emission will be observed if there is strong interaction, while a weak interaction promotes red-shifted emission [217]. Synthetic 6′–alkylated aminoluciferins have been developed as substrates for Ultra-Glo and QuntiLum luciferases. These substrates are significantly brighter than traditional substrates under saturating conditions [208]. Optimization of the luciferase from deep sea shrimp, *Oplophorus,* as well as variants of its luminogenic substrate has been explored. A combination of an engineered luciferase, NanoLuc, with a novel coelenterazine analogue, furimazine, generated brighter luminescence than Fluc or Rluc. Positions 2, 6 and 8 of the imidazopyrazinone core have been modified to produce novel coelenterazine analogues. These substrates produce bright luminescence and exhibit good stability and low background [143]. Two new substrate analogs, EnduRen™ and ViviRen™, have been examined for improved signal, reduced autoluminescence and longer kinetics in a murine model of human glioblastoma expressing *Renilla* luciferase. While EnduRen signal took longer to peak, ViviRen exhibited ~0.5–1.0 log more bioluminescence than coelenterazine. Intraperitoneal administration of substrates took longer to peak and overall produced lower bioluminescent signal output than intravenous administration at the same concentrations and using the same imaging parameters [213]. A total of 23 coelenterazine analogues were examined for substrate specificity with recombinant *Renilla*, *Oplophorus* and recombinant apoaequorin luciferase. Significantly more signal is obtained with e-coelenterazine (7.5 times) and v-coelenterazine (6.4 times) as compared to native coelenterazine [218]. Bis-coelenterazine (bis-CTZ) and 6h-f-coelenterazine (6h-f-CTZ) have been suggested to be better substrates than coelenterazine for nanoKAZ and nanoLuc luminescence assays. The mutant, NanoKAZ displays high luminescence activity with bis-CTZ (112.0 fold) and 6 h-f-CTZ (111.2 fold) as compared to coelenterazine. This improvement is likely in part dependent on the recognition moieties for coelenterazine, and interactions of nanoKAZ with the functional groups at C2- and/or C6-positions [218].

An improved ability to access the luciferase as compared to D-luciferin makes CycLuc1 a better substrate for imaging in vivo. Improving access to intracellular luciferase in live cells in combination with a red-shift in light emission are recommended for improving in vivo imaging [210]. Compact, rigid aminoluciferins were modelled after CycLuc1 and CycLuc2, increasing the total photon flux of near-infrared light over D-luciferin from live luciferase-expressing cells. These synthetic luciferin analogues fuse 5′,6′-membered rings of varying composition. The resulting CycLuc5 and CycLuc6 light emit at longer wavelengths than D-luciferin with CycLuc6 yielding strongly red-shifted bioluminescence (636 nm). CycLuc10 produces an even more red-shifted signal with the peak at 642 nm. These substrates have been tested for bioluminescence imaging in live mice and 20–200 fold less substrate than D-luciferin is required for imaging tumor cells. Higher numbers of red-shifted photons are seen with these substrates along with detection of luciferase expression deep in the brain that cannot be detected with D-luciferin. Coelenterazine analogs were synthesized by making modifications at the C-8 position to produce substrates with brighter signals and red-shifted bioluminescence [219]. The teLuc, a NanoLuc mutant, coupled with diphenylterazine, a coelenterazine analog, displays sustained bioluminescence with a ~40 min half-life and a quantum yield that was twice that of NanoLuc-furimazine. Additionally, 13 times more photons than Fluc-D-luciferin at wavelengths longer than 600 nm are produced. CycLuc1 substrate is a cyclic alkylaminoluciferin that is able to produce improved light emission at a dose of 7.6 mg/kg as compared with the standard dose of 150 mg/kg of D-luciferin for in vivo imaging of cells and animals expressing Luc2 firefly luciferase. Improved cell permeability is reportedly the cause for the brighter signal and not the red-shift [10]. A red-shifted emission maximum for D-luciferin was achieved by replacing the native sulfur atom at position 1 with selenium without altering luciferase recognition [220]. This concept is based on the polar effects of selenium, previously reported to produce a red-shifted emission in fluorophores. Luciferases are known to recognize selenium analogues as well as the natural sulfur-containing substrates. The new substrate displays improved performance for in vivo imaging but is somewhat limited by temperature, perfusion, bio-distribution and clearance. The bioluminescent imaging emission maximum of this substrate is 600 nm, compared to D-luciferin having an emission maximum at 558 nm and aminoluciferin at 588 nm, a potentially significantly longer wavelength, advantageous for in vivo imaging.

A wide array of new substrates for bioluminescence resonance energy transfer (BRET) have been examined that combine luciferases and fluorescent proteins to expand the sensitivity of bioluminescence imaging [221]. Substrates were chosen based on the spectral overlap and brightness to allow for strong transfer of photon energy to the fluorescence protein or BRET. Bioluminescence half-lives of Prolume purple (PPI) or methoxy-eCoelenterazine (me-eCTZ) and Prolume purple II (PPII) or methoxy-eCoelenterazine-methoxy (Me-CTZ-Me) are longer (153 s and 217 s respectively) than coelenterazine, suggesting an advantage for imaging sensitivity. PPI has a 13-fold brighter signal and PPII has a fivefold brighter signal than coelenterazine [221]. An in vivo Z-DEVD-aminoluciferin has been developed as a modified firefly luciferase substrate that is cleaved by caspase-3 to liberate aminoluciferin, which is then consumed by luciferase for light emission [222]. The use of this new substrate for in vivo imaging in two oncology models produced light as early as 24 h to monitor apoptosis in vivo. In addition to significantly shortening the time to determine therapeutic efficacy in these tumor models, this substrate could be used in slow growing models and therapeutic studies in orthotopic and systemic models. Caged luciferins produce luminescence in two steps: first, the caged substrate is cleaved by a specific biological molecule and then luciferase oxidizes the free luciferin to emit light. Thus, the amount of free luciferin and the activity of the enzyme is closely related to light output making these modified probes useful bioluminogenic substrates in detecting small molecule functions or target enzyme activity [223]. Furin probes, acetyl-RVRR-aminoluciferin and acetyl-RYKR-aminoluciferin are hydrolyzed in the presence of furin to release aminoluciferin and generate bioluminescence in combination with firefly luciferase. The greater signal production by acetyl-RVRR-aminoluciferin could allow investigation into the role of furin in hypoxia in vivo [224]. The dynamics of luciferase expression could be studied by changing caged luciferins to uncaged luciferins by photolysis using UV illumination, and detecting bioluminescent signal. Since this method does not use luciferin but caged luciferin, it has the advantage that it can be used to image specific enzymes or small molecules at specific times or locations in tissues of living animals [225]. The need for photoactivatable probes that could be activated by long-wavelength excitation led to the development of a photocaged upconversion nanoparticle consisting of D-luciferin as the reporter, silica-coated lanthanide-doped upconversion nanoparticles (UCNP) and a photoactivatable linker. The uncaging of D-luciferin triggered by D-luciferin-conjugated UCNPs excited by near-infrared light could result in a bioluminescent signal that can be used for deep tissue imaging.

A bright, cyan-excitable, orange-red fluorescent protein was used to build a BRET system using the blue light emitting NanoLuc luciferase [226]. They hypothesized that the combination of an orange-red FP, CyOFP1, serving as the BRET acceptor for NanoLuc could feature a high enzymatic turnover of NanoLuc with a high quantum yield and red-shifted emission of the FP. This system could be used to develop a bioluminescent enzyme that would enable deep tissue imaging in living mice. A synthetic derivative of the native coelenterazine substrate, *coelenterazine-v*, which red-shifts the emission maxima of RLuc by 35 nm was used in a BRET system to identify protein-protein interactions in small animal deep-tissue tumor models. These red-emitting BRET systems produce a bright signal and had enhanced sensitivity for imaging in deep tissues [227]. A list of improved substrates for bioluminescence have is shown in Table 2.

Use of Reporter Enzyme Fluorescence to Improve Imaging

We have developed a novel fluorescence-based imaging technology designated reporter-enzyme fluorescence (REF). The specificity, sensitivity and decreased expense [28, 68] makes this method attractive [232]. Other alternatives include computed tomography (CT) [233], magnetic resonance imaging (MRI) [234] and F-fluorodeoxyglucose positron emission tomography/CT (F-FDG PET/CT) [235], but REF imaging is relatively inexpensive, making it appealing for pre-clinical studies. REF utilizes custom fluorogenic or fluorescence resonance emission transfer (FRET) substrates that upon enzymatic cleavage produce a fluorescent product [28, 49, 69, 236]. Hence, REF does not require recombinant reporter strains [45, 155] that can have an unknown impact on bacterial virulence, but can be carried out in any wild type bacterial strain. We have developed several near-infrared FRET substrates: CNIR4, CNIR5, CNIR9 and CNIR10 by linking a quencher QSY21 or its derivative, to either Cy5 (CNIR4) or Cy5.5 (CNIR5, CNIR9 and CNIR10) through a lactam ring. The first-generation substrate that was most successful, CNIR5, represented a significant breakthrough with a detection threshold of 10^4 CFU in the lungs of live mice [28, 68]. This threshold provides the sensitivity to detect *M. tuberculosis* at levels similar to those in recently infected organs, which could be used to provide new insight into *M. tuberculosis* disease mechanisms. CNIR5 is composed of Cy5.5, with a maximum emission at 680 nm, linked to a quencher, QSY22. This substrate displays a good correlation between bacterial CFU and fluorescence from 10^2 to 10^6 CFU [28]. Maximal fluorescence is observed for CNIR5 at around 48 h post-administration, followed by CNIR10, CNIR4 and CNIR9. CNIR5 has been modified for longer wavelength emission using IRDye800cw that has maximal emission at 789 nm that can be quenched with the QC-1 quencher. The resulting substrate, CNIR800, should allow increased tissue penetration of signal due to reduced absorbance and scattering of light. This most recently modified REF probe has a detection threshold of ~1000 CFU for mouse pulmonary infection with *M. tuberculosis* [69]. REF imaging with CNIR800 gives a good correlation with CFU for a dynamic range of 3–4 logs, which is similar to that of conventional CFU methods and should be sufficient for evaluation of most therapeutics and vaccines. REF probes were originally designed to serve as fluorescence-generating substrates for the constitutively expressed *Mtb* β-lactamase (BlaC) [63, 237]. Bacterial β-lactamases confer resistance to penicillin and cephalosporin through hydrolysis of the β-lactam ring that these antibiotics contain [238–241]. Both *M. tuberculosis* and *M. bovis* BCG naturally express BlaC, an enzyme that belongs to the class A β-lactamase family [63, 64]. Extended spectrum class A β-lactamases can hydrolyze all classes of β-lactam substrates, including cephalosporins. Cephalosporin

Table 2 Substrates improved for bioluminescent imaging

Substrate	Modification	λmax (nm)	Enzyme	Application	Reference
6′-amino-luciferin	Amino analog of D-luciferin substrate	605	Firefly luciferase	Protease activity detection in vitro	[224]
4-methyl-D-luciferin	Methyl derivative of D-luciferin	535	Firefly luciferase	Linking luciferin to other molecules	[228]
N-alkylated 6′-aminoluciferins	Alkylation of 6-amino-2 cyanobenzothiazole	493	Ultra Glo and QuantiLum luciferase	Scaffold for next generation bioluminogenic assays	[208]
Cyclic alkylaminoluciferin	Replacement of phenolic hydroxyl of D-luciferin with alkylamino groups	607	Modified luciferase Ultra-Glo	Improved sensitivity of detection in high-throughput screening applications	[206]
D-napththylluciferin D-quinolylluciferin	Synthesis of 2-cyano-6-methoxy substituted naphthalene and quinolone compounds	524 608	Firefly luciferase	Mechanistic studies	[229]
Coumarylamino-luciferin	3-cyanocouramin derivatives bearing an amino group at the 7-position	530	Firefly luciferase	Application for BRET systems	[207]
Benzothiophene luciferin	Replaced the benzothiazole ring system with benzothiophene	523	Firefly luciferase	Greater sensitivity for analyte detection in applications longer-lived blues-shifted emission	[208]
Adenylated derivatives of D-LH2	Introduction of conjugated double bonds between aromatic parts and thiazoline ring of luciferin	675	Firefly luciferase	Suitable for bio-imaging of deep sites in living animals	[230]
Biphenyl-type luciferin analog	4,5-dihydrothiazoline ring connected directly to biphenyl moiety	675	Firefly luciferase	Stable luciferins that have possible application in deep tissue imaging	[231]
Caged luciferin	A red-shifted luciferin analog containing a selenium atom instead of sulfur atom on the thiazole position	600	Firefly luciferase	Useful for longitudinal studies of enzyme activites	[223]

(continued)

Table 2 (continued)

Substrate	Modification	λmax (nm)	Enzyme	Application	Reference
ViviRenTM & EnduRenTM	These contain small blocking groups that protect the oxygenation site with coelenterazine	480	Renilla luciferase	Orthotropic murine model of human glioblastoma expressing Rluc	[213]
Z-DEVD-aminoluciferin	Conserved recognition sequence caspase-3 and 7, conjugated to aminoluciferin	560	Firefly luciferase	Bioluminescent imaging of caspase activity	[222]
Methoxy-eCoelenterazine (Prolume purple)	A synthetic analog of e-Coelenterazine with an additional methoxy group	405	Renilla luciferase	Image tumors expressing NIR luciferase in mice	[221]
Furimazine	A different motif at position 2 of the imidazopyrazinone core: 2-furanylmethyl-deoxy-coelenterazine	490	NanoLuc	Fusion onto other proteins allows luminescent assays to image localization within cells and metabolism	[143]
Diphenylterazine	A coelenterazine analog which extends the coelenterazine conjugation system through an aromatic ring at C-8	>600	teLuc	Possible applications in the fields of chemistry, biology and biomedicine	[219]

λ_{max} = Emission wavelength

hydrolyzed by β-lactamases leads to a hydrolyzed β-lactam and the loss of a 3′ leaving group [242, 243], making it possible to design both fluorogenic and FRET probes targeted to this enzyme.

The high sensitivity of this approach is due to a combination of the fact that the substrate does not need to gain access to the bacterial cytoplasm, but only to the surface localized BlaC enzyme, and the fluorescent product can build up at the site of infection, enhancing signal. The custom REF probes carry an acetylated D-glucosamine connected to the carboxylate of cysteine through γ-amino-butyric acid, producing a charged molecule, that facilitates uptake into eukaryotic cells through transport via the D-glucosamine [70]. The fluorescent product is less membrane permeable, allowing the dye to be retained within the cell once the probe is within cells. The stability of the fluorescent product ensures proper localization of infected tissue and the ability to follow the site of infection in real-time. Also, probes used in REF are not limited by the number of tagged molecules but continuously produce more signal as long as the substrate is available. Use of BlaC ensures specificity due to its absence in mammals and presence only in tuberculosis-complex bacteria. The fact that BlaC is normally constitutively expressed by all wild type *M. tuberculosis* strains suggests that there are no metabolic impacts due to expression of this biomarker.

Comparison of the crystal structure of the *M. tuberculosis* β-lactamase, BlaC, to that of other similar enzymes, such as the *Escherichia coli* β-lactamase, TEM-1, reveals that BlaC has an unusually large active site pocket, suggesting that substrates with high specificity can be developed [244]. Adjustments in the β-lactam ring structure allowed extremely high specificity for the *M. tuberculosis* β-lactamase active site, generating a probe that can be used in a rapid point-of-care (POC) diagnostic system for TB. This REF system, designated REF-TB can sensitively and specifically detect TB in <10 min using unprocessed suspected TB-patient sputum [245]. REF-TB is promising for use in a true POC diagnostic that can detect as few as 1–10 CFU of *M. tuberculosis* in sputum and other specimens without the need for equipment, technological expertise or the infrastructure of a clinical laboratory. Since REF does not use reporter strains but an endogenous enzyme produced by the pathogen itself, it can be applied directly to sputum, tissue homogenates and any other clinical material. The REF-TB diagnostic probe, CDG-3, has been developed by modifying the structure of the probe to further improve sensitivity and specificity [246]. In a trial with 50 clinical samples, CDG-3 detected *M. tuberculosis* with 90% sensitivity and 73% specificity relative to *M. tuberculosis* culture, demonstrating its potential as a low-cost POC test for use in resource-limited areas. These characteristics, along with the very high catalytic activity of β-lactamase [247] make this enzyme a good choice for development of specific probes to detect TB and for imaging in live animals or patients.

Pharmacokinetics of the REF substrates and cleaved products play an important role in signal production for substrates used in animals and humans. Multiple administration of substrate could increase levels of substrate available and, thereby, signal from cleaved product. In addition, different routes of substrate administration, such as intra-peritoneal or intra-venous may produce somewhat different results in terms of signal. Detailed analysis of serum levels, followed by tissue levels of substrate and product at key time points that correspond to initial, peak and clearing levels can allow greater insight into optimal routes and frequencies of administration. The sensitivity of REF substrates can likely be improved through rational design of their structure structures, combined with analysis of the resulting activity relationships and pharmacokinetics. It has been suggested that large substrates would be tolerated well by BlaC, making it likely that numerous modifications can be evaluated and are expected to produce reasonable activity [244, 245]. Improving the sensitivity of REF substrates would enable this technology to better track *M. tuberculosis* in nearly any organ and at very early time points.

REF imaging can be used for bacterial detection without genetic modifications enabling its direct application to nearly any infection model. REF can be used to detect and image a wide array of pathogens, since fluorogenic substrates can be developed for numerous enzymatic targets other than BlaC, such as proteases, kinases, ureases and β-galactosidases. However, careful thought should be given to the target in order to ensure it displays optimal characteristics for imaging. BlaC represents a good model enzyme to develop REF technologies that will ensure successful application of this strategy, at least to tuberculosis. REF imaging provides an immediate read-out on bacterial load present in lungs during infections, speeding progress in the study of TB pathogenesis, since determination of bacterial numbers normally requires three to 6 weeks, but even in more rapid-growing organisms this approach could save investigators a great deal of time. Furthermore, REF imaging could also be used to discriminate carcinomas from TB, a key problem in diagnosis of nodular lesions in U.S. patients. REF serves as a novel tool to accelerate translational TB imaging and has the potential to be applied to humans, providing a strategy for rapid prediction of therapeutic outcomes.

Summary

Diverse technologies have been developed to facilitate optical imaging of *M. tuberculosis* that are constantly being improved to increase their scope and accuracy. Optical imaging strategies can be divided into three broad categories: (1) recombinant expression of fluorescent proteins, (2) bioluminescent imaging techniques, and (3) fluorescent and colorimetric probes for REF imaging that can be delivered exogenously and do not require genetically engineered markers. Each of these strategies has advantages and disadvantages, which is the most appropriate for a particular purpose requires a good understanding of these differences.

Fluorescent proteins provide a variety of imaging options, both in terms of brightness and wavelength. A variety of newly engineered fluorescent proteins can be used to visualize many bacterial species and/or individually tagged bacterial or host proteins simultaneously. This makes imaging via fluorescent proteins a flexible technique that can be applied to imaging needs in model systems ranging from *C. elegans* and zebrafish to a variety of mammalian hosts. Creation of extremely bright proteins such as tdTomato, the engineering of proteins of variable stability for time sensitive applications, and the development of proteins that fluoresce at near-infrared wavelengths to allow better penetration through mammalian tissues have been critical recent advances in fluorescent proteins. Fluorescent proteins can also be engineered to monitor different cellular processes, such as visualizing protein localization through fluorescent fusion proteins and monitoring gene expression through fluorescent reporter systems. However, all of these techniques require recombinant strains. Model systems also display high levels of auto-fluorescence, increasing the background seen in in vivo experiments and requiring spectral unmixing to differentiate signal from noise. Despite these issues, fluorescent protein imaging is extremely useful and has numerous applications for tuberculosis.

Bioluminescent imaging techniques generally have the advantage of very low background due to the fact that the energy driving luminescence is generated by specific chemical reactions rather than excitation of all tissue by a light source. Bacterial luminescence systems such as the *P. luminescens* Lux cassette have the advantage that there is no need for introduction of a luciferase substrate. Exploitation of insect and aquatic animal bioluminescence systems has allowed development of luminescent constructs that emit light at different wavelengths. The presence of multiple reporters allows for multiple targets to be visualized simultaneously. Similar to fluorescent proteins, most bioluminescent imaging techniques require recombinant engineering of the strain being studied, which limits applicability to strains where these systems have been introduced.

REF has the major advantage that it does not require for genetic engineering to allow optical imaging, since it uses endogenous enzymes as a target combined with a custom fluorogenic substrate. REF substrates are specifically activated upon cleavage of the β-lactam ring by the enzyme BlaC, which is endogenously expressed by all strains of *M. tuberculosis*. The REF technology allows a highly specific fluorescent signal to be emitted only in the presence of the bacteria at a long wavelength, helping to ensure low background and the catalytic nature makes REF more sensitive than fluorescence dependent upon the amount of fluorescent protein present. As a result, REF is likely to have a very low limit of detection. While this technique is relatively new compared to more common fluorescent protein and bioluminescent systems, the sensitivity and specificity of this technique, combined with the ability to apply it to any strain of *M. tuberculosis* without recombinant engineering, suggest that it holds great promise for the future.

Future Directions

Over the past decade, strides have been made in the field of real-time optical imaging improving the sensitivity and specificity of these technologies. However, to fully realize the potential of this technique, further developments are needed. While the development of near-infrared fluorescent proteins has drastically improved in vivo imaging, these proteins may be further optimized to improve brightness and stability in animals. Similarly, the limits of detection for luminescent in vivo imaging could be improved by development of systems that emit light at longer wavelengths. If this could be achieved in a similar system to the bacterial luminescent cassettes where exogenous substrates are not required, the potential of luminescent imaging would be greatly enhanced. Finally, the development of novel fluorescent substrates such as those used in REF imaging that display improved tissue penetration, decreased background, and improved specificity for *M. tuberculosis*, would obviate the need for recombinant strains that can impact virulence.

Arguably the most important long-term goal for real-time optical imaging of TB will be to move this technology from the bench into the clinic by developing novel technologies that can be used to aid in diagnosis and treatment of tuberculosis in patients. While recombinant fluorescent and luminescent strains do not have a clinical application, fluorescent probes such as those used in REF imaging have a number of potential clinical applications. REF imaging is already being tested for use as a diagnostic tool for human sputum with promising additional applications for this technology expected in the future [236]. Since REF has successfully been used to monitor fluorescent in real-time in animal models, it is reasonable to expect that REF can also be applied to diagnostic imaging in humans. REF may be applicable to diagnosis of tuberculosis in pediatric patients where the gold standard diagnostic technique of smear microscopy is ineffective [248]. Combination of REF with fiber-optic microendoscopy, rather than external illumination and signal collection, greatly enhances REF sensitivity, particularly in deep tissues like the lungs [249, 250]. While further development and testing of fluorescent probes and the detection systems is necessary before clinical applications are feasible, the clinical potential of real-time optical imaging will continue to grow as new technologies emerge.

Acknowledgements Support for this work was from the National Heart, Lung, and Blood Institute and the National Institute of Allergy and Infectious Diseases, National Institutes of Health (grants HL115463 [to Y. K.] and AI104960 [to J. D. C.]; and the Bill and Melinda Gates Foundation (grant 48523 to J. D. C.).

References

1. Andreu N, Zelmer A, Sampson SL, Ikeh M, Bancroft GJ, Schaible UE, Wiles S, Robertson BD. Rapid in vivo assessment of drug efficacy against Mycobacterium tuberculosis using an improved firefly luciferase. J Antimicrob Chemother. 2013;68:2118–27.
2. Andreu N, Zelmer A, Wiles S. Noninvasive biophotonic imaging for studies of infectious disease. FEMS Microbiol Rev. 2011;35:360–94.
3. Carroll P, Schreuder LJ, Muwanguzi-Karugaba J, Wiles S, Robertson BD, Ripoll J, Ward TH, Bancroft GJ, Schaible UE, Parish T. Sensitive detection of gene expression in mycobacteria under replicating and non-replicating conditions using optimized far-red reporters. PLoS One. 2010;5:e9823.
4. Hutchens M, Luker GD. Applications of bioluminescence imaging to the study of infectious diseases. Cell Microbiol. 2007;9:2315–22.
5. Jakobs S, Subramaniam V, Schonle A, Jovin TM, Hell SW. EFGP and DsRed expressing cultures of Escherichia coli imaged by confocal, two-photon and fluorescence lifetime microscopy. FEBS Lett. 2000;479:131–5.
6. Kim D, Hung CF, Wu TC. Monitoring the trafficking of adoptively transferred antigen- specific CD8-positive T cells in vivo, using noninvasive luminescence imaging. Hum Gene Ther. 2007;18:575–88.
7. Schweichel D, Steitz J, Tormo D, Gaffal E, Ferrer A, Buchs S, Speuser P, Limmer A, Tuting T. Evaluation of DNA vaccination with recombinant adenoviruses using bioluminescence imaging of antigen expression: impact of application routes and delivery with dendritic cells. J Gene Med. 2006;8:1243–50.
8. Winnard PT Jr, Kluth JB, Raman V. Noninvasive optical tracking of red fluorescent protein-expressing cancer cells in a model of metastatic breast cancer. Neoplasia. 2006;8:796–806.
9. Earl PL, Americo JL, Cotter CA, Moss B. Comparative live bioluminescence imaging of monkeypox virus dissemination in a wild-derived inbred mouse (Mus musculus castaneus) and outbred African dormouse (Graphiurus kelleni). Virology. 2015;475:150–8.
10. Evans MS, Chaurette JP, Adams ST Jr, Reddy GR, Paley MA, Aronin N, Prescher JA, Miller SC. A synthetic luciferin improves bioluminescence imaging in live mice. Nat Methods. 2014;11:393–5.
11. Gross S, Abraham U, Prior JL, Herzog ED, Piwnica-Worms D. Continuous delivery of D-luciferin by implanted micro-osmotic pumps enables true real-time bioluminescence imaging of luciferase activity in vivo. Mol Imaging. 2007;6:121–30.

12. Hiler DJ, Greenwald ML, Geusz ME. Imaging gene expression in live transgenic mice after providing luciferin in drinking water. Photochem Photobiol Sci. 2006;5:1082–5.
13. Lee S, Cha EJ, Park K, Lee SY, Hong JK, Sun IC, Kim SY, Choi K, Kwon IC, Kim K, Ahn CH. A near-infrared-fluorescence-quenched gold-nanoparticle imaging probe for in vivo drug screening and protease activity determination. Angew Chem Int Ed Engl. 2008;47:2804–7.
14. Luker KE, Luker GD. Applications of bioluminescence imaging to antiviral research and therapy: multiple luciferase enzymes and quantitation. Antivir Res. 2008;78:179–87.
15. Rudin M, Weissleder R. Molecular imaging in drug discovery and development. Nat Rev Drug Discov. 2003;2:123–31.
16. Baker M. Whole-animal imaging: the whole picture. Nature. 2010;463:977–80.
17. Weissleder R. A clearer vision for in vivo imaging. Nat Biotechnol. 2001;19:316–7.
18. Xu T, Close D, Handagama W, Marr E, Sayler G, Ripp S. The expanding toolbox of in vivo bioluminescent imaging. Front Oncol. 2016;6:150.
19. Avci P, Karimi M, Sadasivam M, Antunes-Melo WC, Carrasco E, Hamblin MR. In-vivo monitoring of infectious diseases in living animals using bioluminescence imaging. Virulence. 2018;9:28–63.
20. Kim JE, Kalimuthu S, Ahn BC. In vivo cell tracking with bioluminescence imaging. Nucl Med Mol Imaging. 2015;49:3–10.
21. Choy G, Choyke P, Libutti SK. Current advances in molecular imaging: noninvasive in vivo bioluminescent and fluorescent optical imaging in cancer research. Mol Imaging. 2003;2:303–12.
22. Rao J, Dragulescu-Andrasi A, Yao H. Fluorescence imaging in vivo: recent advances. Curr Opin Biotechnol. 2007;18:17–25.
23. Scheuer W, van Dam GM, Dobosz M, Schwaiger M, Ntziachristos V. Drug-based optical agents: infiltrating clinics at lower risk. Sci Transl Med. 2012;4:134ps11.
24. Hoffman RM. Use of fluorescent proteins and color-coded imaging to visualize cancer cells with different genetic properties. Cancer Metastasis Rev. 2016;35:5–19.
25. Licha K, Olbrich C. Optical imaging in drug discovery and diagnostic applications. Adv Drug Deliv Rev. 2005;57:1087–108.
26. Andreu N, Fletcher T, Krishnan N, Wiles S, Robertson BD. Rapid measurement of antituberculosis drug activity in vitro and in macrophages using bioluminescence. J Antimicrob Chemother. 2012;67:404–14.
27. Andreu N, Zelmer A, Fletcher T, Elkington PT, Ward TH, Ripoll J, Parish T, Bancroft GJ, Schaible U, Robertson BD, Wiles S. Optimisation of bioluminescent reporters for use with mycobacteria. PLoS One. 2010;5:e10777.
28. Kong Y, Yao H, Ren H, Subbian S, Cirillo SL, Sacchettini JC, Rao J, Cirillo JD. Imaging tuberculosis with endogenous beta-lactamase reporter enzyme fluorescence in live mice. Proc Natl Acad Sci U S A. 2010;107:12239–44.
29. Ollinger J, Bailey MA, Moraski GC, Casey A, Florio S, Alling T, Miller MJ, Parish T. A dual read-out assay to evaluate the potency of compounds active against *Mycobacterium tuberculosis*. PLoS One. 2013;8:e60531.
30. Singh V, Biswas RK, Singh BN. Double recombinant Mycobacterium bovis BCG strain for screening of primary and rationale-based antimycobacterial compounds. Antimicrob Agents Chemother. 2014;58:1389–96.
31. Vocat A, Hartkoorn RC, Lechartier B, Zhang M, Dhar N, Cole ST, Sala C. Bioluminescence for assessing drug potency against nonreplicating *Mycobacterium tuberculosis*. Antimicrob Agents Chemother. 2015;59:4012–9.
32. Zelmer A, Carroll P, Andreu N, Hagens K, Mahlo J, Redinger N, Robertson BD, Wiles S, Ward TH, Parish T, Ripoll J, Bancroft GJ, Schaible UE. A new in vivo model to test antituberculosis drugs using fluorescence imaging. J Antimicrob Chemother. 2012;67:1948–60.
33. Zhang T, Li SY, Nuermberger EL. Autoluminescent Mycobacterium tuberculosis for rapid, real-time, non-invasive assessment of drug and vaccine efficacy. PLoS One. 2012;7:e29774.
34. Passamaneck YJ, Di Gregorio A, Papaioannou VE, Hadjantonakis AK. Live imaging of fluorescent proteins in chordate embryos: from ascidians to mice. Microsc Res Tech. 2006;69:160–7.

35. Wacker SA, Oswald F, Wiedenmann J, Knochel W. A green to red photoconvertible protein as an analyzing tool for early vertebrate development. Dev Dyn. 2007;236:473–80.
36. Benard EL, van der Sar AM, Ellett F, Lieschke GJ, Spaink HP, Meijer AH. Infection of zebrafish embryos with intracellular bacterial pathogens. J Vis Exp. 2012;(61):e3781. https://doi.org/10.3791/3781.
37. Davis JM, Clay H, Lewis JL, Ghori N, Herbomel P, Ramakrishnan L. Real-time visualization of mycobacterium-macrophage interactions leading to initiation of granuloma formation in zebrafish embryos. Immunity. 2002;17:693–702.
38. van der Sar AM, Musters RJ, van Eeden FJ, Appelmelk BJ, Vandenbroucke-Grauls CM, Bitter W. Zebrafish embryos as a model host for the real time analysis of *Salmonella typhimurium* infections. Cell Microbiol. 2003;5:601–11.
39. Hoffman RM. Advantages of multi-color fluorescent proteins for whole-body and in vivo cellular imaging. J Biomed Opt. 2005;10:41202.
40. Seitz G, Warmann SW, Fuchs J, Mau-Holzmann UA, Ruck P, Heitmann H, Hoffman RM, Mahrt J, Muller GA, Wessels JT. Visualization of xenotransplanted human rhabdomyosarcoma after transfection with red fluorescent protein. J Pediatr Surg. 2006;41:1369–76.
41. Shcherbo D, Merzlyak EM, Chepurnykh TV, Fradkov AF, Ermakova GV, Solovieva EA, Lukyanov KA, Bogdanova EA, Zaraisky AG, Lukyanov S, Chudakov DM. Bright far-red fluorescent protein for whole-body imaging. Nat Methods. 2007;4:741–6.
42. Stewart CN Jr. Go with the glow: fluorescent proteins to light transgenic organisms. Trends Biotechnol. 2006;24:155–62.
43. Muller-Taubenberger A, Anderson KI. Recent advances using green and red fluorescent protein variants. Appl Microbiol Biotechnol. 2007;77:1–12.
44. Shaner NC, Steinbach PA, Tsien RY. A guide to choosing fluorescent proteins. Nat Methods. 2005;2:905–9.
45. Kong Y, Yang D, Cirillo SL, Li S, Akin A, Francis KP, Maloney T, Cirillo JD. Application of fluorescent protein expressing strains to evaluation of anti-tuberculosis therapeutic efficacy in vitro and in vivo. PLoS One. 2016;11:e0149972.
46. Glickman MS, Jacobs WR Jr. Microbial pathogenesis of *Mycobacterium tuberculosis*: dawn of a discipline. Cell. 2001;104:477–85.
47. Smith I. Mycobacterium tuberculosis pathogenesis and molecular determinants of virulence. Clin Microbiol Rev. 2003;16:463–96.
48. Zumla A, Raviglione M, Hafner R, Von Reyn CF. Tuberculosis. N Engl J Med. 2013;368:745–55.
49. Kong Y, Akin AR, Francis KP, Zhang N, Troy TL, Xie H, Rao J, Cirillo SL, Cirillo JD. Whole-body imaging of infection using fluorescence. Curr Protoc Microbiol. 2011; Chapter 2:Unit 2C.3.
50. Wilson T, Hastings JW. Bioluminescence. Annu Rev Cell Dev Biol. 1998;14:197–230.
51. Meighen EA. Molecular biology of bacterial bioluminescence. Microbiol Rev. 1991;55:123–42.
52. Hastings JW, Weber K, Friedland J, Eberhard A, Mitchell GW, Gunsalus A. Structurally distinct bacterial luciferases. Biochemistry. 1969;8:4681–9.
53. Contag CH, Contag PR, Mullins JI, Spilman SD, Stevenson DK, Benaron DA. Photonic detection of bacterial pathogens in living hosts. Mol Microbiol. 1995;18:593–603.
54. Francis KP, Joh D, Bellinger-Kawahara C, Hawkinson MJ, Purchio TF, Contag PR. Monitoring bioluminescent *Staphylococcus aureus* infections in living mice using a novel luxABCDE construct. Infect Immun. 2000;68:3594–600.
55. Francis KP, Yu J, Bellinger-Kawahara C, Joh D, Hawkinson MJ, Xiao G, Purchio TF, Caparon MG, Lipsitch M, Contag PR. Visualizing pneumococcal infections in the lungs of live mice using bioluminescent Streptococcus pneumoniae transformed with a novel gram-positive lux transposon. Infect Immun. 2001;69:3350–8.
56. Lorenz WW, Mccann RO, Longiaru M, Cormier MJ. Isolation and expression of a cDNA encoding *Renilla reniformis* luciferase. Proc Natl Acad Sci U S A. 1991;88:4438–42.

57. de Wet JR, Wood KV, Helinski DR, Deluca M. Cloning of firefly luciferase cDNA and the expression of active luciferase in *Escherichia coli*. Proc Natl Acad Sci U S A. 1985;82:7870–3.
58. Wood KV, Lam YA, Mcelroy WD. Introduction to beetle luciferases and their applications. J Biolumin Chemilumin. 1989;4:289–301.
59. Rice BW, Cable MD, Nelson MB. In vivo imaging of light-emitting probes. J Biomed Opt. 2001;6:432–40.
60. Zhao H, Doyle TC, Coquoz O, Kalish F, Rice BW, Contag CH. Emission spectra of bioluminescent reporters and interaction with mammalian tissue determine the sensitivity of detection in vivo. J Biomed Opt. 2005;10:41210.
61. Troy T, Jekic-Mcmullen D, Sambucetti L, Rice B. Quantitative comparison of the sensitivity of detection of fluorescent and bioluminescent reporters in animal models. Mol Imaging. 2004;3:9–23.
62. Chang M, Anttonen KP, Cirillo SL, Francis KP, Cirillo JD. Real-time bioluminescence imaging of mixed mycobacterial infections. PLoS One. 2014;9:e108341.
63. Flores AR, Parsons LM, Pavelka MS, Jr. Genetic analysis of the beta-lactamases of *Mycobacterium tuberculosis* and *Mycobacterium smegmatis* and susceptibility to beta-lactam antibiotics. Microbiology. 2005;151:521–32.
64. Hugonnet JE, Blanchard JS. Irreversible inhibition of the *Mycobacterium tuberculosis* beta-lactamase by clavulanate. Biochemistry. 2007;46:11998–2004.
65. Ioerger TR, Feng Y, Chen X, Dobos KM, Victor TC, Streicher EM, Warren RM, van Pittius NCG, van Helden PD, Sacchettini JC. The non-clonality of drug resistance in Beijing-genotype isolates of Mycobacterium tuberculosis from the Western Cape of South Africa. BMC Genomics. 2010;11:670.
66. Voladri RK, Lakey DL, Hennigan SH, Menzies BE, Edwards KM, Kernodle DS. Recombinant expression and characterization of the major beta-lactamase of Mycobacterium tuberculosis. Antimicrob Agents Chemother. 1998;42:1375–81.
67. Zlokarnik G, Negulescu PA, Knapp TE, Mere L, Burres N, Feng L, Whitney M, Roemer K, Tsien RY. Quantitation of transcription and clonal selection of single living cells with beta-lactamase as reporter. Science. 1998;279:84–8.
68. Kong Y, Cirillo JD. Reporter enzyme fluorescence (REF) imaging and quantification of tuberculosis in live animals. Virulence. 2010;1:558–62.
69. Yang HJ, Kong Y, Cheng Y, Janagama H, Hassounah H, Xie H, Rao J, Cirillo JD. Real-time imaging of *Mycobacterium tuberculosis*, using a novel near-infrared fluorescent substrate. J Infect Dis. 2017;215:405–14.
70. Xing B, Khanamiryan A, Rao J. Cell-permeable near-infrared fluorogenic substrates for imaging beta-lactamase activity. J Am Chem Soc. 2005;127:4158–9.
71. Siragusa GR, Nawotka K, Spilman SD, Contag PR, Contag CH. Real-time monitoring of Escherichia coli O157:H7 adherence to beef carcass surface tissues with a bioluminescent reporter. Appl Environ Microbiol. 1999;65:1738–45.
72. Wiles S, Pickard KM, Peng K, Macdonald TT, Frankel G. In vivo bioluminescence imaging of the murine pathogen *Citrobacter rodentium*. Infect Immun. 2006;74:5391–6.
73. Xiong YQ, Willard J, Kadurugamuwa JL, Yu J, Francis KP, Bayer AS. Real-time in vivo bioluminescent imaging for evaluating the efficacy of antibiotics in a rat Staphylococcus aureus endocarditis model. Antimicrob Agents Chemother. 2005;49:380–7.
74. Lagendijk EL, Validov S, Lamers GE, De Weert S, Bloemberg GV. Genetic tools for tagging gram-negative bacteria with mCherry for visualization in vitro and in natural habitats, biofilm and pathogenicity studies. FEMS Microbiol Lett. 2010;305:81–90.
75. Lee J, Attila C, Cirillo SL, Cirillo JD, Wood TK. Indole and 7-hydroxyindole diminish *Pseudomonas aeruginosa* virulence. Microb Biotechnol. 2009;2:75–90.
76. Wang X, Li Z, Li B, Chi H, Li J, Fan H, Yao R, Li Q, Dong X, Chen M, Qu H, et al. Bioluminescence imaging of colonization and clearance dynamics of Brucella Suis vaccine strain S2 in mice and guinea pigs. Mol Imaging Biol. 2016;18:519–26.
77. Chen CH, Durand E, Wang J, Zon LI, Poss KD. Zebraflash transgenic lines for in vivo bioluminescence imaging of stem cells and regeneration in adult zebrafish. Development. 2013;140:4988–97.

78. Liang MR, Alestrom P, Collas P. Glowing zebrafish: integration, transmission, and expression of a single luciferase transgene promoted by noncovalent DNA-nuclear transport peptide complexes. Mol Reprod Dev. 2000;55:8–13.
79. Mayerhofer R, Araki K, Szalay AA. Monitoring of spatial expression of firefly luciferase in transformed zebrafish. J Biolumin Chemilumin. 1995;10:271–5.
80. Weger M, Weger BD, Diotel N, Rastegar S, Hirota T, Kay SA, Strahle U, Dickmeis T. Real-time in vivo monitoring of circadian E-box enhancer activity: a robust and sensitive zebrafish reporter line for developmental, chemical and neural biology of the circadian clock. Dev Biol. 2013;380:259–73.
81. Karlsson EA, Meliopoulos VA, Savage C, Livingston B, Mehle A, Schultz-Cherry S. Visualizing real-time influenza virus infection, transmission and protection in ferrets. Nat Commun. 2015;6:6378.
82. Galbadage T, Shepherd TF, Cirillo SL, Gumienny TL, Cirillo JD. The Caenorhabditis elegans p38 MAPK gene plays a key role in protection from mycobacteria. Microbiology. 2016;5:436–52.
83. Galbadage T, Hartman PS. Repeated temperature fluctuation extends the life span of Caenorhabditis elegans in a daf-16-dependent fashion. Mech Ageing Dev. 2008;129:507–14.
84. Tarantal AF, Lee CC. Long-term luciferase expression monitored by bioluminescence imaging after adeno-associated virus-mediated fetal gene delivery in rhesus monkeys (*Macaca mulatta*). Hum Gene Ther. 2010;21:143–8.
85. Tarantal AF, Lee CC, Jimenez DF, Cherry SR. Fetal gene transfer using lentiviral vectors: in vivo detection of gene expression by microPET and optical imaging in fetal and infant monkeys. Hum Gene Ther. 2006;17:1254–61.
86. Greives MR, Aldrich MB, Sevick-Muraca EM, Rasmussen JC. Near-infrared fluorescence lymphatic imaging of a toddler with congenital lymphedema. Pediatrics. 2017;139:e20154456.
87. Marshall MV, Rasmussen JC, Tan IC, Aldrich MB, Adams KE, Wang X, Fife CE, Maus EA, Smith LA, Sevick-Muraca EM. Near-infrared fluorescence imaging in humans with indocyanine green: a review and update. Open Surg Oncol J. 2010;2:12–25.
88. Corlu A, Choe R, Durduran T, Rosen MA, Schweiger M, Arridge SR, Schnall MD, Yodh AG. Three-dimensional in vivo fluorescence diffuse optical tomography of breast cancer in humans. Opt Express. 2007;15:6696–716.
89. Intes X, Ripoll J, Chen Y, Nioka S, Yodh AG, Chance B. In vivo continuous-wave optical breast imaging enhanced with Indocyanine Green. Med Phys. 2003;30:1039–47.
90. Piper SK, Habermehl C, Schmitz CH, Kuebler WM, Obrig H, Steinbrink J, Mehnert J. Towards whole-body fluorescence imaging in humans. PLoS One. 2013;8:e83749.
91. Verjans JW, Jaffer FA. Biological imaging of atherosclerosis: moving beyond anatomy. J Cardiovasc Transl Res. 2013;6:681–94.
92. Mezzanotte L, An N, Mol IM, Löwik CW, Kaijzel EL. A new multicolor bioluminescence imaging platform to investigate NF-kappaB activity and apoptosis in human breast cancer cells. PLoS One. 2014;9:e85550.
93. Subach FV, Verkhusha VV. Chromophore transformations in red fluorescent proteins. Chem Rev. 2012;112:4308–27.
94. Tomosugi W, Matsuda T, Tani T, Nemoto T, Kotera I, Saito K, Horikawa K, Nagai T. An ultramarine fluorescent protein with increased photostability and pH insensitivity. Nat Methods. 2009;6:351–3.
95. Rizzo MA, Springer GH, Granada B, Piston DW. An improved cyan fluorescent protein variant useful for FRET. Nat Biotechnol. 2004;22:445–9.
96. Kremers GJ, Goedhart J, van Munster EB, Gadella TW Jr. Cyan and yellow super fluorescent proteins with improved brightness, protein folding, and FRET Forster radius. Biochemistry. 2006;45:6570–80.
97. Goedhart J, Van Weeren L, Hink MA, Vischer NO, Jalink K, Gadella TW Jr. Bright cyan fluorescent protein variants identified by fluorescence lifetime screening. Nat Methods. 2010;7:137–9.

98. Griesbeck O, Baird GS, Campbell RE, Zacharias DA, Tsien RY. Reducing the environmental sensitivity of yellow fluorescent protein. Mechanism and applications. J Biol Chem. 2001;276:29188–94.
99. Nagai T, Ibata K, Park ES, Kubota M, Mikoshiba K, Miyawaki A. A variant of yellow fluorescent protein with fast and efficient maturation for cell-biological applications. Nat Biotechnol. 2002;20:87–90.
100. Cubitt AB, Woollenweber LA, Heim R. Understanding structure-function relationships in the Aequorea victoria green fluorescent protein. Methods Cell Biol. 1999;58:19–30.
101. Shcherbo D, Souslova EA, Goedhart J, Chepurnykh TV, Gaintzeva A, Shemiakina II, Gadella TW, Lukyanov S, Chudakov DM. Practical and reliable FRET/FLIM pair of fluorescent proteins. BMC Biotechnol. 2009b;9:24.
102. Karasawa S, Araki T, Nagai T, Mizuno H, Miyawaki A. Cyan-emitting and orange-emitting fluorescent proteins as a donor/acceptor pair for fluorescence resonance energy transfer. Biochem J. 2004;381:307–12.
103. Wang L, Jackson WC, Steinbach PA, Tsien RY. Evolution of new nonantibody proteins via iterative somatic hypermutation. Proc Natl Acad Sci U S A. 2004;101:16745–9.
104. Shcherbo D, Murphy CS, Ermakova GV, Solovieva EA, Chepurnykh TV, Shcheglov AS, Verkhusha VV, Pletnev VZ, Hazelwood KL, Roche PM, Lukyanov S, Zaraisky AG, Davidson MW, Chudakov DM. Far-red fluorescent tags for protein imaging in living tissues. Biochem J. 2009a;418:567–74.
105. Lin MZ, Mckeown MR, Ng HL, Aguilera TA, Shaner NC, Campbell RE, Adams SR, Gross LA, Ma W, Alber T, Tsien RY. Autofluorescent proteins with excitation in the optical window for intravital imaging in mammals. Chem Biol. 2009;16:1169–79.
106. Kogure T, Karasawa S, Araki T, Saito K, Kinjo M, Miyawaki A. A fluorescent variant of a protein from the stony coral Montipora facilitates dual-color single-laser fluorescence cross-correlation spectroscopy. Nat Biotechnol. 2006;24:577–81.
107. Volkman HE, Pozos TC, Zheng J, Davis JM, Rawls JF, Ramakrishnan L. Tuberculous granuloma induction via interaction of a bacterial secreted protein with host epithelium. Science. 2010;327:466–9.
108. Cosma CL, Humbert O, Ramakrishnan L. Superinfecting mycobacteria home to established tuberculous granulomas. Nat Immunol. 2004;5:828–35.
109. Tobin DM, Vary JC Jr, Ray JP, Walsh GS, Dunstan SJ, Bang ND, Hagge DA, Khadge S, King MC, Hawn TR, Moens CB. The lta4h locus modulates susceptibility to mycobacterial infection in zebrafish and humans. Cell. 2010;140:717–30.
110. Volkman HE, Clay H, Beery D, Chang JC, Sherman DR, Ramakrishnan L. Tuberculous granuloma formation is enhanced by a mycobacterium virulence determinant. PLoS Biol. 2004;2:e367.
111. Clay H, Davis JM, Beery D, Huttenlocher A, Lyons SE, Ramakrishnan L. Dichotomous role of the macrophage in early *Mycobacterium marinum* infection of the zebrafish. Cell Host Microbe. 2007;2:29–39.
112. Yang CT, Cambier CJ, Davis JM, Hall CJ, Crosier PS, Ramakrishnan L. Neutrophils exert protection in the early tuberculous granuloma by oxidative killing of mycobacteria phagocytosed from infected macrophages. Cell Host Microbe. 2012;12:301–12.
113. Berg RD, Levitte S, O'sullivan MP, O'leary SM, Cambier CJ, Cameron J, Takaki KK, Moens CB, Tobin DM, Keane J, Ramakrishnan L. Lysosomal disorders drive susceptibility to tuberculosis by compromising macrophage migration. Cell. 2016;165:139–52.
114. Bernut A, Nguyen-Chi M, Halloum I, Herrmann JL, Lutfalla G, Kremer L. *Mycobacterium abscessus*-induced granuloma formation is strictly dependent on TNF signaling and neutrophil trafficking. PLoS Pathog. 2016;12:e1005986.
115. Boot M, Jim KK, Liu T, Commandeur S, Lu P, Verboom T, Lill H, Bitter W, Bald D. A fluorescence-based reporter for monitoring expression of mycobacterial cytochrome bd in response to antibacterials and during infection. Sci Rep. 2017;7:10665.
116. Levitte S, Adams KN, Berg RD, Cosma CL, Urdahl KB, Ramakrishnan L. Mycobacterial acid tolerance enables phagolysosomal survival and establishment of tuberculous infection in vivo. Cell Host Microbe. 2016;20:250–8.

117. Smith AM, Mancini MC, Nie S. Bioimaging: second window for in vivo imaging. Nat Nanotechnol. 2009;4:710–1.
118. Pansare V, Hejazi S, Faenza W, Prud'homme RK. Review of long-wavelength optical and NIR imaging materials: contrast agents, fluorophores and multifunctional nano carriers. Chem Mater. 2012;24:812–27.
119. Heim R, Tsien RY. Engineering green fluorescent protein for improved brightness, longer wavelengths and fluorescence resonance energy transfer. Curr Biol. 1996;6:178–82.
120. Miyawaki A, Llopis J, Heim R, Mccaffery JM, Adams JA, Ikura M, Tsien RY. Fluorescent indicators for Ca2+ based on green fluorescent proteins and calmodulin. Nature. 1997;388:882–7.
121. Romoser VA, Hinkle PM, Persechini A. Detection in living cells of Ca2+–dependent changes in the fluorescence emission of an indicator composed of two green fluorescent protein variants linked by a calmodulin-binding sequence. A new class of fluorescent indicators. J Biol Chem. 1997;272:13270–4.
122. Seksek O, Biwersi J, Verkman AS. Direct measurement of trans-Golgi pH in living cells and regulation by second messengers. J Biol Chem. 1995;270:4967–70.
123. Lippincott-Schwartz J, Snapp E, Kenworthy A. Studying protein dynamics in living cells. Nat Rev Mol Cell Biol. 2001;2:444–56.
124. Nehls S, Snapp EL, Cole NB, Zaal KJ, Kenworthy AK, Roberts TH, Ellenberg J, Presley JF, Siggia E, Lippincott-Schwartz J. Dynamics and retention of misfolded proteins in native ER membranes. Nat Cell Biol. 2000;2:288–95.
125. Heim R, Prasher DC, Tsien RY. Wavelength mutations and posttranslational autoxidation of green fluorescent protein. Proc Natl Acad Sci U S A. 1994;91:12501–4.
126. Prendergast FG. Biophysics of the green fluorescent protein. Methods Cell Biol. 1999;58:1–18.
127. Baird GS, Zacharias DA, Tsien RY. Biochemistry, mutagenesis, and oligomerization of DsRed, a red fluorescent protein from coral. Proc Natl Acad Sci U S A. 2000;97:11984–9.
128. Bevis BJ, Glick BS. Rapidly maturing variants of the discosoma red fluorescent protein (DsRed). Nat Biotechnol. 2002;20:83–7.
129. Terskikh A, Fradkov A, Ermakova G, Zaraisky A, Tan P, Kajava AV, Zhao X, Lukyanov S, Matz M, Kim S, Weissman I, Siebert P. "Fluorescent timer": protein that changes color with time. Science. 2000;290:1585–8.
130. Yang F, Moss LG, Phillips GN Jr. The molecular structure of green fluorescent protein. Nat Biotechnol. 1996;14:1246–51.
131. Andresen M, Schmitz-Salue R, Jakobs S. Short tetracysteine tags to beta-tubulin demonstrate the significance of small labels for live cell imaging. Mol Biol Cell. 2004;15:5616–22.
132. Davis SJ, Vierstra RD. Soluble, highly fluorescent variants of green fluorescent protein (GFP) for use in higher plants. Plant Mol Biol. 1998;36:521–8.
133. Sheff MA, Thorn KS. Optimized cassettes for fluorescent protein tagging in *Saccharomyces cerevisiae*. Yeast. 2004;21:661–70.
134. Patterson GH, Knobel SM, Sharif WD, Kain SR, Piston DW. Use of the green fluorescent protein and its mutants in quantitative fluorescence microscopy. Biophys J. 1997;73:2782–90.
135. Triccas JA, Berthet FX, Pelicic V, Gicquel B. Use of fluorescence induction and sucrose counterselection to identify *Mycobacterium tuberculosis* genes expressed within host cells. Microbiology. 1999;145(Pt 10):2923–30.
136. Kong Y, Cirillo JD. Fluorescence imaging of mycobacterial infection in live mice using fluorescent protein-expressing strains. Methods Mol Biol. 2018;1790:75–85.
137. Sharma S, Gelman E, Narayan C, Bhattacharjee D, Achar V, Humnabadkar V, Balasubramanian V, Ramachandran V, Dhar N, Dinesh N. Simple and rapid method to determine antimycobacterial potency of compounds by using autoluminescent *Mycobacterium tuberculosis*. Antimicrob Agents Chemother. 2014;58:5801–8.
138. Hsiang CY, Hseu YC, Chang YC, Kumar KJ, Ho TY, Yang HL. Toona sinensis and its major bioactive compound gallic acid inhibit LPS-induced inflammation in nuclear factor-kappaB transgenic mice as evaluated by in vivo bioluminescence imaging. Food Chem. 2013;136:426–34.

139. Maguire CA, Bovenberg MS, Crommentuijn MH, Niers JM, Kerami M, Teng J, Sena-Esteves M, Badr CE, Tannous BA. Triple bioluminescence imaging for in vivo monitoring of cellular processes. Mol Ther Nucleic Acids. 2013;2:e99.
140. Muranaka T, Kubota S, Oyama T. A single-cell bioluminescence imaging system for monitoring cellular gene expression in a plant body. Plant Cell Physiol. 2013;54:2085–93.
141. Meighen EA. Bacterial bioluminescence: organization, regulation, and application of the lux genes. FASEB J. 1993;7:1016–22.
142. Baldwin TO. Firefly luciferase: the structure is known, but the mystery remains. Structure. 1996;4:223–8.
143. Hall MP, Unch J, Binkowski BF, Valley MP, Butler BL, Wood MG, Otto P, Zimmerman K, Vidugiris G, Machleidt T, Robers MB, Benink HA, Eggers CT, Slater MR, Meisenheimer PL, Klaubert DH, Fan F, Encell LP, Wood KV. Engineered luciferase reporter from a deep sea shrimp utilizing a novel imidazopyrazinone substrate. ACS Chem Biol. 2012;7:1848–57.
144. Heise K, Oppermann H, Meixensberger J, Gebhardt R, Gaunitz F. Dual luciferase assay for secreted luciferases based on Gaussia and NanoLuc. Assay Drug Dev Technol. 2013;11:244–52.
145. Inouye S, Ohmiya Y, Toya Y, Tsuji FI. Imaging of luciferase secretion from transformed Chinese hamster ovary cells. Proc Natl Acad Sci U S A. 1992;89:9584–7.
146. Hastings JW, Potrikus CJ, Gupta SC, Kurfurst M, Makemson JC. Biochemistry and physiology of bioluminescent bacteria. Adv Microb Physiol. 1985;26:235–91.
147. Gahan CG. The bacterial lux reporter system: applications in bacterial localisation studies. Curr Gene Ther. 2012;12:12–9.
148. Demidova TN, Gad F, Zahra T, Francis KP, Hamblin MR. Monitoring photodynamic therapy of localized infections by bioluminescence imaging of genetically engineered bacteria. J Photochem Photobiol B. 2005;81:15–25.
149. Van Staden ADP, Heunis T, Smith C, Deane S, Dicks LM. Efficacy of lantibiotic treatment of *Staphylococcus aureus*-induced skin infections, monitored by in vivo bioluminescent imaging. Antimicrob Agents Chemother. 2016;60:3948–55.
150. Dai T, Tegos GP, Zhiyentayev T, Mylonakis E, Hamblin MR. Photodynamic therapy for methicillin-resistant *Staphylococcus aureus* infection in a mouse skin abrasion model. Lasers Surg Med. 2010;42:38–44.
151. Vecchio D, Dai T, Huang L, Fantetti L, Roncucci G, Hamblin MR. Antimicrobial photodynamic therapy with RLP068 kills methicillin-resistant Staphylococcus aureus and improves wound healing in a mouse model of infected skin abrasion PDT with RLP068/Cl in infected mouse skin abrasion. J Biophotonics. 2013;6:733–42.
152. Branchini BR, Southworth TL, Deangelis JP, Roda A, Michelini E. Luciferase from the Italian firefly *Luciola italica*: molecular cloning and expression. Comp Biochem Physiol B Biochem Mol Biol. 2006;145:159–67.
153. Maguire CA, Van Der Mijn JC, Degeling MH, Morse D, Tannous BA. Codon-optimized *Luciola italica* luciferase variants for mammalian gene expression in culture and in vivo. Mol Imaging. 2012;11:13–21.
154. Andrew PW, Roberts IS. Construction of a bioluminescent mycobacterium and its use for assay of antimycobacterial agents. J Clin Microbiol. 1993;31:2251–4.
155. Heuts F, Carow B, Wigzell H, Rottenberg ME. Use of non-invasive bioluminescent imaging to assess mycobacterial dissemination in mice, treatment with bactericidal drugs and protective immunity. Microbes Infect. 2009;11:1114–21.
156. Zhang T, Li SY, Converse PJ, Almeida DV, Grosset JH, Nuermberger EL. Using bioluminescence to monitor treatment response in real time in mice with *Mycobacterium ulcerans* infection. Antimicrob Agents Chemother. 2011;55:56–61.
157. Hakamata Y, Murakami T, Kobayashi E. "Firefly rats" as an organ/cellular source for long-term in vivo bioluminescent imaging. Transplantation. 2006;81:1179–84.
158. Mcgregor A, Choi KY. Cytomegalovirus antivirals and development of improved animal models. Expert Opin Drug Metab Toxicol. 2011;7:1245–65.

159. Moore HA, Whitmore D. Circadian rhythmicity and light sensitivity of the zebrafish brain. PLoS One. 2014;9:e86176.
160. Kaneko M, Cahill GM. Light-dependent development of circadian gene expression in transgenic zebrafish. PLoS Biol. 2005;3:e34.
161. Lagido C, Mclaggan D, Flett A, Pettitt J, Glover LA. Rapid sublethal toxicity assessment using bioluminescent *Caenorhabditis elegans*, a novel whole-animal metabolic biosensor. Toxicol Sci. 2009;109:88–95.
162. Tarantal AF, Lee CC, Batchelder CA, Christensen JE, Prater D, Cherry SR. Radiolabeling and in vivo imaging of transplanted renal lineages differentiated from human embryonic stem cells in fetal rhesus monkeys. Mol Imaging Biol. 2012;14:197–204.
163. Dalton JP, Uy B, Okuda KS, Hall CJ, Denny WA, Crosier PS, Swift S, Wiles S. Screening of anti-mycobacterial compounds in a naturally infected zebrafish larvae model. J Antimicrob Chemother. 2017;72:421–7.
164. Meighen EA, Dunlap PV. Physiological, biochemical and genetic control of bacterial bioluminescence. Adv Microb Physiol. 1993;34:1–67.
165. Lee CY, Szittner RB, Meighen EA. The lux genes of the luminous bacterial symbiont, *Photobacterium leiognathi*, of the ponyfish. Nucleotide sequence, difference in gene organization, and high expression in mutant *Escherichia coli*. Eur J Biochem. 1991;201:161–7.
166. Eckstein JW, Cho KW, Colepicolo P, Ghisla S, Hastings JW, Wilson T. A time-dependent bacterial bioluminescence emission spectrum in an in vitro single turnover system: energy transfer alone cannot account for the yellow emission of *Vibrio fischeri* Y-1. Proc Natl Acad Sci U S A. 1990;87:1466–70.
167. O'kane DJ, Prasher DC. Evolutionary origins of bacterial bioluminescence. Mol Microbiol. 1992;6:443–9.
168. Cao JG, Meighen EA. Purification and structural identification of an autoinducer for the luminescence system of *Vibrio harveyi*. J Biol Chem. 1989;264:21670–6.
169. Eberhard A, Burlingame AL, Eberhard C, Kenyon GL, Nealson KH, Oppenheimer NJ. Structural identification of autoinducer of *Photobacterium fischeri* luciferase. Biochemistry. 1981;20:2444–9.
170. Engebrecht J, Nealson K, Silverman M. Bacterial bioluminescence: isolation and genetic analysis of functions from *Vibrio fischeri*. Cell. 1983;32:773–81.
171. Engebrecht J, Silverman M. Identification of genes and gene products necessary for bacterial bioluminescence. Proc Natl Acad Sci U S A. 1984;81:4154–8.
172. Rocchetta HL, Boylan CJ, Foley JW, Iversen PW, Letourneau DL, Mcmillian CL, Contag PR, Jenkins DE, Parr TR, Jr. Validation of a noninvasive, real-time imaging technology using bioluminescent *Escherichia coli* in the neutropenic mouse thigh model of infection. Antimicrob Agents Chemother. 2001;45:129–37.
173. Wiles S, Clare S, Harker J, Huett A, Young D, Dougan G, Frankel G. Organ specificity, colonization and clearance dynamics in vivo following oral challenges with the murine pathogen Citrobacter rodentium. Cell Microbiol. 2004;6:963–72.
174. Hardy J, Francis KP, Deboer M, Chu P, Gibbs K, Contag CH. Extracellular replication of *Listeria monocytogenes* in the murine gall bladder. Science. 2004;303:851–3.
175. Sanli G, Blaber SI, Blaber M. Reduction of wobble-position GC bases in Corynebacteria genes and enhancement of PCR and heterologous expression. J Mol Microbiol Biotechnol. 2001;3:123–6.
176. Craney A, Hohenauer T, Xu Y, Navani NK, Li Y, Nodwell J. A synthetic luxCDABE gene cluster optimized for expression in high-GC bacteria. Nucleic Acids Res. 2007;35:e46.
177. Qazi SN, Counil E, Morrissey J, Rees CE, Cockayne A, Winzer K, Chan WC, Williams P, Hill PJ. agr Expression precedes escape of internalized *Staphylococcus aureus* from the host endosome. Infect Immun. 2001;69:7074–82.
178. Ranes MG, Rauzier J, Lagranderie M, Gheorghiu M, Gicquel B. Functional analysis of pAL5000, a plasmid from *Mycobacterium fortuitum*: construction of a "mini" mycobacterium-Escherichia coli shuttle vector. J Bacteriol. 1990;172:2793–7.

179. Stover CK, de la Cruz VF, Fuerst TR, Burlein JE, Benson LA, Bennett LT, Bansal GP, Young JF, Lee MH, Hatfull GF, et al. New use of BCG for recombinant vaccines. Nature. 1991;351:456–60.
180. Bourn WR, Jansen Y, Stutz H, Warren RM, Williamson AL, van Helden PD. Creation and characterisation of a high-copy-number version of the pAL5000 mycobacterial replicon. Tuberculosis (Edinb). 2007;87:481–8.
181. Baggett B, Roy R, Momen S, Morgan S, Tisi L, Morse D, Gillies RJ. Thermostability of firefly luciferases affects efficiency of detection by in vivo bioluminescence. Mol Imaging. 2004;3:324–32.
182. Gupta RK, Patterson SS, Ripp S, Simpson ML, Sayler GS. Expression of the *Photorhabdus luminescens lux* genes (luxA, B, C, D, and E) in Saccharomyces cerevisiae. FEMS Yeast Res. 2003;4:305–13.
183. Close DM, Patterson SS, Ripp S, Baek SJ, Sanseverino J, Sayler GS. Autonomous bioluminescent expression of the bacterial luciferase gene cassette (lux) in a mammalian cell line. PLoS One. 2010;5:e12441.
184. Deluca M, Mcelroy WD. Two kinetically distinguishable ATP sites in firefly luciferase. Biochem Biophys Res Commun. 1984;123:764–70.
185. Seliger HH, Mcelroy WD. The colors of firefly bioluminescence: enzyme configuration and species specificity. Proc Natl Acad Sci U S A. 1964;52:75–81.
186. Bhaumik S, Lewis XZ, Gambhir SS. Optical imaging of Renilla luciferase, synthetic Renilla luciferase, and firefly luciferase reporter gene expression in living mice. J Biomed Opt. 2004;9:578–86.
187. Bowlby MR, Case JF. Ultrastructure and neuronal control of luminous cells in the copepod Gaussia princeps. Biol Bull. 1991;180:440–6.
188. Matthews JC, Hori K, Cormier MJ. Purification and properties of Renilla reniformis luciferase. Biochemistry. 1977;16:85–91.
189. Tannous BA, Kim DE, Fernandez JL, Weissleder R, Breakefield XO. Codon-optimized Gaussia luciferase cDNA for mammalian gene expression in culture and in vivo. Mol Ther. 2005;11:435–43.
190. Santos EB, Yeh R, Lee J, Nikhamin Y, Punzalan B, Punzalan B, La Perle K, Larson SM, Sadelain M, Brentjens RJ. Sensitive in vivo imaging of T cells using a membrane-bound Gaussia princeps luciferase. Nat Med. 2009;15:338–44.
191. Stacer AC, Nyati S, Moudgil P, Iyengar R, Luker KE, Rehemtulla A, Luker GD. NanoLuc reporter for dual luciferase imaging in living animals. Mol Imaging. 2013;12:1–13.
192. Luker GD, Bardill JP, Prior JL, Pica CM, Piwnica-Worms D, Leib DA. Noninvasive bioluminescence imaging of herpes simplex virus type 1 infection and therapy in living mice. J Virol. 2002;76:12149–61.
193. Saxena MT, Aton SJ, Hildebolt C, Prior JL, Abraham U, Piwnica-Worms D, Herzog ED. Bioluminescence imaging of period1 gene expression in utero. Mol Imaging. 2007;6:68–72.
194. Zhao H, Doyle TC, Wong RJ, Cao Y, Stevenson DK, Piwnica-Worms D, Contag CH. Characterization of coelenterazine analogs for measurements of Renilla luciferase activity in live cells and living animals. Mol Imaging. 2004;3:43–54.
195. Pichler A, Prior JL, Piwnica-Worms D. Imaging reversal of multidrug resistance in living mice with bioluminescence: MDR1 P-glycoprotein transports coelenterazine. Proc Natl Acad Sci U S A. 2004;101:1702–7.
196. Riedel CU, Monk IR, Casey PG, Morrissey D, O'sullivan GC, Tangney M, Hill C, Gahan CG. Improved luciferase tagging system for *Listeria monocytogenes* allows real-time monitoring in vivo and in vitro. Appl Environ Microbiol. 2007;73:3091–4.
197. Ur Rahman S, Stanton M, Casey PG, Spagnuolo A, Bensi G, Hill C, Francis KP, Tangney M, Gahan CG. Development of a click beetle luciferase reporter system for enhanced bioluminescence imaging of *Listeria monocytogenes*: analysis in cell culture and murine infection models. Front Microbiol. 2017;8:1797.

198. Fujii H, Noda K, Asami Y, Kuroda A, Sakata M, Tokida A. Increase in bioluminescence intensity of firefly luciferase using genetic modification. Anal Biochem. 2007;366:131–6.
199. Branchini BR, Ablamsky DM, Murtiashaw MH, Uzasci L, Fraga H, Southworth TL. Thermostable red and green light-producing firefly luciferase mutants for bioluminescent reporter applications. Anal Biochem. 2007;361:253–62.
200. Doyle TC, Nawotka KA, Purchio AF, Akin AR, Francis KP, Contag PR. Expression of firefly luciferase in *Candida albicans* and its use in the selection of stable transformants. Microb Pathog. 2006;40:69–81.
201. Enjalbert B, Rachini A, Vediyappan G, Pietrella D, Spaccapelo R, Vecchiarelli A, Brown AJ, D'enfert C. A multifunctional, synthetic Gaussia princeps luciferase reporter for live imaging of Candida albicans infections. Infect Immun. 2009;77:4847–58.
202. Branchini BR, Southworth TL, Khattak NF, Michelini E, Roda A. Red- and green-emitting firefly luciferase mutants for bioluminescent reporter applications. Anal Biochem. 2005;345:140–8.
203. Dorsaz S, Coste AT, Sanglard D. Red-shifted firefly luciferase optimized for *Candida albicans* in vivo bioluminescence imaging. Front Microbiol. 2017;8:1478.
204. Kadurugamuwa JL, Modi K, Coquoz O, Rice B, Smith S, Contag PR, Purchio T. Reduction of astrogliosis by early treatment of pneumococcal meningitis measured by simultaneous imaging, in vivo, of the pathogen and host response. Infect Immun. 2005;73:7836–43.
205. Shinde R, Perkins J, Contag CH. Luciferin derivatives for enhanced in vitro and in vivo bioluminescence assays. Biochemistry. 2006;45:11103–12.
206. Reddy GR, Thompson WC, Miller SC. Robust light emission from cyclic alkylaminoluciferin substrates for firefly luciferase. J Am Chem Soc. 2010;132:13586–7.
207. Takakura H, Sasakura K, Ueno T, Urano Y, Terai T, Hanaoka K, Tsuboi T, Nagano T. Development of luciferin analogues bearing an amino group and their application as BRET donors. Chem Asian J. 2010;5:2053–61.
208. Woodroofe CC, Shultz JW, Wood MG, Osterman J, Cali JJ, Daily WJ, Meisenheimer PL, Klaubert DH. N-Alkylated 6′-aminoluciferins are bioluminescent substrates for Ultra-Glo and QuantiLum luciferase: new potential scaffolds for bioluminescent assays. Biochemistry. 2008;47:10383–93.
209. Harwood KR, Mofford DM, Reddy GR, Miller SC. Identification of mutant firefly luciferases that efficiently utilize aminoluciferins. Chem Biol. 2011;18:1649–57.
210. Mofford DM, Reddy GR, Miller SC. Aminoluciferins extend firefly luciferase bioluminescence into the near-infrared and can be preferred substrates over D-luciferin. J Am Chem Soc. 2014;136:13277–82.
211. Adams ST Jr, Mofford DM, Reddy GS, Miller SC. Firefly luciferase mutants allow substrate-selective bioluminescence imaging in the mouse brain. Angew Chem Int Ed Engl. 2016;55:4943–6.
212. Nishihara R, Abe M, Nishiyama S, Citterio D, Suzuki K, Kim SB. Luciferase-specific coelenterazine analogues for optical contamination-free bioassays. Sci Rep. 2017;7:908.
213. Otto-Duessel M, Khankaldyyan V, Gonzalez-Gomez I, Jensen MC, Laug WE, Rosol M. In vivo testing of Renilla luciferase substrate analogs in an orthotopic murine model of human glioblastoma. Mol Imaging. 2006;5:57–64.
214. Coleman SM, Mcgregor A. A bright future for bioluminescent imaging in viral research. Future Virol. 2015;10:169–83.
215. Luker KE, Schultz T, Romine J, Leib DA, Luker GD. Transgenic reporter mouse for bioluminescence imaging of herpes simplex virus 1 infection in living mice. Virology. 2006;347:286–95.
216. Mezzanotte L, van't Root M, Karatas H, Goun EA, Löwik CW. In vivo molecular bioluminescence imaging: new tools and applications. Trends Biotechnol. 2017;35:640–52.
217. Mezzanotte L, Que I, Kaijzel E, Branchini B, Roda A, Lowik C. Sensitive dual color in vivo bioluminescence imaging using a new red codon optimized firefly luciferase and a green click beetle luciferase. PLoS One. 2011;6:e19277.

218. Inouye S, Shimomura O. The use of Renilla luciferase, Oplophorus luciferase, and apoaequorin as bioluminescent reporter protein in the presence of coelenterazine analogues as substrate. Biochem Biophys Res Commun. 1997;233:349–53.
219. Yeh HW, Karmach O, Ji A, Carter D, Martins-Green MM, Ai HW. Red-shifted luciferase-luciferin pairs for enhanced bioluminescence imaging. Nat Methods. 2017;14:971–4.
220. Conley NR, Dragulescu-Andrasi A, Rao J, Moerner WE. A selenium analogue of firefly D-luciferin with red-shifted bioluminescence emission. Angew Chem Int Ed Engl. 2012;51:3350–3.
221. Rumyantsev KA, Turoverov KK, Verkhusha VV. Near-infrared bioluminescent proteins for two-color multimodal imaging. Sci Rep. 2016;6:36588.
222. Hickson J, Ackler S, Klaubert D, Bouska J, Ellis P, Foster K, Oleksijew A, Rodriguez L, Schlessinger S, Wang B, Frost D. Noninvasive molecular imaging of apoptosis in vivo using a modified firefly luciferase substrate, Z-DEVD-aminoluciferin. Cell Death Differ. 2010;17:1003–10.
223. Li J, Chen L, Du L, Li M. Cage the firefly luciferin! - a strategy for developing bioluminescent probes. Chem Soc Rev. 2013;42:662–76.
224. Dragulescu-Andrasi A, Liang G, Rao J. In vivo bioluminescence imaging of furin activity in breast cancer cells using bioluminogenic substrates. Bioconjug Chem. 2009;20:1660–6.
225. Shao Q, Jiang T, Ren G, Cheng Z, Xing B. Photoactivable bioluminescent probes for imaging luciferase activity. Chem Commun (Camb). 2009;(27):4028–30.
226. Chu J, Oh Y, Sens A, Ataie N, Dana H, Macklin JJ, Laviv T, Welf ES, Dean KM, Zhang F, Kim BB, Tang CT, Hu M, Baird MA, Davidson MW, Kay MA, Fiolka R, Yasuda R, Kim DS, Ng H-L, Lin MZ. A bright cyan-excitable orange fluorescent protein facilitates dual-emission microscopy and enhances bioluminescence imaging in vivo. Nat Biotechnol. 2016;34:760–7.
227. Dragulescu-Andrasi A, Chan CT, De A, Massoud TF, Gambhir SS. Bioluminescence resonance energy transfer (BRET) imaging of protein-protein interactions within deep tissues of living subjects. Proc Natl Acad Sci U S A. 2011;108:12060–5.
228. Farace C, Blanchot B, Champiat D, Couble P, Declercq G, Millet JL. Synthesis and characterization of a new substrate of Photinus pyralis luciferase: 4-methyl-D-luciferin. J Clin Chem Clin Biochem. 1990;28:471–4.
229. Branchini BR, Murtiashaw MH, Magyar RA, Anderson SM. The role of lysine 529, a conserved residue of the acyl-adenylate-forming enzyme superfamily, in firefly luciferase. Biochemistry. 2000;39:5433–40.
230. Iwano S, Sugiyama M, Hama H, Watakabe A, Hasegawa N, Kuchimaru T, Tanaka KZ, Takahashi M, Ishida Y, Hata J, Shimozono S, Namiki K, Fukano T, Kiyama M, Okano H, Kizaka-Kondoh S, Mchugh TJ, Yamamori T, Hioki H, Maki S, Miyawaki A. Single-cell bioluminescence imaging of deep tissue in freely moving animals. Science. 2018;359:935–9.
231. Miura C, Kiyama M, Iwano S, Ito K, Obata R, Hirano T, Maki S, Niwa H. Synthesis and luminescence properties of biphenyl-type firefly luciferin analogs with a new, near-infrared light-emitting bioluminophore. Tetrahedron. 2013;69:9726–34.
232. Skoura E, Zumla A, Bomanji J. Imaging in tuberculosis. Int J Infect Dis. 2015;32:87–93.
233. Lee KS, Im JG. CT in adults with tuberculosis of the chest: characteristic findings and role in management. AJR Am J Roentgenol. 1995;164:1361–7.
234. Hoffman EB, Crosier JH, Cremin BJ. Imaging in children with spinal tuberculosis. A comparison of radiography, computed tomography and magnetic resonance imaging. J Bone Joint Surg Br. 1993;75:233–9.
235. Soussan M, Brillet PY, Mekinian A, Khafagy A, Nicolas P, Vessieres A, Brauner M. Patterns of pulmonary tuberculosis on FDG-PET/CT. Eur J Radiol. 2012;81:2872–6.
236. Sule P, Tilvawala R, Behinaein P, Walkup GK, Cirillo JD. New directions using reporter enzyme fluorescence (REF) as a tuberculosis diagnostic platform. Tuberculosis (Edinb). 2016;101S:S78–82.
237. Hugonnet JE, Tremblay LW, Boshoff HI, Barry CE 3rd, Blanchard JS. Meropenem-clavulanate is effective against extensively drug-resistant *Mycobacterium tuberculosis*. Science. 2009;323:1215–8.

238. Davies J. Inactivation of antibiotics and the dissemination of resistance genes. Science. 1994;264:375–82.
239. Fisher JF, Mobashery S. Three decades of the class A beta-lactamase acyl-enzyme. Curr Protein Pept Sci. 2009;10:401–7.
240. Hermann JC, Ridder L, Holtje HD, Mulholland AJ. Molecular mechanisms of antibiotic resistance: QM/MM modelling of deacylation in a class A beta-lactamase. Org Biomol Chem. 2006;4:206–10.
241. Knox JR, Moews PC, Frere JM. Molecular evolution of bacterial beta-lactam resistance. Chem Biol. 1996;3:937–47.
242. Boyd DB, Lunn WH. Electronic structures of cephalosporins and penicillins. 9. Departure of a leaving group in cephalosporins. J Med Chem. 1979;22:778–84.
243. Faraci WS, Pratt RF. Mechanism of inhibition of the PC1 beta-lactamase of *Staphylococcus aureus* by cephalosporins: importance of the 3′-leaving group. Biochemistry. 1985;24:903–10.
244. Wang F, Cassidy C, Sacchettini JC. Crystal structure and activity studies of the *Mycobacterium tuberculosis* beta-lactamase reveal its critical role in resistance to beta-lactam antibiotics. Antimicrob Agents Chemother. 2006;50:2762–71.
245. Xie H, Mire J, Kong Y, Chang M, Hassounah HA, Thornton CN, Sacchettini JC, Cirillo JD, Rao J. Rapid point-of-care detection of the tuberculosis pathogen using a BlaC-specific fluorogenic probe. Nat Chem. 2012;4:802–9.
246. Cheng Y, Xie H, Sule P, Hassounah H, Graviss EA, Kong Y, Cirillo JD, Rao J. Fluorogenic probes with substitutions at the 2 and 7 positions of cephalosporin are highly BlaC-specific for rapid *Mycobacterium tuberculosis* detection. Angew Chem Int Ed Engl. 2014;53:9360–4.
247. Campbell RE. Realization of beta-lactamase as a versatile fluorogenic reporter. Trends Biotechnol. 2004;22:208–11.
248. Fry S, Barnabas S, Cotton MF. Update on trends in childhood tuberculosis. Curr Opin Pediatr. 2018;30:152–60.
249. Mufti N, Kong Y, Cirillo JD, Maitland KC. Fiber optic microendoscopy for preclinical study of bacterial infection dynamics. Biomed Opt Express. 2011;2:1121–34.
250. Nooshabadi F, Yang HJ, Cheng Y, Durkee MS, Xie H, Rao J, Cirillo JD, Maitland KC. Intravital excitation increases detection sensitivity for pulmonary tuberculosis by whole-body imaging with beta-lactamase reporter enzyme fluorescence. J Biophotonics. 2017;10:821–9.

Mycobacteria Infection and Lipid Droplets: Host and Pathogen Stealing, Sharing and Storing Fat

Richard M. Armstrong and Thomas C. Zahrt

Abstract *Mycobacterium tuberculosis* is an acid-fast intracellular pathogen of macrophages and the etiological agent of the human respiratory disease tuberculosis (TB). A key aspect of the *M. tuberculosis* lifecycle is its ability to establish long-term persistent (i.e. latent) infection within the lungs of infected individuals. During latency, *M. tuberculosis* produces, stores, and utilizes lipid droplets containing the neutral fatty acid triacylglycerol. In many organisms including *M. tuberculosis,* lipid droplets have been shown to function as a long-term energy storage depots, providing energy for key metabolic pathways, and serving as a carbon source for the generation of important biosynthetic precursors. Failure of *M. tuberculosis* to generate, maintain, or utilize triacylglycerol stored within lipid droplets leads to reduced survival of the bacterium in in vitro and in vivo models of persistence. These findings implicate lipid droplets as central organelles vital to the physiology and pathogenesis of *M. tuberculosis* within the host. In this chapter, the persistence of *M. tuberculosis* in the context of lipid droplet biogenesis, storage, and utilization is discussed.

Keywords *Mycobacterium tuberculosis* · Tuberculosis · Granulomas · Foamy macrophages · Non-replicating persistence · Lipid droplets · Triacylglycerol · Phospholipid monolayer · Fatty acids · Phage shock protein A

Introduction

Mycobacterium tuberculosis is responsible for more than 10.4 million new cases of active TB and 1.8 million deaths annually worldwide [1]. This bacterium is transmitted person-to-person through the aerosolization of bacilli contained within the sputum of individuals possessing active disease. It is currently estimated that ~2

R. M. Armstrong · T. C. Zahrt (✉)
Department of Microbiology and Immunology, Center for Infectious Disease Research, Medical College of Wisconsin, Milwaukee, WI, USA
e-mail: ramstrong@mcw.edu; tzahrt@mcw.edu

J. D. Cirillo, Y. Kong (eds.), *Tuberculosis Host-Pathogen Interactions*,
https://doi.org/10.1007/978-3-030-25381-3_9

billion people are infected with *M. tuberculosis*, the vast majority of which harbor an asymptomatic, latent infection in which the bacteria persists within host-generated granulomatous lesions [1, 2]. Reactivation of *M. tuberculosis* from latency, and consequently re-transmission of the organism to others, can occur at any time but is usually associated with conditions or factors leading to immunosuppression within the host [3, 4] (reviewed in [5]). The ability to establish, maintain, and reactivate from latency is an important aspect of the *M. tuberculosis* lifecycle. Furthermore, bacilli persisting during latent states of infection exhibit increased resistance to anti-TB antibiotics, increasing the time necessary to sterilize the infection, as well as the time available to develop resistance against the antibiotics. Because of these and other reasons, understanding the mechanisms by which *M. tuberculosis* persists within the host remains an important goal within the TB field.

M. tuberculosis Encounters a Stressful Environment Within the Granuloma

Following infection, *M. tuberculosis* associates with host alveoli in the lungs where bacteria are phagocytosed by resident alveolar macrophages [6]. Within the macrophage, *M. tuberculosis* inhibits key steps in the phagosome maturation process and resists lysosome-mediated killing [7–9]. While *M. tuberculosis* replicates largely unimpeded within infected macrophages during the early stages of infection, replication is eventually curtailed later on following the emergence of a productive adaptive immune response and formation of granulomatous lesions at sites of infection [10–15]. Granulomas are organized immunological structures comprised of various host cell types including macrophages, dendritic cells, and lymphocytes [15, 16] (reviewed in [17–19]). While it was once thought that granulomas were static structures acting to trap infecting organism and prevent their growth and subsequent dissemination, granulomas are now recognized as being highly dynamic, allowing immune cells to enter and exit, and infecting organisms contained within these cells to traffic from the granuloma to the draining lymph node and extrapulmonary sites [11]. Although granulomas are capable of maintaining their integrity for the entire lifetime of the host, these structures also undergo necrotic caseation, a process that leads to lung cavitation and secondary transmission of *M. tuberculosis* to new susceptible hosts. Thus, granulomas are an important immunological product of *M. tuberculosis* infection, and are a primary site of interaction between the bacterium and the host.

A variety of adverse conditions are present within the granuloma that are thought to restrict important cellular processes or damage essential constituents of the bacterium. For example, the core of the mature granuloma has an extremely low oxygen tension, even reaching an anaerobic state, despite being located in the lungs [20] (reviewed in [21]). This poses a significant challenge for *M. tuberculosis* which is an obligate aerobe. Other adverse environmental and/or physiological stressors within the granuloma are also present and include low pH, reactive oxygen and nitrogen species [22], low nutrient availability [23], and compounds capable of perturbing the cell envelope of the bacteria [24, 25]. To counteract the potentially detrimental environment within the granuloma, *M. tuberculosis* utilizes multiple, and often interconnected, stress-response networks to sense and correspondingly alter gene expression programs to facilitate long-term survival and establishment of a latent infection [26–30] (reviewed in [31–33]). A subset of stress response networks activated within the granuloma are regulated by two-component signal transduction systems (TCSS), extracytoplasmic function (ECF) sigma factors, serine-threonine protein kinases (STPK), and/or other transcription factors (reviewed in [31–33]). Two of the better characterized TCSS that participate in aspects of *M. tuberculosis* persistence during latency are MprAB and DosRST. MprAB is a sensor of misfolded proteins in the extracytoplasmic compartment, and this system is responsible for controlling the expression of a regulon that includes >300 genes [28, 34–37]. Inactivation of the MprA response regulator sensitizes *M. tuberculosis* to cell envelope stressors [28, 36], and attenuates survival of the bacterium during persistent stages of infection when assessed using a murine model of TB [38]. Similarly, DosRST is a two-component system that possesses two paralogous sensors, DosS and DosT [39–42]. This system recognizes and responds to redox stress and hypoxia, respectively, and regulates expression of ~50 downstream effector determinants [40, 42–44]. Inactivation of components of the DosRST system alters the ability of *M. tuberculosis* to establish non-replicating persistence in vitro [29, 43, 45], and attenuates survival of *M. tuberculosis* in animal models capable of producing mature granulomatous lesions that are most similar to those seen in humans, including guinea pigs, rabbits, and rhesus macaques [29, 46–48].

M. tuberculosis Associates with Foamy Macrophages Within the Granuloma

A predominant cell type that has been observed in histological sections of *M. tuberculosis*-induced granulomas are foamy macrophages (Fig. 1) [10, 12–14, 49]. These host cells contain a high abundance of lipid droplets (LDs), quasi-organelles that are produced by almost all eukaryotic cells (reviewed in [50–52]). LDs are unique in biology in that they represent the only naturally occurring single phospholipid monolayer boundary between aqueous and organic phases, and as such offer a unique environment for biophysical interactions. LDs are comprised of a neutral lipid core surrounded by a single monolayer of phospholipids as well as surface-associated proteins. These organelles range in size from tens of nanometers to well over 100 μm in white adipocytes (reviewed in [53]). LDs are thought to function primarily as energy storage vessels (reviewed in [52, 54]); however, recent studies indicate that LDs participate in other biological processes including lipid recycling and modification, cell signaling, antioxidant generation, and protein sequestration during development [55–60] (reviewed in [61, 62]). In eukaryotes,

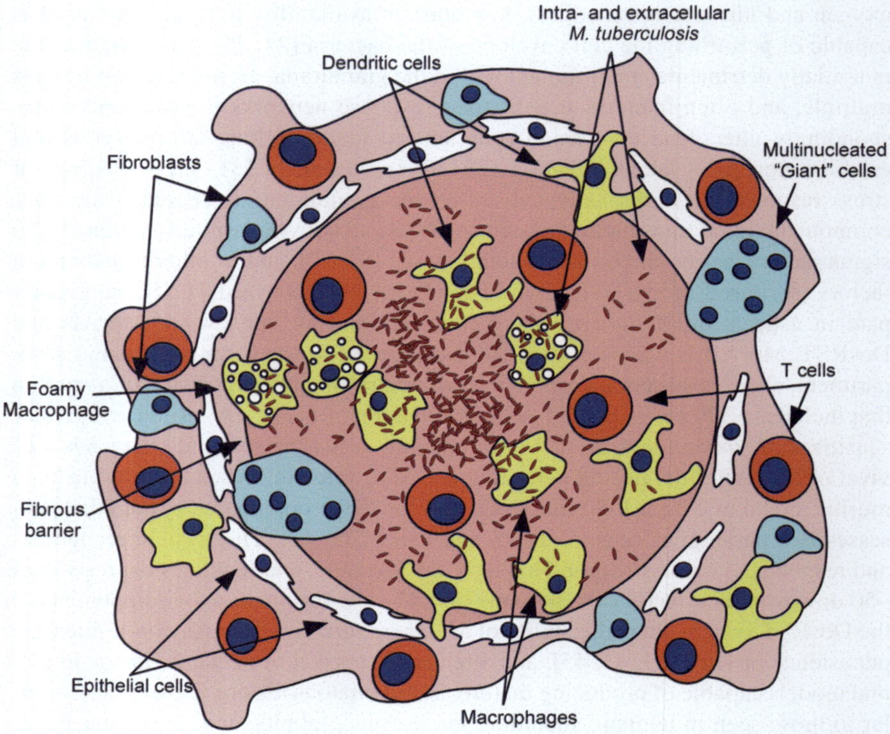

Fig. 1 *M. tuberculosis* establishes persistent infection within the granuloma. The granuloma is a host-generated structure comprised of numerous immune and ancillary cell types including macrophages, dendritic cells, and lymphocytes. Upon maturation, the granuloma becomes partially encased within a calyx of extracellular matrix that is produced by recruited fibroblasts. While a strong T cell response is necessary for initial formation of the granuloma, $CD4^+$ and $CD8^+$ lymphocytes that are positioned both adjacent to and within the granuloma core also function to restrict *M. tuberculosis* growth and further dissemination. A key cell associated with the granuloma is the foamy macrophage. This cell type contains an abundance of lipid droplet within its cytoplasm. For years, the granuloma was assumed to be a relatively static structure; however, recent evidence indicates that granulomas are highly dynamic structures. Importantly, granulomas are capable of maintaining their integrity for the entire lifetime of the host, effectively walling off the tubercle bacilli from the rest of the lung and other infection sites

LDs are generated from the endoplasmic reticulum via an as-of-yet unknown mechanism. Once formed, they are expanded in the cytoplasm by introduction of more neutral lipids into the core simultaneously with the addition of phospholipids to the outer layer.

LDs are capable of storing various neutral fatty acids for the cell, including triacylglycerol (TAG) [63, 64], cholesterol esters (CE) [65, 66], wax esters (WE) [67, 68], and poly(hydoxyalkanoates) (PHA) [69, 70] (reviewed in [71]). Adipocytes, the major fat-storing eukaryotic cell, generates such abundant LDs that these organelles occupy the majority of the cell's cytoplasm. During periods of high nutrient availability, adipocytes import fatty acids and synthesize neutral lipids including CE and TAG, storing these high-energy molecules within LDs. However, when the organism faces conditions of starvation, these triglycerides are then hydrolyzed and used as substrates in the β-oxidation pathway to produce acetyl-CoA for the TCA cycle. Through this process, adipocytes function as energy depots for organisms, allowing for continuation of glycolytic energy generation despite the lack of outside energy sources.

Under normal conditions, macrophages do not typically produce LDs in any significant quantity. However, the oxygen-limiting environment within the granuloma downregulates expression of β-oxidation machinery and upregulates fatty-acid synthesis metabolic pathways, leading to formation of LDs within cells [72]. More recently, it has been shown that infection with *M. tuberculosis*, as well as other *Mycobacterium* species, induces macrophages to become foamy, a process that involves diverting host glycolysis towards ketone body synthesis [14, 73–76]. Interestingly, phagosomes containing *Mycobacterium* are seen closely associated with LDs following infection into foamy macrophages [77], indicating that there is a close association between *Mycobacterium* and LDs within physiologically relevant environments.

Mycobacterium Also Produce Self-Intracytoplasmic Lipid Droplets Under Stressful Conditions

Although *Mycobacterium* induce macrophages to produce LDs and become foamy, *Mycobacterium* themselves are also able to produce LDs in their cytoplasm when grown under conditions of stress (Fig. 2) [78]. The mechanism by which LDs are formed in prokaryotes is largely unknown; however, it is widely accepted that bacterial LDs originate from the inner plasma membrane and bleb off into the cytoplasmic compartment during LD maturation [53, 79, 80]. Like eukaryotic LDs, *Mycobacterium* LDs also contain a fatty acid core comprised primarily of TAG surrounded by a single phospholipid monolayer; however, the proteomic composition of bacterial LDs differs from their eukaryotic counterparts (reviewed in [50, 71, 81]). Interestingly, many bacteria are able to store neutral lipids as an energy reservoir; however, *M. tuberculosis* are among the few pathogenic bacteria known to rely on these organelles [50, 71, 81–83].

A variety of in vitro and in vivo studies indicate that LD production in *Mycobacterium* is important and may contribute to the survival, reactivation, and/or transmission of these bacteria following infection. First, *Mycobacterium* produce LDs in vitro when grown under conditions likely to be encountered within the granuloma, including low oxygen tension, nitric oxide, acidic pH, low iron, cell envelope-perturbing agents, and/or nutrient limitation [10, 84–89]. Second, *Mycobacterium* accumulate LDs within their cytoplasm following infection of foamy macrophages in vitro [77]. Interestingly, fatty acid labeling studies indicate

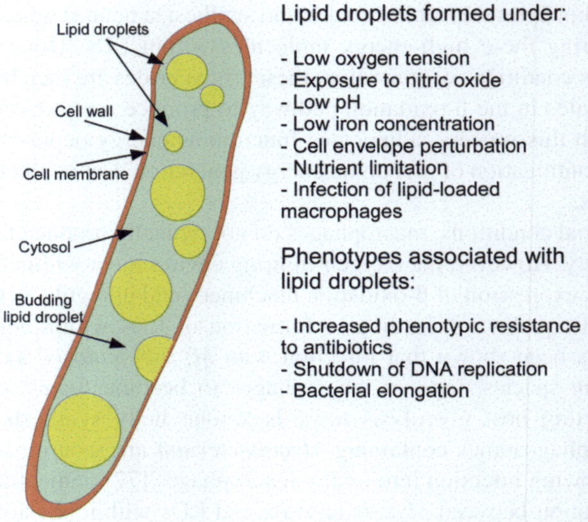

Fig. 2 *M. tuberculosis* produces intracytoplasmic lipid droplets under physiologically relevant conditions. *M. tuberculosis* imports fatty acids directly from host cells (i.e. foamy macrophages), or produces them de novo through various biosynthetic or catabolic pathways, to generate lipid droplets (LDs) within the bacterial cytoplasm. LDs are comprised of a neutral fatty acid core such as triacylglycerol surrounded by a phospholipid monolayer and proteins. LDs range in size from 10 to 20 nm to hundreds of nanometers in diameter, and their production can be stimulated following exposure of *M. tuberculosis* to various physiologically relevant conditions including low oxygen tension, acidic pH, reactive oxygen or nitrogen species, limited nutrient availability, and macrophage infection. Recent evidence indicates that *M. tuberculosis* produce LDs during the transition into non-replicating persistence to establish latency. Conversely, LDs are mobilized for use as an energy source to mediate survival during latency and for reactivation of the bacteria from non-replicating persistence

that the TAG core of *Mycobacterium* LDs is derived, at least in part, from fatty acids that have been usurped from host LDs [12, 64, 77]. Third, accumulation of LDs within the *Mycobacterium* cytoplasm leads to an inhibition in bacterial replication and other phenotypes that mirror those seen following transition of these bacteria into non-replicating persistence [77]. In particular, *Mycobacterium avium* accumulates intracytoplasmic LDs following infection of macrophages that have been pretreated with very low density lipoprotein (vLDL) to induce host LD production [77]. Moreover, these bacteria arrest replication and elongate. In contrast, removal of vLDL from culture medium reverses host and bacterial LD production, and leads to re-initiation of *M. avium* replication [77]. Lastly, mutants of *M. tuberculosis* that are compromised in the ability to synthesize TAG are altered for entrance into non-replicating persistence, while *M. tuberculosis* mutants attenuated in their ability to hydrolyze TAG are defective for resuscitation from non-replicating persistence [64, 89, 90]. Thus, LD production and mobilization is closely associated with the transition of *Mycobacterium* into and out of non-replicating persistence [77, 88].

Determinants Contributing to Intracytoplasmic Lipid Droplet Production and/or Mobilization in *Mycobacterium*

M. tuberculosis encodes ~4500 proteins, a subset of which are involved in LD production, maintenance, and/or mobilization (Table 1) (Fig. 3) [91]. There are ~250 distinct enzymes thought to facilitate the metabolism of fatty acids in *M. tuberculosis*, compared to only 50 in *Escherichia coli* [91]. In addition, *M. tuberculosis* encodes a multitude of lipolytic enzymes, giving it the capacity to produce a large number of lipophilic molecules, including some that are typically seen in plants, yeast, or mammals [91]. While the study of LDs in bacteria remains in its infancy, initial studies have started to identify proteins needed for LD/TAG-based processes within the *Mycobacterium*.

Uptake of Exogenous Fatty Acids Derived from Host Triacylglycerol

Mycobacterium possess the ability to usurp TAG from within host LDs, and transport the resulting fatty acid products across the bacterial membrane for inclusion into self-generated intracytoplasmic LDs. Although the specific proteins essential for these processes remains undefined, the transport of fatty acids from the external environment into the bacterial cytoplasm is typically mediated by the activities of ABC transport systems and acyl-CoA synthetases (ACS). *M. tuberculosis* encodes four predicted ABC transport complexes (Mce1–4). Each system is encoded within a similarly arranged operon of eight genes (*yrbEA*, *yrbEB*, *mceA*, *mceB*, *mceC*, *mceD*, *mceE*, *mceF*); *yrbEA* and *yrbEB* encode for integral membrane proteins that have homology to the permease subunits of ABC transporters, while *mceA-F* encode for proteins that are predicted to be secreted or cell surface-localized [92]. Energy needed to mediate substrate translocation through each of the four systems is thought to be provided by MceG, an ATPase that is located distally from the Mce locus [93]. The Mce4 complex has been shown to regulate the import of cholesterol. Mce4A is capable of binding cholesterol directly [94], while Mce4A, MceG, and OmamA, an Mce-associated membrane protein, are needed for cholesterol uptake and/or utilization under conditions in which cholesterol is the sole carbon source [95, 96]. Similarly, the Mce1 locus is thought to mediate the uptake of mycolic acids, long chain fatty acids that are common in members of the *Mycobacterium* family. For example, *mce1* mutants of *M. tuberculosis* accumulate free mycolic acids in their cell envelope, and are unable to grow in medium containing mycolic acid as the sole carbon source [97, 98]. The substrates transported by the Mce2 and Mce3 loci have yet to be defined.

Another class of proteins involved in fatty acid import, and likely in the downstream synthesis of TAG in *Mycobacterium*, are the ACS. These determinants are prototypical transmembrane proteins which import fatty acids across the membrane

Table 1 Mycobacterium proteins involved in LD production and/or mobilization

Rv#	Name	Synonyms	Description	*M. avium*	*M. bovis* BCG pasteur	*M. leprae*	*M. marinum*	*M. smegmatis*
Rv0217c	LipW	–	Possible esterase LipW	MAV_4954	BCG_0254c	–	MMAR_2621	MSMEG_0280
Rv0220	LipC	–	Probable lipoate biosynthesis protein C LipC	MAV_4953	BCG_0257	–	MMAR_3656	MSMEG_0289
Rv0221	Rv0221	–	Conserved hypothetical protein. Possible triacylglycerol synthase	MAV_4952	BCG_0258	–	MMAR_0464	MSMEG_0290
Rv0467	ICL1	AceA/ICL	Catalyzes breakdown of isocitrate into succinate and glyoxylate	MAV_4682	BCG_0507	(ML2462c)	MMAR_0792	MSMEG_0911
Rv0646c	LipG	–	Probable esterase/lipase LipG	MAV_4515	BCG_0695c	ML1899	MMAR_0981	MSMEG_1352
Rv0655	MceG	Mkl	Possible ribonucleotide-transport ATP-binding protein ABC transporter	MAV_4504	BCG_0704	ML1892	MMAR_0994	MSMEG_1366
Rv0859	FadA	–	Probable acyl-CoA thiolase FadA. A subunit of *Mycobacteria* trifunctional enzyme in beta-oxidation	MAV_0980	BCG_0911	ML2162	MMAR_4677	MSMEG_5721
Rv0860	FadB	–	Probable fatty acid oxidation protein FadB. B subunit of *Mycobacteria* trifunctional enzyme in beta-oxidation	MAV_0981	BCG_0912	ML2161	MMAR_4676	MSMEG_5720
Rv0895	Rv0895	–	Conserved hypothetical protein. Possible triacylglycerol synthase	–	BCG_0947	–	–	–
Rv0981	MprA	–	Response regulator of extracellular stress sensor, MprAB	MAV_1094	BCG_1036	ML0174	MMAR_4529	MSMEG_5488
Rv0982	MprB	–	Sensor kinase of extracellular stress sensor, MprAB	MAV_1095	BCG_1037	ML0175	MMAR_4528	MSMEG_5487
Rv1039c	MPER1	PPE15	Probable mycobacterial perilipin	–	BCG_1097c	–	MMAR_452	–
Rv1076	LipU	–	Possible lipase LipU	MAV_1200	BCG_1134	ML0314	MMAR_4391	MSMEG_5271
Rv1109c	Rv1109c	–	Protein of unknown function, localizes to lipid droplets in BCG	MAV_1229	BCG_1169c	ML1939	MMAR_4356	MSMEG_5225

Rv1169c	LipX	–	PE family protein. Possible lipase	–	BCG_1232c	–	–	–
Rv1206	FacL6	FadD6	Probable fatty-acid-CoA ligase	MAV_1351	BCG_1266	(ML1062)	MMAR_4232	MSMEG_5086
Rv1399c	LipH	–	Probable lipase LipH	–	BCG_1460c	(ML0545c)	MMAR_2208	–
Rv1400c	LipI	–	Probable lipase LipI	MAV_3377	BCG_1461c	(ML0546c)	MMAR_2209	MSMEG_3059
Rv1425	Rv1425	–	Conserved hypothetical protein. Possible triacylglycerol synthase	MAV_3352	BCG_1486	(ML0566)	MMAR_2231	–
Rv1426	LipO	–	Probable esterase LipO	MAV_3350	BCG_1487c	–	MMAR_2232	MSMEG_0302
Rv1428c	Rv1482c	–	Protein of unknown function, localizes to lipid droplets in BCG	MAV_3296	BCG_1489c	–	–	MSMEG_5642
Rv1497	LipL	–	Probable esterase LipL	MAV_3275	BCG_1560	(ML1797c)	MMAR_2305	–
Rv1683	Rv1683	–	Bifunctional enzyme: long-chain acyl-CoA synthase and lipase	MAV_3089	BCG_1721	ML1346	MMAR_1389	MSMEG_3767
Rv1760	Rv1760	–	Conserved hypothetical protein. Possible triacylglycerol synthase	MAV_3015	BCG_1801	–	MMAR_2634	MSMEG_4297
Rv1834	LipZ	–	Probable hydrolase	MAV_2139	BCG_1869	–	MMAR_2711	MSMEG_2777
Rv1837c	GlcB	–	Catalyzes addition of acetyl-CoA to glyoxylate to form malate	MAV_2880	BCG_1872c	ML2069	MMAR_2713	MSMEG_3640
Rv1900c	LipJ	–	Probable lignin peroxidase LipJ	MAV_5228	BCG_1939c	(ML2016)	MMAR_0286	MSMEG_4477
Rv1915	AceAa[a]	ICL2a	Catalyzes breakdown of isocitrate into succinate and glyoxylate (gene interrupted in H37Rv, a-subunit)	–	–	ML1985c	–	–
Rv1916	AceAb[a]	ICL2b	Catalyzes breakdown of isocitrate into succinate and glyoxylate (gene interrupted in H37Rv, b-subunit)	MAV_2781	BCG_1954	–	MMAR_2821	MSMEG_3706
Rv1923	LipD	–	Probable lipase LipD	–	BCG_1962	–	MMAR_2828	MSMEG_3162
Rv2027c	DosT	–	Sensor kinase of DosRST hypoxia/oxidative stress sensor system	–	BCG_2046c	–	–	MSMEG_5241

(continued)

Table 1 (continued)

Rv#	Name	Synonyms	Description	*M. avium*	*M. bovis* BCG pasteur	*M. leprae*	*M. marinum*	*M. smegmatis*
Rv2031c	HspX	acr	Stress-responsive protein chaperone, induced by hypoxia, under regulation of DosRST	–	BCG_2050c	ML1795	MMAR_3484	MSMEG_3932
Rv2045c	LipT	–	Probable carboxylesterase LipT	MAV_2466	BCG_2064c	(ML1434c)	MMAR_3020	MSMEG_3848
Rv2217	LipB	–	Probable lipoate biosynthesis protein B LipB	MAV_2271	BCG_2233	ML0859	MMAR_3285	MSMEG_4285
Rv2218	LipA	–	Probable lipoate biosynthesis protein A LipA	MAV_2270	BCG_2234	ML0858	MMAR_3286	MSMEG_4286
Rv2245	KasA	AceE	Member of FasII fatty-acid synthetase, catalyzes the condensation of fatty acid synthesis	MAV_2192	BCG_2262	ML1655	MMAR_3338	MSMEG_4327
Rv2284	LipM	–	Probable esterase LipL	MAV_2146	BCG_2299	–	MMAR_3429	–
Rv2285	Rv2285	–	Conserved hypothetical protein. Possible triacylglycerol synthase	–	BCG_2300	–	MMAR_3431	–
Rv2463	LipP	–	Probable esterase/lipase LipP	MAV_1709	BCG_2483	(ML1482)	MMAR_3810	MSMEG_4680
Rv2484c	Rv2484c	–	Conserved hypothetical protein. Possible triacylglycerol synthase	MAV_1686	BCG_2502c	ML1244	MMAR_3835	MSMEG_4705
Rv2485c	LipQ	–	Probable carboxylesterase LipQ	MAV_1685	BCG_2503c	ML1243	MMAR_3836	–
Rv2524c	Fas	FasI	Fatty acid synthetase catalyzes the formation of long-chain fatty acids	MAV_1650	BCG_2545c	ML1191	MMAR_3962	MSMEG_4757
Rv2744c	PspA	35kD_Ag	PspA family member, localizes to lipid droplets	MAV_3635	BCG_2760c	ML0981	MMAR_1971	MSMEG_2695
Rv2970c	LipN	–	Probable lipase/esterase LipN	MAV_3814	BCG_2991c	ML1668c	MMAR_1746	MSMEG_2409
Rv3084	LipR	–	Probable acetyl-hydrolase/esterase LipR	–	BCG_3109	–	–	MSMEG_3010
Rv3087	Rv3087	–	Conserved hypothetical protein. Possible triacylglycerol synthase	–	BCG_3112	–	MMAR_2599	–

Rv3088	Tgs4	–	Triacylglycerol synthase	–	BCG_3113	–	MMAR_2598	–
Rv3097c	LipY	PE_ PGRS63	Triacylglycerol lipase, responsible for primary breakdown of stored TAG in lipid droplets	–	BCG_3122c	–	MMAR_1547	–
Rv3130c	Tgs1	–	Triacylglycerol synthase	–	BCG_3153c	–	MMAR_1519	MSMEG_3948
Rv3132c	DosS	DevS	Sensor kinase of DosRS hypoxia/oxidative stress sensor system	MAV_4108	BCG_3155c	–	MMAR_1517	–
Rv3133c	DosR	DevR	Response regulator of DosRST hypoxia/ oxidative stress sensor system	MAV_4109	BCG_3156c	–	MMAR_1516	MSMEG_5244
Rv3203	LipV	–	Possible lipase LipV	MAV_4150	BCG_3229	ML0820c	MMAR_1355	MSMEG_1940
Rv3233c	Rv3233c[b]	–	Conserved hypothetical protein. Possible triacylglycerol synthase	–	–	ML0785	–	–
Rv3234c	Tgs3[b]	–	Triacylglycerol synthase	MAV_4196	BCG_3263c	ML0784	MMAR_1311	MSMEG_1882
Rv3371	Rv3371	–	Conserved hypothetical protein. Possible triacylglycerol synthase	MAV_4336	BCG_3443	ML0415c	MMAR_1157	–
Rv3480c	Rv3480c	–	Conserved hypothetical protein. Possible triacylglycerol synthase	–	BCG_3544c	–	MMAR_4955	–
Rv3487c	LipF	–	Probable esterase/lipase LipF	–	BCG_3551c	–	–	–
Rv3734c	Tgs2	–	Triacylglycerol synthase	MAV_0355	BCG_3794c	–	MMAR_5271	MSMEG_6322
Rv3740c	Rv3740c	–	Conserved hypothetical protein. Possible triacylglycerol synthase	–	BCG_3799c	–	MMAR_5278	–
Rv3775	LipE	–	Probable lipase LipE	MAV_0246	BCG_3837	ML0119	MMAR_5330	MSMEG_6575
Rv3804c	Ag85a	FbpA	Bifunctional enzyme both in mycolate synthesis and as a diacylglycerol-acyl-CoA transferase	MAV_0214	BCG_3866c	ML0097	MMAR_5368	MSMEG_6398
N/A	Mce1	–	Mce1 operon, responsible for uptake of mycolic acids	–	Complete	Complete	Complete	–

(continued)

Table 1 (continued)

Rv#	Name	Synonyms	Description	*M. avium*	*M. bovis* BCG pasteur	*M. leprae*	*M. marinum*	*M. smegmatis*
N/A	Mce2	–	Mce2 operon, substrate unknown	Complete	Complete	–	Partial	Partial+
N/A	Mce3	–	Mce3 operon, substrate unknown	Partial	–	–	Complete	Complete
N/A	Mce4	–	Mce4 operon, responsible for uptake of cholesterol	Partial	Complete	Partial	Complete	Complete

For the Mce operon comparisons: reviewing each individual gene would have greatly extended the length of the table, so instead, the authors resolved to simplify the readout. To this end, the following shorthand designations were used: *Complete* a complete set of the core eight genes comprising an mce operon are present, *Partial* at least one of the core eight genes is absent/translocated to a different chromosomal locus, *Partial+* this indicates that there are multiple genes within the *M. smegmatis* genome which resemble the corresponding genes in *M. tuberculosis* H37Rv genome's mce2 operon, suggesting duplications of the operon within the species' genome

Parentheses surrounding a gene "()" indicates the presence of a homologous pseudogene in *M. leprae*

[a]The Isocitrate lyase two gene is annotated in *M. tuberculosis* H37Rv as two genes interrupted by a frameshift mutation, whereas in all other evaluated *Mycobacterium* species, it was a single gene. All species presented here contain a complete *ICL2* gene, however some are designated as AceAa versus AceAb homologues

[b]The genes encoding Tgs3 and Rv3233c appear to have diverged from other *Mycobacterium* species. In this case, the two genes appear to separately encode the N- and C-terminal portions of the complete Tgs3 gene observed in the other organisms listed here. Interestingly this gene interruption is also present in the *M. tuberculosis* strains Erdmann and CDC1551, indicating an earlier divergence of the locus

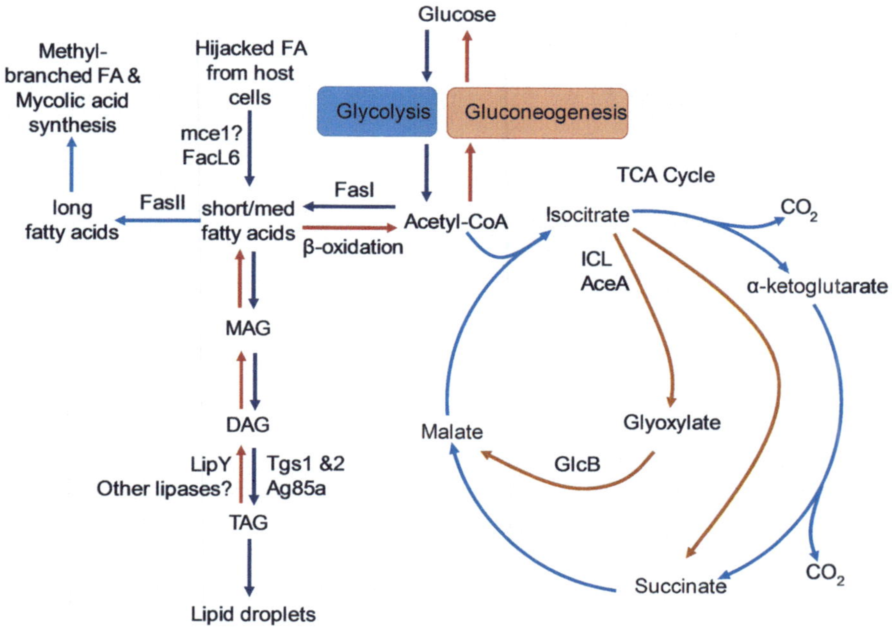

Fig. 3 Energetics of triacylglycerol catabolism through β-oxidation and the glyoxylate shunt. Under conditions of nutrient availability, *M. tuberculosis* utilizes sugars and other readily available carbon sources to generate energy (glycolysis, tricarboxcylic acid (TCA) cycle, oxidative phosphorylation) and essential precursors needed for macromolecule biosynthesis. However, upon conditions of nutrient starvation, *M. tuberculosis* accesses TAG stored within lipid droplets for use in energy-generating pathways. In particular, TAG is processed through the activity of lipases and esterases into fatty acid products capable of generating acetyl-CoA through the process of β-oxidation. Acetyl-CoA then feeds into a variant of the traditional TCA known as the glyoxylate shunt, where acetyl-CoA is converted into glyoxylate and then malate through the activity of isocitrate lyase (ICL/AceA) and malate synthase (GlcB). This metabolic bypass allows retention of the two carbons that would otherwise be lost as CO_2 during a single round of the TCA cycle, and generation of complex macromolecules from these carbon molecules. *FA* fatty acids, *mce1* operon encoding a possible fatty-acid transporter complex, *FacL6* acyl-CoA sythetase, *FasI & FasII* fatty acid synthase I & II, *MAG/DAG/TAG* mono/di/tri-acylglycerol, respectively, *LipY* lipase Y, *Tgs1 & 2* triglyceride synthase 1 & 2, *Ag85a* bi-functional diacylglycerol acyl-CoA transferase

while also mediating the covalent attachment of these fatty acids to coenzyme-A (CoA) [99]. ACS utilize ATP to activate the acyl-group of the fatty acid and join it via a high energy bond to CoA. Once activated, the newly synthesized acyl-CoA can be utilized by other metabolic proteins (discussed below) for the generation of mono-,di-, and tri-glycerides, and subsequent storage of these determinants into bacterial LDs. FacL6 (Rv1206) is an ACS that is upregulated in *M. tuberculosis* under conditions of non-replicating persistence. Furthermore, this protein facilitates the uptake of fatty acids [100], and is needed for the production of TAG in *M. tuberculosis* following transition into non-replicating persistence in vitro [100].

De Novo Fatty Acid Synthesis

De novo fatty acid synthesis within *M. tuberculosis* is mediated principally by two fatty-acid synthetases (Fas). *fasI* encodes a single polypeptide of over 3000 residues that possesses all of the necessary functional domains, including an acyl-carrier protein domain, needed to fully synthesize medium-chain fatty acids (C_{16}–C_{20}) from acetyl-CoA [101]. In contrast, FasII is a multimeric complex of proteins that is able to extend the length of smaller acyl-CoA molecules to produce long (C_{24-65}) precursors needed for the synthesis of complex fatty acids, including mycolic acids [91].

Synthesis of Triacylglycerol

TAG is synthesized through the sequential addition of acyl chains to a glycerol backbone. First, acyl chains are generated either through de novo biosynthesis, through the activity of the fatty-acid synthesis pathway, or by the conjugation of imported fatty acids onto CoA via ACS. Next, CoA-conjugated acyl chains are esterified sequentially onto *sn*-glycerol-3-phosphate. Formation of monoacylglycerol (MAG)-3 phosphate is mediated by the activity of a glycerol-3-phosphate O-acyltransferase, while diacylglycerol (DAG)-3 phosphate is formed by the addition of an acyl chain onto MAG-3 phosphate via acylglycerol-3-phosphate acyltransferases (reviewed in [82, 102–104]). The terminal addition of an acyl group onto DAG is mediated by diacylglycerol-acyltransferases, also known as triacylglycerol synthases (Tgs). *M. tuberculosis* encodes at least 15 determinants that exhibit Tgs activity when expressed in *E. coli*, including *Rv0221*, *Rv0895*, *Rv1425*, *Rv1760*, *Rv2285*, *Rv2484c*, *Rv3087*, *Rv3088* (*tgs4*), *Rv3130c* (*tgs1*), *Rv3233c*, *Rv3234c* (*tgs3*), *Rv3371*, *Rv3480c*, *Rv3734c* (*tgs2*), and *Rv3740c* [105] (Table 1). Expression of several of these genes is upregulated following exposure of *M. tuberculosis* to conditions present within the granuloma, or following the growth of *M. tuberculosis* under conditions promoting intracytoplasmic LD production [64, 87, 89, 105]. While both Tgs1 and Tgs2 localize to *Mycobacterium* LDs [106], the subcellular localization of the other Tgs proteins remains undefined. Several lines of evidence indicate that Tgs 1 may be the principle Tgs responsible for TAG production within *M. tuberculosis*. Deletion of *tgs1* renders the tubercle bacillus unable to produce appreciable amounts of TAG and LDs [86, 89, 105, 107]. Furthermore, *tgs1* mutants of *M. tuberculosis* are attenuated in their ability to enter into non-replicating persistence, and are significantly more sensitive to anti-TB antibiotics including isoniazid, rifampicin, streptomycin, ciprofloxacin, ethambutol, and pyrazinamide compared to their wild-type counterparts [10, 86, 87]. Interestingly, *tgs1* expression is under the control of DosRST, providing further evidence that LD/TAG production is closely tied to stress responses and transition of *M. tuberculosis* into and out of non-replicating persistence [107, 108]. Unfortunately, no studies have yet assessed the importance of the other Tgs for TAG and/or LD production in *Mycobacterium*. Apart from the Tgs described above, additional enzymes may also be capable of facilitating the final step in TAG synthesis. Ag85a (aka FbpA or Rv3804c), is a mycolyl-transferase that normally functions to affix mycolic acid groups to the arabinogalactan layer surrounding the peptidoglycan in the *M. tuberculosis* cell envelope [109]. However, Ag85a exhibits diglyceride acyltransferase activity, and is also able to regulate intracytoplasmic LD production in *Mycobacterium smegmatis* [110].

Lipid Droplet Mobilization

TAG contained within intracytoplasmic LDs, or that is present within host LDs, is hydrolyzed through the activity of *Mycobacterium* lipases/esterases. Resulting fatty acid products are then fed into various catabolic pathways, including the β-oxidation pathway, to produce energy needed for survival during latency or for reactivation from non-replicating persistence [91, 111–114]. *M. tuberculosis* encodes 24 predicted lipases or esterases, including *lipA* (*Rv2218*), *lipB* (*Rv2217*), *lipC* (*Rv0220*), *lipD* (*Rv1923*), *lipE* (*Rv3775*), *lipF* (*Rv3487c*), *lipG* (*Rv0646c*), *lipH* (*Rv1399c*), *lipI* (*Rv1400c*), *lipJ* (*Rv1900c*), *lipL* (*Rv1497*), *lipM* (*Rv2284*), *lipN* (*Rv2970c*), *lipO* (*Rv1426*), *lipP* (*Rv2463*), *lipQ* (*Rv2485c*), *lipR* (*Rv3084*), *lipT* (*Rv2045c*), *lipU* (*Rv1076*), *lipV* (*Rv3203*), *lipW* (*Rv0217c*), *lipX* (*Rv1169c*), *lipY* (*Rv3097c*), and *lipZ* (*Rv1834*) [91, 115] (Table 1). Additionally, a number of other determinants possessing the α/β-hydrolase fold characteristic of lipases are also encoded within the *M. tuberculosis* genome [116, 117]. A variety of in vitro and/or in vivo studies indicate that *lip* determinants may contribute to the hydrolysis of TAG within *M. tuberculosis*. For example, lysates from *E. coli* strains producing LipY, LipC, LipL, LipX, LipK, LipG, LipP, LipE, LipT, LipW, LipD, LipJ, LipZ, LipO, LipQ, LipR, and LipS are capable of hydrolyzing the triglyceride triolein [115]. Furthermore, *lipY*, *lipE*, *lipC*, *lipZ*, *lipL*, and *lipT* are all induced for expression when *M. tuberculosis* is grown under conditions of nutrient stress during which stored TAG is mobilized [115]. LipY contains an N-terminal PE-domain that normally functions in protein export and localization, and a C-terminal domain that exhibits similarity to hormone-sensitive lipases [115]. Consistent with this domain architecture, LipY is present in the cytoplasm but is also secreted and localizes to the bacterial surface [118]. It is currently thought that LipY may be one of the predominant lipases utilized for the hydrolysis of TAG in *M. tuberculosis*. First, a *lipY* mutant exhibits reduced ability to hydrolyze intracellular TAG under conditions of nutrient starvation [115]. In contrast, overproduction of LipY in *M. smegmatis* (a mycobacterial species that does not possess a LipY homolog) reduces the amount of TAG available for storage within LDs [119]. Second, *lipY* mutants are attenuated in their ability to reactivate from non-replicating persistence within a human TB in vitro granuloma model [10]. Finally, small molecular inhibitors of LipY abrogate *M. tuberculosis* growth in vitro under conditions of hypoxia in which TAG from intracytoplasmic LDs is normally mobilized as an energy source [120].

Metabolic Pathways That Use Products Generated from Triacylglycerol Hydrolysis

During normal cellular respiration, carbon sources are taken up by the organism and broken down into two-carbon pieces—acetyl-CoA in this case—through glycolysis, β-oxidation, and other catabolic process. When complex carbon molecules such as sugars are plentiful, organisms freely utilize them for both energy generation and biosynthetic processes, including the production of amino acids, nucleic acids, and structural sugar moieties. However, under conditions of nutrient limitation, organisms may turn to the catabolism of alternative carbon sources such as TAG to generate energy and carbon intermediates important for various processes [90, 121].

β-Oxidation Pathway

M. tuberculosis encodes ~100 genes thought to be involved in fatty-acid degradation (i.e. β-odixation), a catabolic pathway that requires only five reactions to complete [91]. The primary steps of fatty acid degradation are as follows: (1) Activation of the fatty acid by an acyl-CoA synthetase (generally FadD enzymes in *Mycobacterium*); (2) Dehydrogenation of the fatty acid between the C2 and C3 position, resulting in a double bond between these two carbons. This activity is catalyzed by an acyl-CoA dehydrogenase; (3) The newly-formed double bond is then hydrated to form a hydroxyacyl-CoA intermediate, an activity facilitated by enoyl-CoA hydratases; (4) The hydroxyl group is dehydrated to form a ketoacyl-CoA group. This activity is carried out by 3-hydroxyacyl-CoA dehydrogenases; and (5) Thiolysis between the C2 and C3 carbon by thiolases, releasing a free molecule of acetyl-CoA and resulting in an acyl-CoA molecule that is shortened by two carbon units. *M. tuberculosis* encodes numerous individual enzymes likely to be capable of performing these enzymatic steps. For example, there are 36 predicted acyl-CoA synthetases, and an additional 36 predicted acyl-CoA dehydrogenases encoded within the genome [91]. However, in addition to these individual determinants, *M. tuberculosis* also encodes a β-oxidation enzyme complex that consists of FadA (Rv0859) and FadB (Rv0860) [91]. These enzymes form a canonical $\alpha_2\beta_2$ heterotetramer, similar to β-oxidation enzyme complexes in other prokaryotes [122]. The FadA/FadB heterotetramer facilitates three of the four steps of β-oxidation following activation of the acyl group by a FadD enzyme [91, 122].

Glyoxylate Shunt

The glyoxylate shunt, as illustrated in Fig. 3, is a modification of the tricarboxylic acid (TCA) cycle. It is a pathway commonly found in prokaryotes, plants, and fungi [123, 124]. The glyoxylate shunt utilizes the enzymes isocitrate lyase (ICL) and malate synthase (MS) to bypass the carbon-loss steps of the TCA cycle under conditions of oxygen limitation and nutrient depletion. Using this pathway, reducing factors in the form of NADH and $FADH_2$ are retained, and acetyl-CoA can be expanded into more complex carbon moieties. Importantly, ICL is not present in mammals and therefore is a putative drug target for *M. tuberculosis* (Fig. 4).

Isocitrate Lyase

ICL was first described in the 1950's [111, 123]. It was not until several decades later until *M. tuberculosis* was recognized to possess ICL activity [113, 114]. *M. tuberculosis* encodes two ICLs: *icl1* (*Rv0467*) and *icl2* (*Rv1915*/*Rv1916*). The gene encoding *icl2* was originally annotated as two separate hypothetical transcripts (*aceAa* and *aceAb*) in strain H37Rv due to the presence of a frameshift mutation; however, other sequenced strains of *M. tuberculosis*, including CDC1551 and Erdman, lack this frameshift and therefore encode a single intact *icl2* allele. Icl1 and Icl2 both possess ICL activity in vitro, although Icl1 appears to be more active than Icl2 [125]. Interestingly, deletion of either *icl1* or *icl2* alone does not alter

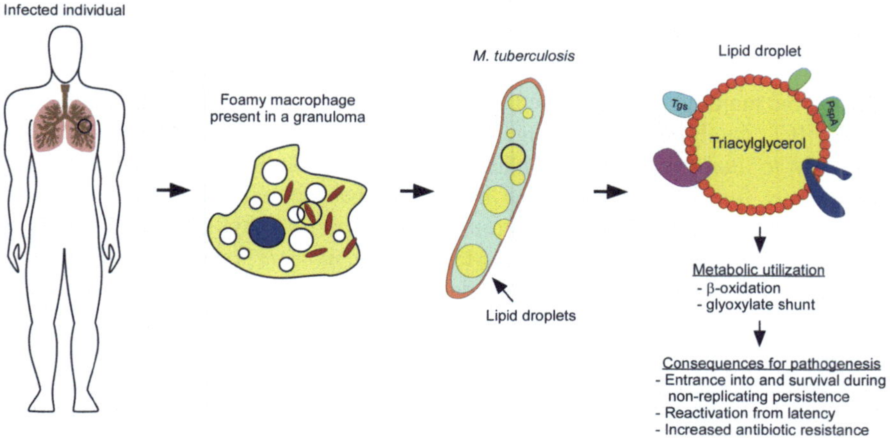

Fig. 4 Summary of the impact of lipid droplets on *M. tuberculosis*-host interactions. Following infection into the lungs of a susceptible individual, *M. tuberculosis* persists within macrophages that are contained within granulomatous lesions generated by the host. Within these structures, *M. tuberculosis* causes infected macrophages to produce lipid droplets and become "foamy". Through an as-of-yet unknown mechanism, *M. tuberculosis* usurps triacylglycerol contained within host lipid droplets, and utilizes the resulting host fatty acid products for incorporation into its own lipid droplets which reside in the cytoplasm but are thought to bud from the plasma membrane. Triacylglycerol contained within the core of *M. tuberculosis* lipid droplets are used for energy production by supplying fatty acids that feed into the β-oxidation pathway and the glyoxylate shunt. In particular, mobilization of lipid droplets facilitates entrance of *M. tuberculosis* into and survival during non-replicating persistence, reactivation from latency, and increased phenotypic resistance to anti-tuberculosis antibiotics

M. tuberculosis growth in vitro in medium containing fatty acids as the sole carbon source [126]. In contrast, *M. tuberculosis* is unable to grow on fatty acids as the sole carbon source following deletion of both *icl1* and *icl2* [126]. ICL is also required for aspects of *M. tuberculosis* physiology and pathogenesis in macrophages and in vivo. For example, *icl1* mutants of *M. tuberculosis* are attenuated for survival in cultured macrophages [127]. Additionally, *M. tuberculosis* mutants deleted in *icl1* exhibit moderate survival defects in the lungs of mice during persistent stages of infection [126, 127], and correspondingly these mice exhibit reduced tissue pathology [126, 127]. In contrast, loss of *icl2* does not alter the growth kinetics, survival, or ability of *M. tuberculosis* to induce tissue pathology when assessed in macrophages in vitro or within mice [126]. Interestingly, *M. tuberculosis* mutants deleted in both *icl1* and *icl2* exhibit impaired growth/survival in macrophages in vitro, and are cleared from the lungs and spleen of infected mice shortly after infection [126]. Furthermore, these mice exhibit no signs of pathology in the lungs or spleens, indicating that ICL activity is essential for growth and/or survival of *M. tuberculosis* in vivo [126]. More recently, it has been shown that exposure of *M. tuberculosis* to key frontline anti-tubercular drugs including rifampicin, isoniazid, and streptomycin induces ICL activity [128], and that loss of *icl1* increases sensitivity to these antibiotics.

Malate Synthase

The second major enzyme involved in the glyoxylate pathway is MS. As mentioned above, ICL catalyzes the cleavage of isocitrate into succinate and glyoxylate. However, to retain as much carbon as possible under conditions in which the TCA cycle is not functioning, glyoxylate is recycled back into TCA components. MS catalyzes the addition of an acetyl group, in the form of acetyl-CoA, to the newly-formed glyoxylate to generate malate. MS in *M. tuberculosis* is encoded by *Rv1837c*. Although the enzyme encoded by this determinant has been examined structurally as a possible drug target [129, 130], some have argued ICL may be the more attractive target of the two enzymes for inhibiting the glyoxylate shunt [131]. Regardless, the entire glyoxylate pathway merits further study to assess the potential for drug development against *M. tuberculosis* when the bacterium is utilizing fatty acids for survival during non-replicating persistence.

Other Proteins Associated with the Lipid Droplet Surface

While a number of enzymes important for the synthesis or hydrolysis of TAG have been shown to localize to the LD surface, very little is known about the identity of other determinants comprising the bacterial LD proteome. In eukaryotes, hundreds of different proteins have been identified on the LD surface [132–135]. While the ability of proteins to localize to LDs remains an area of intense investigation, recent studies indicate that proteins likely associate with LDs via one of three primary mechanisms: (1) hairpin helices on proteins insert into the neutral lipid core, (2) amphipathic helices present on the surface of proteins interact with hydrophobic regions resulting from packing defects of phospholipids on the LD surface, and (3) lipidation of proteins—directly anchoring a lipid moiety to the protein and tethering of the protein to the LD surface (reviewed in [136]). Of the proteins identified on eukaryotic LDs, the most prototypical and well-studied are the Perilipin family (previously the PAT family) [137, 138] (reviewed in [139, 140]). These proteins contain multiple amphipathic and hydrophobic repeat domains which are thought to confer specific and high affinity interactions with LDs. Though not yet understood, it stands to reason that the association of bacterial proteins with LDs may be mediated using similar mechanisms.

Recent work has begun to elucidate the proteomic composition of bacterial LDs. Proteins associated with the LDs from *Mycobacterium bovis* BCG include triacylglycerol synthases Tgs1 and Tgs2, long-chain acyl-CoA synthase and lipase BCG1721, heat-shock chaperone HspX (Acr), protein of unknown function BCG1169c, and acylglycerol-phosphate acyltransferase BCG1489c [106]. PspA (Rv2744c) is another protein that has been found to associate with LDs produced in *M. tuberculosis* and *M. smegmatis* [141]. PspA is a member of a broadly-conserved, stress-responsive protein family in bacteria and plants [142–149]. In most bacteria, PspA localizes to the cytosolic face of the plasma membrane under conditions of stress where it is thought to prevent loss of proton-motive force [150]. However, in *M. tuberculosis*, PspA localizes to the surface of LDs where it functions in an unknown way to regulate LD homeostasis [141]. In particular, PspA regulates the number and size distribution of LDs. Furthermore, *M. tuberculosis* mutants altered in PspA production exhibit reduced survival during non-replicating persistence. Interestingly, PspA is encoded from within a locus (*clgR-Rv2744c*(*pspA*)*-Rv2743c-Rv2742c*) that is a major point of signal integration within the cell envelope stress response network of *M. tuberculosis*. In particular, this locus is regulated by the MprAB TCSS, the SigE extracytoplasmic function sigma factor, the PknB serine-threonine protein kinase, and the first determinant in this operon, ClgR [30, 151–155]. Finally, a mycobacterial perilipin-like protein was recently identified by Daniel et. al. [156]. This protein, PPE15 (encoded by *Rv1039c*, later re-designated as Mycobacterial PERilipin-1—MPER1), was found to be upregulated in vitro during dormancy-stimulating conditions [156]. Deletion of *Rv1039c* reduces the ability of *M. tuberculosis* to produce LDs and store TAG when assessed using various model systems including an in vitro granuloma model [156]. Furthermore, the *Rv1039c* mutant exhibits increased susceptibility to the drug rifampicin. When taken together, currently available data on *Mycobacterium* LDs, albeit limited, indicates that these organelles harbor proteins able to synthesize and hydrolyze TAG within the LD core, and regulate LD structure and/or homeostasis. Given the overall number and functional diversity of proteins known to comprise LDs from eukaryotes, the small number of *Mycobacterium* LD-associated proteins identified thus far likely represents only a minor subset of determinants comprising the LD proteome in bacteria.

Conclusions

The lifecycle of *M. tuberculosis* within the host is complex and multifaceted. While *M. tuberculosis* is capable of causing active primary disease, infection by *M. tuberculosis* most commonly results in the establishment of a life-long latent infection. The decision between active vs. latent infection is regulated both by the virulence strategies employed by the bacterium, and the corresponding host responses generated during the infection. The granuloma is a primary site where *M. tuberculosis* and the host engage one another, and it is widely thought that the outcome of infection, in part, is facilitated through the interactions that occur within these structures. Specific environmental conditions and host cell types encountered by *M. tuberculosis* within the mature granuloma initiate signaling pathways that cause the bacteria to produce intracytoplasmic LDs containing TAG, initiating transition of the bacterium into non-replicating persistence that can last the lifetime of the host. While the importance of LDs (and TAG) for *M. tuberculosis* physiology and pathogenesis is only beginning to be understood, disruption of enzymes facilitating TAG production or hydrolysis negatively impacts the *M. tuberculosis* lifecycle within the host, altering the ability of the organism to establish, maintain, and reactivate from latency. Thus, the continued circulation of *M. tuberculosis* within the human population is intimately linked to the formation of granulomas, the production of intracytoplasmic LDs, and the synthesis and hydrolysis of TAG.

Despite the fact that much is known about the synthesis, composition, and function of LDs in eukaryotes, the field of prokaryotic LDs, in particular *Mycobacterium* LDs, remains in its infancy. For *M. tuberculosis*, much of this is due to the biosafety issues and technical challenges of isolating and purifying LDs from this organism. For example, *M. tuberculosis* is a Risk Group 3 pathogen and as such requires manipulation within a Biosafety Level 3 (BSL3) facility to prevent transmission of aerosols. Unfortunately, purification of LDs requires the use of specialized equipment that is aerosol-generating. In particular, *M. tuberculosis* must be lysed using a French press rather than a bead beater so that LD integrity can be maintained. Similarly, isolation of LDs requires that total cell lysates be fractionated by differential ultracentrifugation. As a consequence, investigators interested in studying LDs in *M. tuberculosis* have been limited to using attenuated derivatives and/or non-pathogenic *Mycobacterium* surrogates. In addition, conditions required to induce the production of LDs in *Mycobacterium* species requires the use of specialized growth medium, extensive incubation times, and/or large volume cultures. Going forward, the continued study of *Mycobacterium* LDs, including the mechanisms by which these organelles are formed, maintained, and mobilized for use in energy-generating pathways, will undoubtedly lead to exciting new insights into the processes regulating *M. tuberculosis* physiology, pathogenesis, and drug resistance.

References

1. WHO. Global tuberculosis report. 2016.
2. WHO. TB report 2014. 2014.
3. Selwyn PA, Hartel D, Lewis VA, Schoenbaum EE, Vermund SH, Klein RS, Walker AT, Friedland GH. A prospective study of the risk of tuberculosis among intravenous drug users with human immunodeficiency virus infection. N Engl J Med. 1989;320(9):545–50. https://doi.org/10.1056/NEJM198903023200901.
4. van Rie A, Warren R, Richardson M, Victor TC, Gie RP, Enarson DA, Beyers N, van Helden PD. Exogenous reinfection as a cause of recurrent tuberculosis after curative treatment. N Engl J Med. 1999;341(16):1174–9. https://doi.org/10.1056/NEJM199910143411602.
5. Khan FA, Minion J, Pai M, Royce S, Burman W, Harries AD, Menzies D. Treatment of active tuberculosis in HIV-coinfected patients: a systematic review and meta-analysis. Clin Infect Dis. 2010;50(9):1288–99. https://doi.org/10.1086/651686.
6. Schlesinger LS. Macrophage phagocytosis of virulent but not attenuated strains of *Mycobacterium tuberculosis* is mediated by mannose receptors in addition to complement receptors. J Immunol. 1993;150(7):2920–30.
7. Armstrong JA, Hart PDA. Response of cultured macrophages to *Mycobacterium tuberculosis*, with observation on fusion of lysosomes with phagosomes. J Exp Med. 1971;134(3):713–40. https://doi.org/10.1084/jem.134.3.713.
8. Clemens DL, Horwitz MA. Characterization of the *Mycobacterium tuberculosis* phagosome and evidence that phagosomal maturation is inhibited. J Exp Med. 1995;181(1):257.
9. Goren MB, D'Arcy Hart P, Young MR, Armstrong JA. Prevention of phagosome-lysosome fusion in cultured macrophages by sulfatides of *Mycobacterium tuberculosis*. Proc Natl Acad Sci U S A. 1976;73(7):2510–4.
10. Kapoor N, Pawar S, Sirakova TD, Deb C, Warren WL, Kolattukudy PE. Human granuloma in vitro model, for TB dormancy and resuscitation. PLoS One. 2013;8(1):e53657. https://doi.org/10.1371/journal.pone.0053657.
11. Lin PL, Ford CB, Coleman MT, Myers AJ, Gawande R, Ioerger T, Sacchettini J, Fortune SM, Flynn JL. Sterilization of granulomas is common in active and latent tuberculosis despite within-host variability in bacterial killing. Nat Med. 2014;20(1):75–9. https://doi.org/10.1038/nm.3412.. http://www.nature.com/nm/journal/v20/n1/abs/nm.3412.html#supplementary-information
12. Peyron P, Vaubourgeix J, Poquet Y, Levillain F, Botanch C, Bardou F, Daffé M, Emile J-F, Marchou B, Cardona P-J, de Chastellier C, Altare F. Foamy macrophages from tuberculous patients' granulomas constitute a nutrient-rich reservoir for *M. tuberculosis* persistence. PLoS Pathog. 2008;4(11):e1000204. https://doi.org/10.1371/journal.ppat.1000204.
13. Ridley DS, Ridley MJ. Rationale for the histological spectrum of tuberculosis. A basis for classification. Pathology. 1987;19(2):186–92.
14. Russell DG, Cardona P-J, Kim M-J, Allain S, Altare F. Foamy macrophages and the progression of the human tuberculosis granuloma. Nat Immunol. 2009;10(9):943–8. https://doi.org/10.1038/ni.1781.
15. Vandiviere HM, Loring WE, Melvin IG, Willis HS. The treated pulmonary lesion and its tubercle bacillus. II. The death and resurrection. Am J Med Sci. 1956;232(1):30–7.
16. Kennedy HE, Vandiviere HM, Melvin IG, Willis HS. The treated pulmonary lesion and its tubercle bacillus. III. Drug susceptibility studies. Am J Med Sci. 1957;233(6):676–84.
17. Gengenbacher M, Kaufmann SHE. *Mycobacterium tuberculosis*: success through dormancy. FEMS Microbiol Rev. 2012;36(3):514–32. https://doi.org/10.1111/j.1574-6976.2012.00331.x.
18. Gomez JE, McKinney JD. *M. tuberculosis* persistence, latency, and drug tolerance. Tuberculosis. 2004;84(1–2):29–44. https://doi.org/10.1016/j.tube.2003.08.003.
19. Silva Miranda M, Breiman A, Allain S, Deknuydt F, Altare F. The tuberculous granuloma: an unsuccessful host defence mechanism providing a safety shelter for the bacteria? Clin Dev Immunol. 2012;2012:14. https://doi.org/10.1155/2012/139127.

20. Wayne LG, Hayes LG. An in vitro model for sequential study of shiftdown of *Mycobacterium tuberculosis* through two stages of nonreplicating persistence. Infect Immun. 1996;64(6):2062–9.
21. Wayne LG, Sohaskey CD. Nonreplicating persistence of *Mycobacterium tuberculosis*. Annu Rev Microbiol. 2001;55:139–63. https://doi.org/10.1146/annurev.micro.55.1.139.
22. Hu Y, Butcher PD, Mangan JA, Rajandream M-A, Coates ARM. Regulation of hmp gene transcription in *Mycobacterium tuberculosis*: effects of oxygen limitation and nitrosative and oxidative stress. J Bacteriol. 1999;181(11):3486–93.
23. Nyka W. Studies on the effect of starvation on Mycobacteria. Infect Immun. 1974;9(5):843–50.
24. Rivas-Santiago B, Hernandez-Pando R, Carranza C, Juarez E, Contreras JL, Aguilar-Leon D, Torres M, Sada E. Expression of cathelicidin LL-37 during *Mycobacterium tuberculosis* infection in human alveolar macrophages, monocytes, neutrophils, and epithelial cells. Infect Immun. 2008;76(3):935–41. https://doi.org/10.1128/iai.01218-07.
25. Sturgill-Koszycki S, Schlesinger P, Chakraborty P, Haddix P, Collins H, Fok A, Allen R, Gluck S, Heuser J, Russell D. Lack of acidification in *Mycobacterium* phagosomes produced by exclusion of the vesicular proton-ATPase. Science. 1994;263(5147):678–81. https://doi.org/10.1126/science.8303277.
26. Dutta NK, Mehra S, Kaushal D. A *Mycobacterium tuberculosis* sigma factor network responds to cell-envelope damage by the promising anti-mycobacterial thioridazine. PLoS One. 2010;5(4):e10069. https://doi.org/10.1371/journal.pone.0010069.
27. Fontán PA, Aris V, Alvarez ME, Ghanny S, Cheng J, Soteropoulos P, Trevani A, Pine R, Smith I. *Mycobacterium tuberculosis* sigma factor E regulon modulates the host inflammatory response. J Infect Dis. 2008;198(6):877–85.
28. He H, Hovey R, Kane J, Singh V, Zahrt TC. MprAB is a stress-responsive two-component system that directly regulates expression of sigma factors SigB and SigE in Mycobacterium tuberculosis. J Bacteriol. 2006;188(6):2134–43.
29. Malhotra V, Sharma D, Ramanathan VD, Shakila H, Saini DK, Chakravorty S, Das TK, Li Q, Silver RF, Narayanan PR, Tyagi JS. Disruption of response regulator gene, *devR*, leads to attenuation in virulence of *Mycobacterium tuberculosis*. FEMS Microbiol Lett. 2004;231(2):237–45. https://doi.org/10.1016/s0378-1097(04)00002-3.
30. McGillivray A, Golden NA, Gautam US, Mehra S, Kaushal D. The *Mycobacterium tuberculosis* Rv2745c plays an important role in responding to redox stress. PLoS One. 2014;9(4):e93604. https://doi.org/10.1371/journal.pone.0093604.
31. Bretl DJ, Demetriadou C, Zahrt TC. Adaptation to environmental stimuli within the host: two-component signal transduction systems of Mycobacterium tuberculosis. Microbiol Mol Biol Rev. 2011;75(4):566–82. https://doi.org/10.1128/mmbr.05004-11.
32. Bretl DJ, Zahrt TC. Regulation of envelope stress responses by Mycobacterium tuberculosis. In: Regulation of bacterial virulence. Washington: American Society of Microbiology; 2013. https://doi.org/10.1128/9781555818524.ch24.
33. Sachdeva P, Misra R, Tyagi AK, Singh Y. The sigma factors of Mycobacterium tuberculosis: regulation of the regulators. FEBS J. 2010;277(3):605–26. https://doi.org/10.1111/j.1742-4658.2009.07479.x.
34. Bretl DJ, Bigley TM, Terhune SS, Zahrt TC. The MprB extracytoplasmic domain negatively regulates activation of the Mycobacterium tuberculosis MprAB two-component system. J Bacteriol. 2014;196(2):391–406. https://doi.org/10.1128/JB.01064-13.
35. Pang X, Howard ST. Regulation of the α-crystallin gene acr2 by the MprAB two-component system of Mycobacterium tuberculosis. J Bacteriol. 2007;189(17):6213–21. https://doi.org/10.1128/JB.00492-07.
36. Pang X, Vu P, Byrd TF, Ghanny S, Soteropoulos P, Mukamolova GV, Wu S, Samten B, Howard ST. Evidence for complex interactions of stress-associated regulons in an mprAB deletion mutant of Mycobacterium tuberculosis. Microbiology. 2007;153(4):1229–42. https://doi.org/10.1099/mic.0.29281-0.
37. Zahrt TC, Wozniak C, Jones D, Trevett A. Functional analysis of the Mycobacterium tuberculosis MprAB two-component signal transduction system. Infect Immun. 2003;71(12):6962–70. https://doi.org/10.1128/IAI.71.12.6962-6970.2003.

38. Zahrt TC, Deretic V. Mycobacterium tuberculosis signal transduction system required for persistent infections. Proc Natl Acad Sci. 2001;98(22):12706–11. https://doi.org/10.1073/pnas.221272198.
39. Boon C, Li R, Qi R, Dick T. Proteins of Mycobacterium bovis BCG induced in the Wayne dormancy model. J Bacteriol. 2001;183(8):2672–6. https://doi.org/10.1128/JB.183.8.2672-2676.2001.
40. Dasgupta N, Kapur V, Singh KK, Das TK, Sachdeva S, Jyothisri K, Tyagi JS. Characterization of a two-component system, devR-devS, of *Mycobacterium tuberculosis*. Tuber Lung Dis. 2000;80(3):141–59. https://doi.org/10.1054/tuld.2000.0240.
41. Roberts DM, Liao RP, Wisedchaisri G, Hol WGJ, Sherman DR. Two sensor kinases contribute to the hypoxic response of *Mycobacterium tuberculosis*. J Biol Chem. 2004;279(22):23082–7. https://doi.org/10.1074/jbc.M401230200.
42. Saini DK, Malhotra V, Dey D, Pant N, Das TK, Tyagi JS. DevR–DevS is a bona fide two-component system of *Mycobacterium tuberculosis* that is hypoxia-responsive in the absence of the DNA-binding domain of DevR. Microbiology. 2004;150(4):865–75. https://doi.org/10.1099/mic.0.26218-0.
43. Boon C, Dick T. *Mycobacterium bovis* BCG response regulator essential for hypoxic dormancy. J Bacteriol. 2002;184(24):6760–7. https://doi.org/10.1128/JB.184.24.6760-6767.2002.
44. Park H-D, Guinn KM, Harrell MI, Liao R, Voskuil MI, Tompa M, Schoolnik GK, Sherman DR. Rv3133c/dosR is a transcription factor that mediates the hypoxic response of *Mycobacterium tuberculosis*. Mol Microbiol. 2003;48(3):833–43.
45. Leistikow RL, Morton RA, Bartek IL, Frimpong I, Wagner K, Voskuil MI. The *Mycobacterium tuberculosis* DosR regulon assists in metabolic homeostasis and enables rapid recovery from nonrespiring dormancy. J Bacteriol. 2010;192(6):1662–70. https://doi.org/10.1128/JB.00926-09.
46. Converse PJ, Karakousis PC, Klinkenberg LG, Kesavan AK, Ly LH, Allen SS, Grosset JH, Jain SK, Lamichhane G, Manabe YC, McMurray DN, Nuermberger EL, Bishai WR. Role of the dosR-dosS two-component regulatory system in *Mycobacterium tuberculosis* virulence in three animal models. Infect Immun. 2009;77(3):1230–7. https://doi.org/10.1128/iai.01117-08.
47. Mehra S, Dutta NK, Mollenkopf H-J, Kaushal D. *Mycobacterium tuberculosis* MT2816 encodes a key stress-response regulator. J Infect Dis. 2010;202(6):943–53. https://doi.org/10.1086/654820.
48. Mehra S, Foreman TW, Didier PJ, Ahsan MH, Hudock TA, Kissee R, Golden NA, Gautam US, Johnson A-M, Alvarez X, Russell-Lodrigue KE, Doyle LA, Roy CJ, Niu T, Blanchard JL, Khader SA, Lackner AA, Sherman DR, Kaushal D. The DosR regulon modulates adaptive immunity and is essential for *Mycobacterium tuberculosis* persistence. Am J Respir Crit Care Med. 2015;191(10):1185–96. https://doi.org/10.1164/rccm.201408-1502OC.
49. Barros U, Ladiwala U, Birdi TJ, Antia NH. Localization and retention of mycobacterial antigen in lymph nodes of leprosy patients. Br J Exp Pathol. 1987;68(5):733–41.
50. Murphy DJ. The biogenesis and functions of lipid bodies in animals, plants and microorganisms. Prog Lipid Res. 2001;40(5):325–438. https://doi.org/10.1016/S0163-7827(01)00013-3.
51. Thiam AR, Farese RV Jr, Walther TC. The biophysics and cell biology of lipid droplets. Nat Rev Mol Cell Biol. 2013;14(12):775–86. https://doi.org/10.1038/nrm3699.
52. Walther TC, Farese RV. Lipid droplets and cellular lipid metabolism. Annu Rev Biochem. 2012;81:687–714. https://doi.org/10.1146/annurev-biochem-061009-102430.
53. Fujimoto T, Parton RG. Not just fat: the structure and function of the lipid droplet. Cold Spring Harb Perspect Biol. 2011;3(3):a004838. https://doi.org/10.1101/cshperspect.a004838.
54. Mak HY. Lipid droplets as fat storage organelles in Caenorhabditis elegans: thematic review series: lipid droplet synthesis and metabolism: from yeast to man. J Lipid Res. 2012;53(1):28–33. https://doi.org/10.1194/jlr.R021006.
55. Bailey AP, Koster G, Guillermier C, Hirst Elizabeth MA, MacRae James I, Lechene Claude P, Postle Anthony D, Gould Alex P. Antioxidant role for lipid droplets in a stem cell niche of *Drosophila*. Cell. 2015;163(2):340–53. https://doi.org/10.1016/j.cell.2015.09.020.

56. Bartz R, Zehmer JK, Zhu M, Chen Y, Serrero G, Zhao Y, Liu P. Dynamic activity of lipid droplets: protein phosphorylation and GTP-mediated protein translocation. J Proteome Res. 2007;6(8):3256–65. https://doi.org/10.1021/pr070158j.
57. Li Z, Johnson MR, Ke Z, Chen L, Welte MA. Drosophila lipid droplets buffer the H2Av supply to protect early embryonic development. Curr Biol. 2014;24(13):1485–91. https://doi.org/10.1016/j.cub.2014.05.022.
58. Ohsaki Y, Cheng J, Fujita A, Tokumoto T, Fujimoto T. Cytoplasmic lipid droplets are sites of convergence of proteasomal and autophagic degradation of apolipoprotein B. Mol Biol Cell. 2006;17(6):2674–83. https://doi.org/10.1091/mbc.E05-07-0659.
59. Souza SC, Muliro KV, Liscum L, Lien P, Yamamoto MT, Schaffer JE, Dallal GE, Wang X, Kraemer FB, Obin M, Greenberg AS. Modulation of hormone-sensitive lipase and protein kinase A-mediated lipolysis by perilipin A in an adenoviral reconstituted system. J Biol Chem. 2002;277(10):8267–72. https://doi.org/10.1074/jbc.M108329200.
60. Velikkakath AKG, Nishimura T, Oita E, Ishihara N, Mizushima N. Mammalian Atg2 proteins are essential for autophagosome formation and important for regulation of size and distribution of lipid droplets. Mol Biol Cell. 2012;23(5):896–909. https://doi.org/10.1091/mbc.E11-09-0785.
61. Arrese EL, Saudale FZ, Soulages JL. Lipid droplets as signaling platforms linking metabolic and cellular functions. Lipid Insight. 2014;7:7–16. https://doi.org/10.4137/LPI.S11128.
62. Farese RV, Walther TC. Lipid droplets finally get a little R-E-S-P-E-C-T. Cell. 2009;139(5):855–60. https://doi.org/10.1016/j.cell.2009.11.005.
63. Alvarez HM, Mayer F, Fabritius D, Steinbuchel A. Formation of intracytoplasmic lipid inclusions by *Rhodococcus opacus* strain PD630. Arch Microbiol. 1996;165(6):377–86.
64. Daniel J, Maamar H, Deb C, Sirakova TD, Kolattukudy PE. Mycobacterium tuberculosis uses host triacylglycerol to accumulate lipid droplets and acquires a dormancy-like phenotype in lipid-loaded macrophages. PLoS Pathog. 2011;7(6):e1002093. https://doi.org/10.1371/journal.ppat.1002093.
65. Mahlberg FH, Glick JM, Jerome WG, Rothblat GH. Metabolism of cholesteryl ester lipid droplets in a J774 macrophage foam cell model. Biochim Biophys Acta. 1990;1045(3):291–8.
66. Shio H, Haley NJ, Fowler S. Characterization of lipid-laden aortic cells from cholesterol-fed rabbits. III. Intracellular localization of cholesterol and cholesteryl ester. Lab Investig. 1979;41(2):160–7.
67. Bredemeier R, Hulsch R, Metzger JO, Berthe-Corti L. Submersed culture production of extracellular wax esters by the marine bacterium Fundibacter jadensis. Mar Biotechnol. 2003;5(6):579–83. https://doi.org/10.1007/s10126-003-0012-x.
68. Fixter LM, Fewson CA. The accumulation of waxes by *Acinetobacter calcoaceticus*. Biochem Soc Trans. 1974;2(5):944–5. https://doi.org/10.1042/bst0020944.
69. Anderson AJ, Dawes EA. Occurrence, metabolism, metabolic role, and industrial uses of bacterial polyhydroxyalkanoates. Microbiol Rev. 1990;54(4):450–72.
70. Pötter M, Müller H, Reinecke F, Wieczorek R, Fricke F, Bowien B, Friedrich B, Steinbüchel A. The complex structure of polyhydroxybutyrate (PHB) granules: four orthologous and paralogous phasins occur in Ralstonia eutropha. Microbiology. 2004;150(7):2301–11. https://doi.org/10.1099/mic.0.26970-0.
71. Wältermann M, Steinbüchel A. Neutral lipid bodies in prokaryotes: recent insights into structure, formation, and relationship to eukaryotic lipid depots. J Bacteriol. 2005;187(11):3607–19. https://doi.org/10.1128/jb.187.11.3607-3619.2005.
72. Boström P, Magnusson B, Svensson P-A, Wiklund O, Borén J, Carlsson LMS, Ståhlman M, Olofsson S-O, Hultén LM. Hypoxia converts human macrophages into triglyceride-loaded foam cells. Arterioscler Thromb Vasc Biol. 2006;26(8):1871–6. https://doi.org/10.1161/01.ATV.0000229665.78997.0b.
73. Kim JY, Shakow A, Castro A, Vande C, Farmer P. WHO trade, foreign policy, diplomacy and health report, 3. Tuberculosis control. 2010.
74. Podinovskaia M, Lee W, Caldwell S, Russell DG. Infection of macrophages with Mycobacterium tuberculosis induces global modifications to phagosomal function. Cell Microbiol. 2013;15(6):843–59. https://doi.org/10.1111/cmi.12092.

75. Singh V, Jamwal S, Jain R, Verma P, Gokhale R, Rao Kanury VS. Mycobacterium tuberculosis-driven targeted recalibration of macrophage lipid homeostasis promotes the foamy phenotype. Cell Host Microbe. 2012;12(5):669–81. https://doi.org/10.1016/j.chom.2012.09.012.
76. Smith I. Mycobacterium tuberculosis pathogenesis and molecular determinants of virulence. Clin Microbiol Rev. 2003;16(3):463–96. https://doi.org/10.1128/CMR.16.3.463-496.2003.
77. Caire-Brändli I, Papadopoulos A, Malaga W, Marais D, Canaan S, Thilo L, de Chastellier C. Reversible lipid accumulation and associated division arrest of Mycobacterium avium in lipoprotein-induced foamy macrophages may resemble key events during latency and reactivation of tuberculosis. Infect Immun. 2014;82(2):476–90. https://doi.org/10.1128/iai.01196-13.
78. Nishino N, Tamori Y, Tateya S, Kawaguchi T, Shibakusa T, Mizunoya W, Inoue K, Kitazawa R, Kitazawa S, Matsuki Y, Hiramatsu R, Masubuchi S, Omachi A, Kimura K, Saito M, Amo T, Ohta S, Yamaguchi T, Osumi T, Cheng J, Fujimoto T, Nakao H, Nakao K, Aiba A, Okamura H, Fushiki T, Kasuga M. FSP27 contributes to efficient energy storage in murine white adipocytes by promoting the formation of unilocular lipid droplets. J Clin Invest. 2008;118(8):2808–21. https://doi.org/10.1172/JCI34090.
79. Ding Y, Yang L, Zhang S, Wang Y, Du Y, Pu J, Peng G, Chen Y, Zhang H, Yu J, Hang H, Wu P, Yang F, Yang H, Steinbüchel A, Liu P. Identification of the major functional proteins of prokaryotic lipid droplets. J Lipid Res. 2012;53(3):399–411. https://doi.org/10.1194/jlr.M021899.
80. Ding Y, Zhang S, Yang L, Na H, Zhang P, Zhang H, Wang Y, Chen Y, Yu J, Huo C, Xu S, Garaiova M, Cong Y, Liu P. Isolating lipid droplets from multiple species. Nat Protoc. 2013;8(1):43–51.
81. Wältermann M, Hinz A, Robenek H, Troyer D, Reichelt R, Malkus U, Galla H-J, Kalscheuer R, Stöveken T, Von Landenberg P, Steinbüchel A. Mechanism of lipid-body formation in prokaryotes: how bacteria fatten up. Mol Microbiol. 2005;55(3):750–63. https://doi.org/10.1111/j.1365-2958.2004.04441.x.
82. Alvarez H, Steinbüchel A. Triacylglycerols in prokaryotic microorganisms. Appl Microbiol Biotechnol. 2002;60(4):367–76. https://doi.org/10.1007/s00253-002-1135-0.
83. Burdon KL. Fatty material in bacteria and fungi revealed by staining dried, fixed slide preparations. J Bacteriol. 1946;52(6):665–78.
84. Bacon J, Dover LG, Hatch KA, Zhang Y, Gomes JM, Kendall S, Wernisch L, Stoker NG, Butcher PD, Besra GS, Marsh PD. Lipid composition and transcriptional response of Mycobacterium tuberculosis grown under iron-limitation in continuous culture: identification of a novel wax ester. Microbiology. 2007;153(5):1435–44. https://doi.org/10.1099/mic.0.2006/004317-0.
85. Bacon J, Marsh PD. Transcriptional responses of Mycobacterium tuberculosis exposed to adverse conditions in vitro. Curr Mol Med. 2007;7(3):277–86.
86. Baek S-H, Li AH, Sassetti CM. Metabolic regulation of Mycobacterial growth and antibiotic sensitivity. PLoS Biol. 2011;9(5):e1001065. https://doi.org/10.1371/journal.pbio.1001065.
87. Deb C, Lee C-M, Dubey VS, Daniel J, Abomoelak B, Sirakova TD, Pawar S, Rogers L, Kolattukudy PE. A novel in vitro multiple-stress dormancy model for Mycobacterium tuberculosis generates a lipid-loaded, drug-tolerant, dormant pathogen. PLoS One. 2009;4(6):e6077. https://doi.org/10.1371/journal.pone.0006077.
88. Garton NJ, Waddell SJ, Sherratt AL, Lee S-M, Smith RJ, Senner C, Hinds J, Rajakumar K, Adegbola RA, Besra GS, Butcher PD, Barer MR. Cytological and transcript analyses reveal fat and lazy persister-like bacilli in tuberculous sputum. PLoS Med. 2008;5(4):e75. https://doi.org/10.1371/journal.pmed.0050075.
89. Sirakova TD, Dubey VS, Deb C, Daniel J, Korotkova TA, Abomoelak B, Kolattukudy PE. Identification of a diacylglycerol acyltransferase gene involved in accumulation of triacylglycerol in *Mycobacterium tuberculosis* under stress. Microbiology. 2006;152(9):2717–25. https://doi.org/10.1099/mic.0.28993-0.

90. Low KL, Rao PSS, Shui G, Bendt AK, Pethe K, Dick T, Wenk MR. Triacylglycerol utilization is required for regrowth of in vitro hypoxic nonreplicating *Mycobacterium bovis* bacillus Calmette-Guerin. J Bacteriol. 2009;191(16):5037–43. https://doi.org/10.1128/jb.00530-09.
91. Cole ST, Brosch R, Parkhill J, Garnier T, Churcher C, Harris D, Gordon SV, Eiglmeier K, Gas S, Barry CE, Tekaia F, Badcock K, Basham D, Brown D, Chillingworth T, Connor R, Davies R, Devlin K, Feltwell T, Gentles S, Hamlin N, Holroyd S, Hornsby T, Jagels K, Krogh A, McLean J, Moule S, Murphy L, Oliver K, Osborne J, Quail MA, Rajandream MA, Rogers J, Rutter S, Seeger K, Skelton J, Squares R, Squares S, Sulston JE, Taylor K, Whitehead S, Barrell BG. Deciphering the biology of *Mycobacterium tuberculosis* from the complete genome sequence. Nature. 1998;393(6685):537–44.
92. Casali N, Riley LW. A phylogenomic analysis of the *Actinomycetales mce* operons. BMC Genomics. 2007;8(1):60. https://doi.org/10.1186/1471-2164-8-60.
93. Joshi SM, Pandey AK, Capite N, Fortune SM, Rubin EJ, Sassetti CM. Characterization of mycobacterial virulence genes through genetic interaction mapping. Proc Natl Acad Sci U S A. 2006;103:11760. https://doi.org/10.1073/pnas.0603179103.
94. Khan S, Islam A, Hassan MI, Ahmad F. Purification and structural characterization of Mce4A from Mycobacterium tuberculosis. Int J Biol Macromol. 2016;93(Part A):235–41. https://doi.org/10.1016/j.ijbiomac.2016.06.059.
95. Pandey AK, Sassetti CM. Mycobacterial persistence requires the utilization of host cholesterol. Proc Natl Acad Sci. 2008;105(11):4376–80. https://doi.org/10.1073/pnas.0711159105.
96. Perkowski EF, Miller BK, McCann JR, Sullivan JT, Malik S, Allen IC, Godfrey V, Hayden JD, Braunstein M. An orphaned Mce-associated membrane protein of Mycobacterium tuberculosis is a virulence factor that stabilizes Mce transporters. Mol Microbiol. 2016;100(1):90–107. https://doi.org/10.1111/mmi.13303.
97. Cantrell SA, Leavell MD, Marjanovic O, Iavarone AT, Leary JA, Riley LW. Free mycolic acid accumulation in the cell wall of the mce1 operon mutant strain of Mycobacterium tuberculosis. J Microbiol. 2013;51(5):619–26. https://doi.org/10.1007/s12275-013-3092-y.
98. Forrellad MA, McNeil M, Santangelo MP, Blanco FC, García E, Klepp LI, Huff J, Niederweis M, Jackson M, Bigi F. Role of the Mce1 transporter in the lipid homeostasis of Mycobacterium tuberculosis. Tuberculosis. 2014;94(2):170–7. https://doi.org/10.1016/j.tube.2013.12.005.
99. Coleman RA, Lewin TM, Van Horn CG, Gonzalez-Baró MR. Do long-chain acyl-CoA synthetases regulate fatty acid entry into synthetic versus degradative pathways? J Nutr. 2002;132(8):2123–6.
100. Daniel J, Sirakova T, Kolattukudy P. An acyl-CoA synthetase in Mycobacterium tuberculosis involved in triacylglycerol accumulation during dormancy. PLoS One. 2014;9(12):e114877. https://doi.org/10.1371/journal.pone.0114877.
101. Fernandes ND, Kolattukudy PE. Cloning, sequencing and characterization of a fatty acid synthase-encoding gene from Mycobacterium tuberculosis var. bovis BCG. Gene. 1996;170(1):95–9. https://doi.org/10.1016/0378-1119(95)00842-X.
102. Alvarez HM. Triacylglycerol and wax ester-accumulating machinery in prokaryotes. Biochimie. 2016;120:28–39. https://doi.org/10.1016/j.biochi.2015.08.016.
103. Coleman RA, Lee DP. Enzymes of triacylglycerol synthesis and their regulation. Prog Lipid Res. 2004;43(2):134–76. https://doi.org/10.1016/S0163-7827(03)00051-1.
104. Yen C-LE, Stone SJ, Koliwad S, Harris C, Farese RV. DGAT enzymes and triacylglycerol biosynthesis. J Lipid Res. 2008;49(11):2283–301. https://doi.org/10.1194/jlr.R800018-JLR200.
105. Daniel J, Deb C, Dubey VS, Sirakova TD, Abomoelak B, Morbidoni HR, Kolattukudy PE. Induction of a novel class of diacylglycerol acyltransferases and triacylglycerol accumulation in *Mycobacterium tuberculosis* as it goes into a dormancy-like state in culture. J Bacteriol. 2004;186(15):5017–30. https://doi.org/10.1128/JB.186.15.5017.
106. Low KL, Shui G, Natter K, Yeo WK, Kohlwein SD, Dick T, Rao SPS, Wenk MR. Lipid droplet-associated proteins are involved in the biosynthesis and hydrolysis of triacylglycerol in *Mycobacterium bovis* bacillus Calmette-Guerin. J Biol Chem. 2010;285(28):21662–70. https://doi.org/10.1074/jbc.M110.135731.

107. Chauhan S, Tyagi JS. Powerful induction of divergent tgs1-Rv3131 genes in *Mycobacterium tuberculosis* is mediated by DevR interaction with a high-affinity site and an adjacent cryptic low-affinity site. J Bacteriol. 2009;191(19):6075–81. https://doi.org/10.1128/jb.00310-09.
108. Reed MB, Gagneux S, DeRiemer K, Small PM, Barry CE. The W-Beijing lineage of *Mycobacterium tuberculosis* overproduces triglycerides and has the DosR dormancy regulon constitutively upregulated. J Bacteriol. 2007;189(7):2583–9. https://doi.org/10.1128/jb.01670-06.
109. Puech V, Guilhot C, Perez E, Tropis M, Armitige LY, Gicquel B, Daffé M. Evidence for a partial redundancy of the fibronectin-binding proteins for the transfer of mycoloyl residues onto the cell wall arabinogalactan termini of *Mycobacterium tuberculosis*. Mol Microbiol. 2002;44(4):1109–22. https://doi.org/10.1046/j.1365-2958.2002.02953.x.
110. Elamin AA, Stehr M, Spallek R, Rohde M, Singh M. The *Mycobacterium tuberculosis* Ag85A is a novel diacylglycerol acyltransferase involved in lipid body formation. Mol Microbiol. 2011;81(6):1577–92. https://doi.org/10.1111/j.1365-2958.2011.07792.x.
111. Kornberg HL, Madsen NB. Synthesis of C4-dicarboxylic acids from acetate by a "glyoxylate bypass" of the tricarboxylic acid cycle. Biochim Biophys Acta. 1957;24:651–3. https://doi.org/10.1016/0006-3002(57)90268-8.
112. Muñoz-Elías EJ, Upton AM, Cherian J, McKinney JD. Role of the methylcitrate cycle in *Mycobacterium tuberculosis* metabolism, intracellular growth, and virulence. Mol Microbiol. 2006;60(5):1109–22. https://doi.org/10.1111/j.1365-2958.2006.05155.x.
113. Murthy PS, Sirsi M, Ramakrishnan T. Effect of age on the enzymes of tricarboxylic acid and related cycles in *Mycobacterium tuberculosis* H37Rv. Am Rev Respir Dis. 1973;108(3):689–90. https://doi.org/10.1164/arrd.1973.108.3.689.
114. Wayne LG, Lin KY. Glyoxylate metabolism and adaptation of *Mycobacterium tuberculosis* to survival under anaerobic conditions. Infect Immun. 1982;37(3):1042–9.
115. Deb C, Daniel J, Sirakova TD, Abomoelak B, Dubey VS, Kolattukudy PE. A novel lipase belonging to the hormone-sensitive lipase family induced under starvation to utilize stored triacylglycerol in *Mycobacterium tuberculosis*. J Biol Chem. 2006;281(7):3866–75. https://doi.org/10.1074/jbc.M505556200.
116. Hotelier T, Renault L, Cousin X, Negre V, Marchot P, Chatonnet A. ESTHER, the database of the α/β-hydrolase fold superfamily of proteins. Nucleic Acids Res. 2004;32:D145–7. https://doi.org/10.1093/nar/gkh141.
117. Sultana R, Tanneeru K, Guruprasad L. The PE-PPE domain in *Mycobacterium* reveals a serine α/β hydrolase fold and function: an in-silico analysis. PLoS One. 2011;6(2):e16745. https://doi.org/10.1371/journal.pone.0016745.
118. Daleke MH, Cascioferro A, de Punder K, Ummels R, Abdallah AM, van der Wel N, Peters PJ, Luirink J, Manganelli R, Bitter W. Conserved pro-Glu (PE) and pro-pro-Glu (PPE) protein domains target LipY lipases of pathogenic Mycobacteria to the cell surface via the ESX-5 pathway. J Biol Chem. 2011;286(21):19024–34. https://doi.org/10.1074/jbc.M110.204966.
119. Mishra KC, de Chastellier C, Narayana Y, Bifani P, Brown AK, Besra GS, Katoch VM, Joshi B, Balaji KN, Kremer L. Functional role of the PE domain and immunogenicity of the *Mycobacterium tuberculosis* triacylglycerol hydrolase LipY. Infect Immun. 2008;76(1):127–40. https://doi.org/10.1128/iai.00410-07.
120. Saxena AK, Roy KK, Singh S, Vishnoi SP, Kumar A, Kashyap VK, Kremer L, Srivastava R, Srivastava BS. Identification and characterisation of small-molecule inhibitors of Rv3097c-encoded lipase (LipY) of *Mycobacterium tuberculosis* that selectively inhibit growth of bacilli in hypoxia. Int J Antimicrob Agents. 2013;42(1):27–35. https://doi.org/10.1016/j.ijantimicag.2013.03.007.
121. Singh VK, Srivastava M, Dasgupta A, Singh MP, Srivastava R, Srivastava BS. Increased virulence of *Mycobacterium tuberculosis* H37Rv overexpressing LipY in a murine model. Tuberculosis. 2014;94(3):252–61. https://doi.org/10.1016/j.tube.2014.02.001.
122. Venkatesan R, Wierenga RK. Structure of Mycobacterial β-oxidation trifunctional enzyme reveals its altered assembly and putative substrate channeling pathway. ACS Chem Biol. 2013;8(5):1063–73. https://doi.org/10.1021/cb400007k.

123. Kornberg HL, Beevers H. A mechanism of conversion of fat to carbohydrate in castor beans. Nature. 1957;180(4575):35–6.
124. Tolbert NE. The C2 oxidative photosynthetic carbon cycle. Annu Rev Plant Physiol Plant Mol Biol. 1997;48(1):1–25. https://doi.org/10.1146/annurev.arplant.48.1.1.
125. Höner Zu Bentrup K, Miczak A, Swenson DL, Russell DG. Characterization of activity and expression of isocitrate lyase in *Mycobacterium avium* and *Mycobacterium tuberculosis*. J Bacteriol. 1999;181(23):7161–7.
126. Munoz-Elias EJ, McKinney JD. *Mycobacterium tuberculosis* isocitrate lyases 1 and 2 are jointly required for in vivo growth and virulence. Nat Med. 2005;11(6):638–44.. http://www.nature.com/nm/journal/v11/n6/suppinfo/nm1252_S1.html
127. McKinney JD, zu Bentrup KH, Munoz-Elias EJ, Miczak A, Chen B, Chan W-T, Swenson D, Sacchettini JC, Jacobs WR, Russell DG. Persistence of *Mycobacterium tuberculosis* in macrophages and mice requires the glyoxylate shunt enzyme isocitrate lyase. Nature. 2000;406(6797):735–8.
128. Nandakumar M, Nathan C, Rhee KY. Isocitrate lyase mediates broad antibiotic tolerance in Mycobacterium tuberculosis. Nat Commun. 2014;5:4306. https://doi.org/10.1038/ncomms5306.. http://www.nature.com/articles/ncomms5306#supplementary-information
129. Anstrom DM, Remington SJ. The product complex of M. tuberculosis malate synthase revisited. Protein Sci. 2006;15(8):2002–7. https://doi.org/10.1110/ps.062300206.
130. Smith CV, Huang C-c, Miczak A, Russell DG, Sacchettini JC, Höner zu Bentrup K. Biochemical and structural studies of malate synthase from *Mycobacterium tuberculosis*. J Biol Chem. 2003;278(3):1735–43. https://doi.org/10.1074/jbc.M209248200.
131. May EE, Leitão A, Tropsha A, Oprea TI. A systems chemical biology study of malate synthase and isocitrate lyase inhibition in *Mycobacterium tuberculosis* during active and NRP growth. Comput Biol Chem. 2013;47:167–80. https://doi.org/10.1016/j.compbiolchem.2013.07.002.
132. Brasaemle DL, Dolios G, Shapiro L, Wang R. Proteomic analysis of proteins associated with lipid droplets of basal and lipolytically stimulated 3 T3-L1 adipocytes. J Biol Chem. 2004;279(45):46835–42. https://doi.org/10.1074/jbc.M409340200.
133. Fujimoto Y, Itabe H, Sakai J, Makita M, Noda J, Mori M, Higashi Y, Kojima S, Takano T. Identification of major proteins in the lipid droplet-enriched fraction isolated from the human hepatocyte cell line HuH7. Biochim Biophys Acta (BBA) Mol Cell Res. 2004;1644(1):47–59. https://doi.org/10.1016/j.bbamcr.2003.10.018.
134. Liu P, Ying Y, Zhao Y, Mundy DI, Zhu M, Anderson RGW. Chinese hamster ovary K2 cell lipid droplets appear to be metabolic organelles involved in membrane traffic. J Biol Chem. 2004;279(5):3787–92. https://doi.org/10.1074/jbc.M311945200.
135. Umlauf E, Csaszar E, Moertelmaier M, Schuetz GJ, Parton RG, Prohaska R. Association of stomatin with lipid bodies. J Biol Chem. 2004;279(22):23699–709. https://doi.org/10.1074/jbc.M310546200.
136. Kory N, Farese RV Jr, Walther TC. Targeting fat: mechanisms of protein localization to lipid droplets. Trends Cell Biol. 2016;26(7):535–46. https://doi.org/10.1016/j.tcb.2016.02.007.
137. Greenberg AS, Egan JJ, Wek SA, Garty NB, Blanchette-Mackie EJ, Londos C. Perilipin, a major hormonally regulated adipocyte-specific phosphoprotein associated with the periphery of lipid storage droplets. J Biol Chem. 1991;266(17):11341–6.
138. Kimmel AR, Brasaemle DL, McAndrews-Hill M, Sztalryd C, Londos C. Adoption of PERILIPIN as a unifying nomenclature for the mammalian PAT-family of intracellular lipid storage droplet proteins. J Lipid Res. 2010;51(3):468–71. https://doi.org/10.1194/jlr.R000034.
139. Bickel PE, Tansey JT, Welte MA. PAT proteins, an ancient family of lipid droplet proteins that regulate cellular lipid stores. Biochim Biophys Acta (BBA) Mol Cell Biol Lipids. 2009;1791(6):419–40. https://doi.org/10.1016/j.bbalip.2009.04.002.
140. Kimmel AR, Sztalryd C. The perilipins: major cytosolic lipid droplet–associated proteins and their roles in cellular lipid storage, mobilization, and systemic homeostasis. Annu Rev Nutr. 2016;36(1):471–509. https://doi.org/10.1146/annurev-nutr-071813-105410.

141. Armstrong RM, Adams KL, Zilisch JE, Bretl DJ, Sato H, Anderson DM, Zahrt TC. Rv2744c is a PspA ortholog that regulates lipid droplet homeostasis and nonreplicating persistence in *Mycobacterium tuberculosis*. J Bacteriol. 2016;198(11):1645–61. https://doi.org/10.1128/jb.01001-15.
142. Bidle K, Kirkland PA, Nannen JL, Maupin-Furlow J. Proteomic analysis of Haloferax volcanii reveals salinity-mediated regulation of the stress response protein PspA. Microbiology. 2008;154(Pt 5):1436–43. https://doi.org/10.1099/mic.0.2007/015586-0.
143. Joly N, Burrows PC, Engl C, Jovanovic G, Buck M. A lower-order oligomer form of phage shock protein A (PspA) stably associates with the hexameric AAA(+) transcription activator protein PspF for negative regulation. J Mol Biol. 2009;394(4):764–75. https://doi.org/10.1016/j.jmb.2009.09.055.
144. Jovanovic G, Engl C, Buck M. Physical, functional and conditional interactions between ArcAB and phage shock proteins upon secretin-induced stress in *Escherichia coli*. Mol Microbiol. 2009;74(1):16–28. https://doi.org/10.1111/j.1365-2958.2009.06809.x.
145. Jovanovic G, Lloyd LJ, Stumpf MPH, Mayhew AJ, Buck M. Induction and function of the phage shock protein extracytoplasmic stress response in *Escherichia coli*. J Biol Chem. 2006;281(30):21147–61. https://doi.org/10.1074/jbc.M602323200.
146. Kobayashi R, Suzuki T, Yoshida M. Escherichia coli phage-shock protein A (PspA) binds to membrane phospholipids and repairs proton leakage of the damaged membranes. Mol Microbiol. 2007;66(1):100–9. https://doi.org/10.1111/j.1365-2958.2007.05893.x.
147. McDonald C, Jovanovic G, Ces O, Buck M. Membrane stored curvature elastic stress modulates recruitment of maintenance proteins PspA and Vipp1. MBio. 2015;6(5):e01188–15. https://doi.org/10.1128/mBio.01188-15.
148. Standar K, Mehner D, Osadnik H, Berthelmann F, Hause G, Lünsdorf H, Brüser T. PspA can form large scaffolds in *Escherichia coli*. FEBS Lett. 2008;582(25–26):3585–9. https://doi.org/10.1016/j.febslet.2008.09.002.
149. Vrancken K, van Mellaert L, Anné J. Characterization of the *Streptomyces lividans* PspA response. J Bacteriol. 2008;190(10):3475–81. https://doi.org/10.1128/JB.01966-07.
150. Jovanovic G, Mehta P, McDonald C, Davidson AC, Uzdavinys P, Ying L, Buck M. The N-terminal amphipathic helices determine regulatory and effector functions of phage shock protein A (PspA) in *Escherichia coli*. J Mol Biol. 2014;426(7):1498–511. https://doi.org/10.1016/j.jmb.2013.12.016.
151. Barik S, Sureka K, Mukherjee P, Basu J, Kundu M. RseA, the SigE specific anti-sigma factor of *Mycobacterium tuberculosis*, is inactivated by phosphorylation-dependent ClpC1P2 proteolysis. Mol Microbiol. 2010;75(3):592–606. https://doi.org/10.1111/j.1365-2958.2009.07008.x.
152. Estorninho M, Smith H, Thole J, Harders-Westerveen J, Kierzek A, Butler RE, Neyrolles O, Stewart GR. ClgR regulation of chaperone and protease systems is essential for *Mycobacterium tuberculosis* parasitism of the macrophage. Microbiology. 2010;156(Pt 11):3445–55. https://doi.org/10.1099/mic.0.042275-0.
153. Manganelli R, Voskuil MI, Schoolnik GK, Smith I. The *Mycobacterium tuberculosis* ECF sigma factor σE: role in global gene expression and survival in macrophages. Mol Microbiol. 2001;41(2):423–37. https://doi.org/10.1046/j.1365-2958.2001.02525.x.
154. Sherrid AM, Rustad TR, Cangelosi GA, Sherman DR. Characterization of a Clp protease gene regulator and the reaeration response in *Mycobacterium tuberculosis*. PLoS One. 2010;5(7):e11622. https://doi.org/10.1371/journal.pone.0011622.
155. White MJ, Savaryn JP, Bretl DJ, He H, Penoske RM, Terhune SS, Zahrt TC. The HtrA-like serine protease PepD interacts with and modulates the *Mycobacterium tuberculosis* 35-kDa antigen outer envelope protein. PLoS One. 2011;6(3):e18175. https://doi.org/10.1371/journal.pone.0018175.
156. Daniel J, Kapoor N, Sirakova T, Sinha R, Kolattukudy P. The perilipin-like PPE15 protein in *Mycobacterium tuberculosis* is required for triacylglycerol accumulation under dormancy-inducing conditions. Mol Microbiol. 2016;101(5):784–94. https://doi.org/10.1111/mmi.13422.

Potential Immunology, Transcriptomics and Epigenomic Prediction Tools of the Future to Improve tuberculosis Control

Andrew DiNardo and Anna M. Mandalakas

Abstract *Mycobacterium tuberculosis* (*Mtb*) continues to be a global scourge with 10.4 million cases of TB and 1.7 million deaths each year. The burgeoning molecular biology is both clarifying *Mtb*-induced pathology, but also raising new questions with many major challenges remaining: Immune correlates of protection are still to be clarified. Clinical biomarkers that predict disease progression are needed. Non-sputum quantitative means to monitor treatment efficacy are needed. Herein, we briefly review the spectrum of *Mtb* infection and pathology and then discuss how novel studies in immunology, transcriptomics and epigenomics could be translated into clinical care.

Keywords Tuberculosis · Latent tuberculosis infection · Transmission · Contact score · Tuberculosis elimination · Diagnostics · Biomarkers · Immunology · Transcriptomics · Epigenomics

Introduction

The END TB strategy aims to bring global levels of tuberculosis (TB) down to converge with those already attained by many wealthy countries, amounting to 90% reduction in TB incidence, deaths reduced by 95%, and no affected families facing catastrophic costs from TB [1]. The strategy focuses on early detection and treatment of TB and notably adds preventive treatment as a core strategy. In 2015, globally an estimated 4.3 million TB patients may have gone undetected and untreated, highlighting the need for expanding case finding among those most at risk but also giving a vivid illustration of the challenges faced by TB control programs in high TB-burden settings [2]. Extensive evidence demonstrates that preventive therapy, recommended for child contacts [3], effectively reduces individual risk of TB [4–7].

A. DiNardo · A. M. Mandalakas (✉)
The Global Tuberculosis Program, Section of Global and Immigrant Health, Department of Pediatrics, Baylor College of Medicine and Texas Children's Hopsital, Houston, TX, USA
e-mail: anna.mandalakas@bcm.edu

J. D. Cirillo, Y. Kong (eds.), *Tuberculosis Host-Pathogen Interactions*,
https://doi.org/10.1007/978-3-030-25381-3_10

Nevertheless, in 2015, only 7% of eligible children received preventive treatment following TB exposure providing more evidence of limited health system capacity to implement current guidelines which broadly recommend preventive treatment based on exposure and risk of disease progression. Scale up of preventive treatment is hampered by poor ability to predict who will develop TB after exposure. Even among tuberculin skin test or interferon-gamma release assay positive individuals, no more than 2.7% will develop TB within 2 years. Thus, at least 37 individuals must be treated to prevent a single case of TB [8]. Very few countries have the resources to support such high numbers of individuals needing treatment to prevent additional TB cases. Hence, better prediction of TB disease progression is therefore essential for reaching the END TB targets.

In 2010, 15.3 million children in the world shared a household with an individual with infectious TB resulting in 7.6 million children becoming infected with *Mycobacterium tuberculosis (M. tuberculosis)* in that year alone [9]. Modeling estimates further suggest that cumulative exposure has resulted in a prevalence of over 50 million *M. tuberculosis* infected children in the 22 high TB-burden countries in 2010. This unique model is the only current source of these estimates and provides critically important information to understand the potential impact of preventive treatment. Although treatment of tuberculosis infection decreases subsequent tuberculosis morbidity and mortality among adult contacts [10, 11] and markedly reduces risk in child contacts [7, 12], 10.4 million people combatted TB and 1.3 million died of TB in 2016 alone [2, 13]. In that same year, only 7% of eligible children received preventive therapy following close exposure to an infectious tuberculosis case [2]. The harsh reality of these numbers further emphasizes the dire need to better predict who among these many contacts will actually progress to TB. Such predictive capacity would allow TB control programs to provide preventive treatment to a smaller number of targeted people making preventive treatment a tenable and more cost-effective strategy.

The past decade has enjoyed an explosion of knowledge emerging from the fields of immunology, transcriptomics and epigenomics. Application of this knowledge in the study of tuberculosis has improved our understanding of the pathophysiology of *M.tuberculosis* infection and disease progression. In this chapter, we highlight new knowledge that could potentially improve tuberculosis control and support strides toward elimination, if successfully transformed into front line point of care applications.

Pathophysiology of *M. tuberculosis* Infection

The development of TB was historically thought to involve three key pathophysiologic events: (1) *M. tuberculosis* exposure, (2) *M. tuberculosis* infection, and (3) TB disease. Exposure implies that a person has had significant contact with a contagious TB case. In high TB-burden countries, more than 60% of children exposed to *M. tuberculosis* in their homes will develop a "latent" tuberculosis infection [14–16] which has been classically characterized by a positive tuberculin skin test or interferon-γ release assay result but no TB symptoms or radiographic abnormalities [17]. The course of *M.tuberculosis* infection is influenced largely by the host's immune response to the organism [17–20]. Although individuals have been thought to progress from no infection to infection to disease in a linear, unidirectional fashion, a growing body of evidence suggests that a more complex, dynamic bidirectional continuum of responses exist, leading to a spectrum of tuberculosis infection and disease states [21] (Fig. 1). The host response has previously been hypothesized to be associated with the magnitude of the mycobacterial load harbored by the host. In this theory, *M.tuberculosis* infection progresses from a transient state to a persistent but controlled state, and in some hosts, to a more severe disease state. In parallel, the mycobacterial load increases and the host immune response evolves from an innate response to an acquired response. Progression from infection to disease is complex, nuanced and still poorly understood with a balanced immune response necessary for control of infection [22–26]. Improved understanding of this dynamic interplay is vital in the development of strategies to risk stratify contacts to guide targeted preventive treatment.

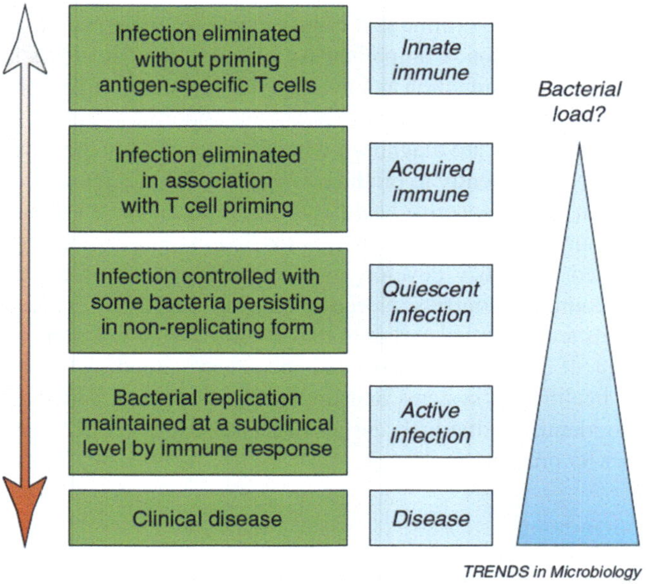

Fig. 1 A spectrum of responses to *M. tuberculosis* infection. The host response has been hypothesized to be associated with the magnitude of the mycobacterial load harbored by the host. During the first two weeks of *M.tuberculosis* infection, the host immune response is driven by innate immunity with adaptive immunity only contributing to the response thereafter. Early *M.tuberculosis* infection in the first two weeks is due to innate immunity with adaptive immunity starting thereafter. The necessary interplay between innate and adaptive immunity requisite for control of infection is yet to be determined

After aerosolization of *M.tuberculosis* into alveolar space, the development of adaptive immunity requires dendritic cells to phagocytize the bacilli and transport it to the draining lymph node for antigen presentation to T cells and development of TB-specific antigen presenting T cells. Recently developed theories, similar to the one described in figure one, raise the possibility that a "primed" or "trained" innate immune response may eliminate *M.tuberculosis* bacilli before dissemination to the draining lymph node and avert subsequent development of adaptive immunity. Unfortunately, improved understanding of the dynamic interplay between the host and *M.tuberculosis* is hindered by several critical limitations which build upon each other. First, despite our ability to measure the presence of *M.tuberculosis* once the host has progressed to a disease state, there is no available method to directly measure *M.tuberculosis* during the state of infection. Hence, it is impossible to quantify the *M.tuberculosis* burden and estimate the burden of infection in the absence of disease. Further, without the capacity to measure and quantify *M.tuberculosis* infection, it is impossible to determine if a robust innate immune response can rid the host of "transient" infection. All current tests of infection are indirect measures of host adaptive immunity. Hence, there is no acceptable "gold" reference standard to directly measure *M.tuberculosis* infection. It is therefore impossible to quantify the *M.tuberculosis* burden and estimate the burden of infection in the absence of disease [27]. Further, without the capacity to measure and quantify *M.tuberculosis* infection, it is impossible to determine if a robust innate immune response can rid the host of "transient" infection. Comprehensive elucidation of host mechanisms that eliminate *M.tuberculosis* infection and avert the development of persistent infection would yield a plethora of preventive and treatment opportunities.

In practice, individuals are diagnosed with TB disease once the burden of infection has progressed sufficiently to produce symptoms that are relevant enough to be recognized within their respective health system. In many high TB burden settings with limited resources and weak health systems, individuals combatting TB disease are not diagnosed until they develop severe manifestations of disease and have likely infected countless contacts. Nevertheless, TB control efforts are more effective if individuals are identified earlier in the cascade of care when interventions can prevent subsequent disease and associated secondary spread of infection (Fig. 2). Strengthening health care systems and improving diagnostic and prognostic tests that are able to identify individuals earlier in this cascade will decease the number of individuals who progress to disease.

Epidemiology of *M. tuberculosis* Infection

Many factors are associated with the risk for acquiring *M. tuberculosis* infection, including those related to the infectious case, the host, the organism and the environment. The extent of contact with the infectious case, the burden of organisms in the sputum and the frequency of cough in the index case are all directly associated with risk of infection [28]. Adults with acid-fast sputum smear-positive pulmonary

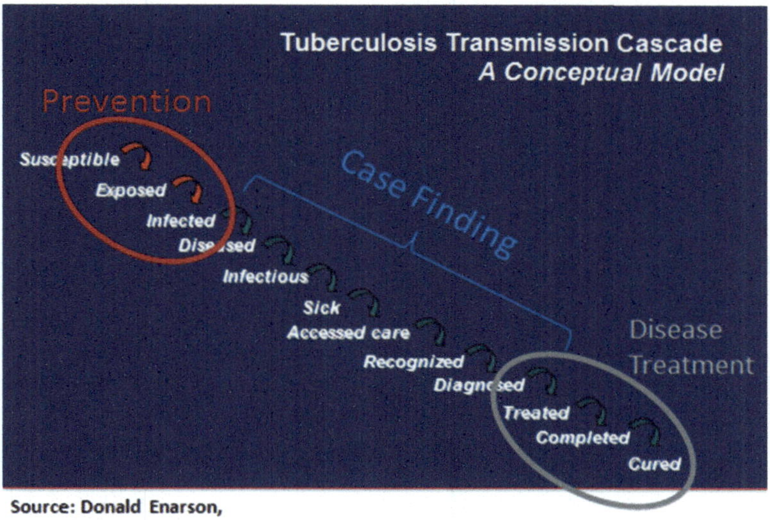

Source: Donald Enarson,
scientific director for the IUATLD, 1992 – 2012

Fig. 2 TB control opportunities along the TB Cascade of Care. The cascade of tuberculosis transmission begins with a host who is susceptible to disease and progresses through the key pathophysiologic events including *M. tuberculosis* exposure, infection and disease. Thereafter, a subset of individuals will progress to develop disease and potentially access care within their health system. The ability of the health system to diagnose disease early and provide effective treatment influences the individual's course through the cascade and impacts the ability of the individual to infect additional contacts thereby propagating the epidemic

tuberculosis are more likely to transmit infection. Risk of infection to adult and child contacts increases as the sputum smear grade of the case increases. Sputum smear grade is a measure of the density of organisms present in the sputum. Nevertheless, it is estimated that 10% of smear negative cases have the capacity to transmit *M. tuberculosis*. In addition, the risk for transmission is directly correlated with the degree of contact with a contagious case. And, although most transmission to young children occurs in their homes [14], a growing body of evidence suggests that significant exposure may happen within some communities and among older contacts [29]. A child's risk of infection is directly correlated with tuberculosis in the primary caregiver, sleep proximity and exposure to the index case, infectiousness of the index case, and having multiple cases of tuberculosis in the home [30]. Markers of close contact such as urban living and overcrowding also correlate with risk of infection in all age groups [31]. An increased risk for infection has been demonstrated in institutional settings, including nursing homes, schools, correctional institutions, homeless shelters, orphanages, and refugee camps [32–34]. The quality and amount of air circulation in the environment is another important factor; generally low air quality in homes compared with commercial buildings is a part of the reason why transmission tends to be greater in the home. The general risk for acquiring infection increases with age from infancy to early adulthood, likely because of increasing contacts with infectious persons.

The risk of TB disease progression is greatest during the first year following infection [35]. The risk of disease progression is inversely related to age, suggesting that an immature or inappropriate immune response favors disease progression [35]. Classic evidence demonstrates that the estimated lifetime risk of TB disease among individuals with a TST ≥10 mm is 10–20% in HIV-uninfected children ≤5 years of age, 5–10% among adolescents, and steadily decreases with increasing age such that the risk is <5% among those older than 35 years of age [36]. The risk in all ages groups increases dramatically in the presence of depressed cellular immunity due to young age, HIV infection or malnutrition and may be modulated by environmental factors [37]. Of HIV-uninfected infants (<1 year of age), 50% will progress TB disease following *M.tuberculosis* infection in the absence of isoniazid preventive therapy (IPT) [35]. The risk of TB in HIV-coinfected children is increased up to 25-fold [38, 39]. However, even in high TB-burden settings, the majority of people with TB are HIV-uninfected [40].

Prediction of *M. tuberculosis* Infection and TB Disease

Well-recognized epidemiologic risk factors for TB currently inform international and national recommendation guiding TB preventive programs such as contact tracing and preventive treatment. When compared to the general population in their communities, young and HIV-infected contacts have a greater risk of *M. tuberculosis* infection and TB disease. This risk is associated with a greater current and future risk of morbidity and mortality. Hence, the presence of *M. tuberculosis* infection in young and HIV-infected contacts is considered significant and treated as relevant disease for which preventive TB treatment is indicated [41]. Nevertheless, as the majority of these contacts will not progress to TB disease, a considerable amount of resources are expended providing preventive treatment to individuals who may not benefit from the intervention. Further, in high TB-burden countries, resources do not exist to support delivery of preventive treatment to such a large target population. Hence, a major research agenda is to develop pragmatic and feasible approaches to identify smaller groups of contacts with the highest risk of *M. tuberculosis* infection and TB disease, and therefore, the greatest potential gain of preventive treatment.

A seminal study conducted among South African children living in a setting with extremely high burdens of TB and HIV developed a standardized, reliable measure of household TB exposure that considered child-specific risk factors [42]. Children were considered *M. tuberculosis* infected if two of three tests of infection were positive. The study employed the traditional tuberculin skin test and two interferon gamma release assays. Principal component analysis was used to identify a discrete set of components that collectively described TB exposure and contributed to a composite contact score. Four components were identified that described 68% of data variance: (1) maternal TB and sleep proximity, (2) index case infectivity, (3) duration of exposure, and (4) exposure to multiple index cases. Components were

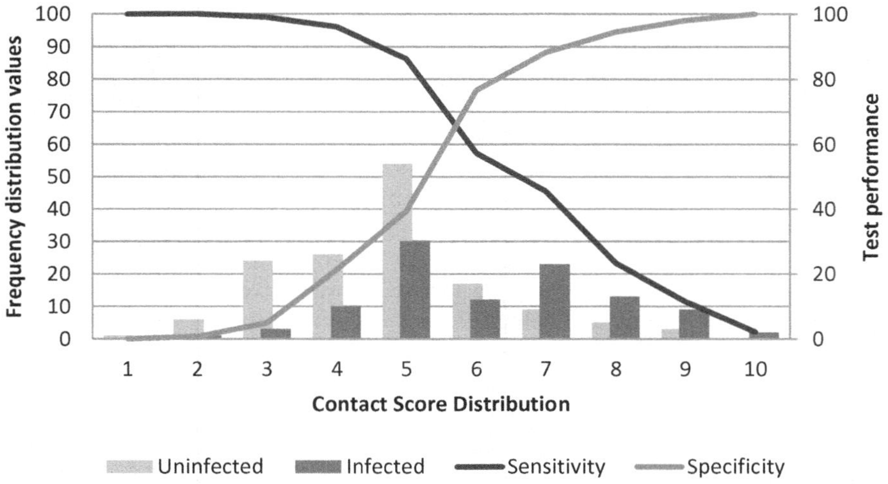

Fig. 3 *M.tuberculosis* contact score distribution stratified by infection status and test performance. The distribution of the *M.tuberculosis* contact score among children less than 6 years of age with and without *M.tuberculosis* infection is illustrated in the frequency distribution graph. The sensitivity and specificity of the contact score at sequential contact score cut-off points are represented by black and grey lines, respectively

derived from 10 binary questions that contributed to a contact score (range 1–10, median 5, 25th–75th interquartile range [IQR] 4–7). Among children aged 3 months to 6 years with household exposure, the odds of being M. tuberculosis infected increased by 74% (OR 1.74, 95%CI 1.42–2.12) with each 1-point increase in the contact score. Although the score was better suited to assess risk of infection among younger children, the study demonstrated that well-quantified TB exposure is a good surrogate measure of *M. tuberculosis* infection in child household contacts in a high-burden setting, and *could* guide targeted preventive treatment in children at highest risk of development of *M. tuberculosis* infection. A prospective, randomized control trial evaluating the well-quantified TB exposure score's capacity to identify, treat and prevent TB progression is needed (Fig. 3).

Retrospective analysis of data on TB cases and contacts from the Taiwan National Surveillance Network of Communicable Disease, a centralized, internet-based TB case management system, was used to develop and validate an eight point score predictive of TB disease among Taiwanese child contacts [43]. The predictive score integrated data routinely collected in contact investigations by public health nurses, such as TST results of the contacts, smear-positivity of the index cases, and residence and sex of the index cases, in a systematic way. Among contacts in the derivation cohort, the observed risk for being a prevalent TB case decreased as the risk score decreased (P, 0.001, Cochran-Armitage trend test). Specifically, a contact with a score of 7 was 12.5 times more likely to be a prevalent case than a contact with a score of 1. Similarly, the observed risk for a contact to develop incident TB increased as the contact score increased (P, 0.001, Cochran-Armitage trend test); a contact with a score of 7 was 7 times more likely to become an incident case than a contact with a score of 1. Further, the number of individuals that needed to be treated (NNT) with Isoniazid preventive therapy to avert one active TB case during the 3-year follow-up dramatically decreased as the contact score increased. Of note, the NNT ranged from 1260 for contacts with a risk score of 2 to one for contacts with a risk score of 7. This predictive score has been deployed as a field assessment tool to guide prioritization of contact tracing. Priority is assigned to child contacts who have a high score (5–7), to ensure all of these high-risk children can receive comprehensive evaluation and a complete course of preventive therapy as clinically indicated. This promising tool demonstrates the ability of setting specific risk factors to predict TB disease among contacts. Nevertheless, reliance on the Tuberculin skin test limits the ability of this particular tool to be adapted to many high TB burden settings as the test and required human resources are not readily available.

While the interactions between host and pathogen that determines progression from infection to disease remain unclear, higher bacillary burdens are associated with increased risk of progression. *M.tuberculosis* has long been known to be spread through aerosolization of infectious sputa via the coughing process. Typically the infectious aerosolized droplets are less than <10 mm in diameter. Hence, droplets reach the lung's alveoli when inhaled. Emerging evidence has demonstrated correlation between cough aerosols and risk of secondary transmission. In a study in Uganda, individuals with contagious TB were asked to cough into a tube with a device inside that contains agar and small filters used as a method of quantifying cough aerosols. Contacts exposed to TB diseased patients with high cough aerosol measures were more likely to develop infection and later disease compared to patients with lower cough aerosol measures [44]. Further, secondary transmission risk was more strongly associated with cough aerosol measures than sputum smear positivity [45, 46]. As an inoculum effect is common in most infectious diseases, this evidence has been interpreted to suggest that there is a greater likelihood of more progressive TB disease with greater magnitudes of inhaled infectious aerosol. This is likely further related to host immune response, but other factors being equal, the authors further hypothesize that a measurement of index case inhaled dose could predict progression in TB contacts.

Immune Signatures for Infection-Disease Discrimination and Progression

There is extensive evidence that the host immune response is critical in determining the spectrum of clinical outcomes from asymptomatic, "latent" infection to overt disease. Specifically, individuals with defects in cellular mediated immunity specific to the IL-12-IFN-γ axis as found in Mendelian Susceptibility of Mycobacterial Diseases (MSMD), HIV-infection and the use of TNF inhibitors are at increased risk of TB disease progression. When macrophages are polarized with IFN-γ (or TNF, FSL-1, GM-CSF or LPS), they develop a "classically activated, or M1 phenotype, with more than 290 genes induced resulting in cellular changes in chemokine receptor, cell activation markers, MHC expression, caspase production, proteasome formation, and protein ubiquitination. These IFN-γ-induced phenotypic changes improve macrophage phago-lysosome maturation, lysosome acidification, NO and ROS production with resultant improvement in intracellular killing of mycobacteria [47–51]. Spoiler alert: despite extensive *in vitro* studies showing multiple mechanisms by which IFN-γ improves macrophage *Mtb* killing capacity, IFN-γ levels in murine models or human studies do not correlate with *Mtb* killing or disease protection, respectively [52]. Elucidating the complex pathophysiology why IFN-γ induces macrophage killing of *Mtb in vivo* but not *in vitro* is a likely prerequisite to improved diagnostics and prognostics.

The identification of genomic regions of *Mtb* not found in BCG (region of differentiation; RD-1) and subsequent identification of proteins (ESAT-6, CFP-10 and TB 10.4) coded by this region led to the development of Interferon Gamma Release Assays (IGRAs). There are two commercially available IGRAs, the ELISA based Quantiferon (QFT; Quest Diagnostics) and ELISPOT-based T-SPOT (Oxford Immunotech), both, which quantifies IFN-γ production after immune cells are stimulated with TB-specific peptides ESAT-6 and CFP-10. While the IGRAs offer improved specificity over TSTs, they are unable to discriminate infection and disease. Historically, it was also thought that these tests are unable to predict progression from infection to disease, however a recent study challenges that paradigm. Among ~2500 HIV-uninfected children part of a TB vaccine trial, a QFT value >4 IU/mL was associated with increased rate of TB progression compared to individuals with positive QFT values between 0.35–4.0 IU/mL [53]. As HIV infection is known to decrease the host's ability to produce IFN-γ, validating this study with HIV-infected children will be important. Further, much attention has been focused on the apparent contradiction that ex vivo IFN-γ improves *M.tuberculosis* killing, while in vivo elevated IFN-γ levels are associated with disease progression. Elucidation of the mechanisms that produce this paradox is a major research agenda as this critical information will likely improve TB diagnostics and prognostics. Despite these gaps in our understanding of the pathophysiology of *M.tuberculosis* infection, an emerging body of evidence has capitalized on IGRA testing and demonstrated that BCG vaccination is associated with a decreased risk of *M.tuberculosis* infection [54, 55]. This intriguing evidence lends support to modeling work completed by the WHO suggesting that TB elimination will not be achieved without introduction of an improved vaccine.

Since measurement of IFN-γ alone has historically not been sufficient to discriminate infection from disease or predict progression form infection to disease, investigators have turned to alternative approaches such as multi-parameter flow cytometry for predictive biomarker signature. By evaluating the *Mtb*-specific production of IFN-γ, TNF and IL-2 simultaneously, discrimination of infection and disease was feasible (sensitivity ~67% and specificity 92%); infection was characterized by an increase in production of all three markers while disease was characterized by single-positive TNF production [56]. Adding immune activation markers CD38 and HLA-DR and cell proliferation marker Ki-67 to TNF and IFN-γ further improved specificity and sensitivity in discriminating infection and disease [57]. It is critical that these biomarker signatures be prospectively evaluated for capacity to identify individuals at increased risk for TB progression. In one such study, ex vivo BCG stimulation of perinatal BCG vaccinated children, multi-parameter investigation of IL-2, TNF, IL-17 and IFN-γ by CD4, CD8 and γϱ T cells were unable to discriminate children who would go on to develop TB from those without disease. One possible explanation for the inability of these biomarkers to predict disease progression is that the blood was collected before TB exposure. Alternatively evaluation of a mix of pro-inflammatory and anti-inflammatory immune markers may be necessary to predict disease progression [24]. Similarly, the predominance of immune investigation to date has focused on lymphocyte from peripheral blood. With improving fluorescent and mass-spectroscopy technology that allows for simultaneous evaluation of >30 immune markers [58], future studies should evaluate the role of site-specific immunity, non-lymphocytes (dendritic cells, monocytes, mast cells, basophils, etc.), transcription factors, phosphorylation marks and anti-inflammatory cytokines to improve discriminatory and predictive capacity.

It must be reiterated that the complexities of host-pathogen interactions that determine TB disease progression remain to be elucidated [24]. Of note, recent years have documented the necessity of a balanced immune response with studies showing that both a suppressed and an effusive immune response can lead to *M. tuberculosis* growth. Too little TNF leads to intracellular *Mtb* growth, while too much TNF leads to macrophage necroptosis and extracellular *Mtb* growth [25, 26]. Too little IFN-γ leads to intracellular Mtb growth, but excess IFN-γ results in an exuberant immune response with collateral host inflammatory lung pathology [22]. A new paradigm, the Goldilocks paradigm, suggests that a balance of inflammatory and anti-inflammatory immunity is needed for *M. tuberculosis* control. With improved quantitative measurements of *M. tuberculosis* bacillary burden [59], and improved technologies allowing for simultaneous measurement of the balance of the innate and adaptive immune response, prospective studies are needed to identify the requisite balance that correlates with infection control versus disease progression.

Transcriptomic Approaches to Discrimination and Prognostication

In an alternative approach for TB biomarkers discovery, investigators have explored gene expression signatures. In one such study, whole blood, dominated by myeloid cell influence, was able to discriminate TB from latent infection and other active infections (Still's disease, lupus, Staphylococcal and streptococcal infection). In particular, the Type I and Type II interferon signaling pathway in whole blood, neutrophils and monocytes was up-regulated in TB. This 393-transcript signature was parsed down to an 86-transcript signature while retaining discriminatory capacity. In a different evaluation of >2000 children being worked up for pulmonary TB, a 51-gene signature was able to discriminate infection and disease with 83% sensitivity and specificity [60]. To evaluate a transcription signature that could predict TB disease progression, a study of >10,000 latently infected individuals first performed data mining on RNA-sequencing (RNA-seq). From the RNA-seq training set, a 16-gene RT-PCR signature was able identify TB progression with sensitivity 39–53% and specificity of 81–90% [61]. Using a data mining approach examining publicly available datasets, a 3-gene signature was able to discriminate TB from asymptomatic infection and other diseases with excellent sensitivity and specificity depending on cutoffs. Considering the existing near point of care PCR capacity and developing technology that will bring PCR to point of care (POC) clinical utility, these gene expression signatures promise to improve current diagnosis and prognosis. Alternatively, next generation sequencing has been combined with nanopore technology resulting in a portable, but not yet affordable, sequencing modality that has the potential for POC utility [62]. It will be interesting if a combined approach simultaneously evaluating host transcription signature combined with direct *M tuberculosis* detection by Gene Xpert will yield a high enough negative predictive value to rule out TB.

Epigenetics Link Transcriptomics and Immunology; Potential Diagnostic and Prognostic Improvements?

A cell's phenotype is determined more by the regulated expression of its genes than its genetic information. While each cell in the body has the same genome, the regulation of gene transcription into protein determines its phenotype. Epigenetics is the study of how gene expression is modified without alterations in the genetic code. For example, by adding a methyl to the 5′ carbon of cytosine, DNA is less accessible to transcription factor binding and gene transcription. Epigenetic mechanisms occur in concert: DNA methylation induces recruitment methyl-CpG binding domain proteins (MBD) "readers" that recruit histone deacetylases (HDACs) that remove acetyl groups from histone tails (Fig. 4). Further, DNA methyltransferases (DNMT) collude with the Polycomb Repressive Complex protein EZH2 to induce epigenetically silencing via the addition of three methyl groups to histone 3 at lysine 27 (H3K27Me3).

Immune cells in particular must stay responsive to fluctuating environments and must be both tailored and measured to address diverse pathogenic challenges without inducing a pro-inflammatory response with excess host collateral damage. For example, an IFN-γ characterized Type 1 immune response to large invading helminth infection would induce excessive collateral host hepatocyte and alveolar tissue damage [63, 64]. Therefore, both the innate and adaptive immune arms are

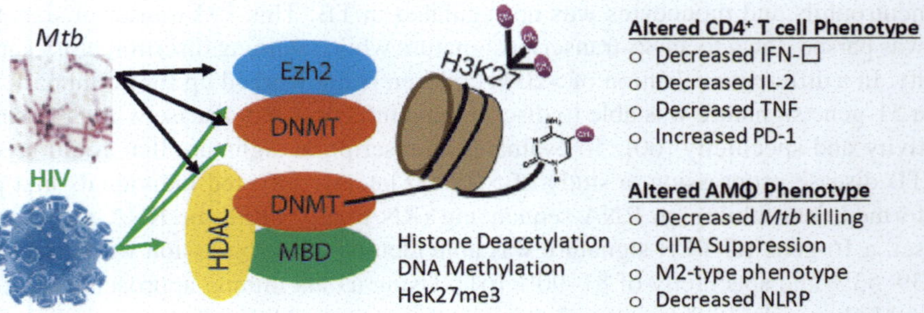

Fig. 4 TB and HIV-induced chronic inflammation induces epigenetic changes in DNA methyltransferases (DNMT), Polycomb Repressive Complex EZH2 and Histone deacetylase (HDAC)-mediated immune silencing. Future studies are needed to elucidate if these epigenetic changes can augment existing TB diagnosis or prognosis

epigenetically regulated to deliver targeted, measured and "trained" responses [65, 66]. In the field of oncology, clarifications of epigenetic biomarker signatures and mechanisms have transformed disease prognostication, treatment determination and novel drug discovery [67]. Future studies will disclose if similar revelations and revolutions await tuberculosis care.

For example, BCG vaccination has recently been discovered to induce long-term innate immune training of monocytes and macrophages. After vaccination of healthy students, BCG induced increased histone methylation (increases in H3K4me3) at the *tnf* and *IL6* promoter sites in monocytes and macrophages resulting in increased monocyte killing of *Mtb*, as well as *Staphylococcal aureus* and candida up to three months after vaccination [65]. Now that BCG induced epigenetic mediated "innate immune training" has been demonstrated in healthy controls, it is vital for studies to seek innate epigenetic biomarker signatures that have capacity to either discriminate infection from disease or to identify individuals at high risk of infection to disease progression [68, 69].

The adaptive immune response is incredibly dynamic, starting with hypomethylation of *RAG* and RAG-mediated TCR rearrangement [70]. To remain nimble to an ever-changing environment, T cells develop into an ever-increasing number of distinct immune phenotypes (Th1, Th2, Th9, Th17, etc.), frequently using epigenetic modifications to respond to environmental cues [71–73]. For example to become a Th1 T cell, the *IFNG* promoter must de-methylate and the IL-4 loci is suppressed via repressive histone modifications [74–76]. The evidence suggests that in response to stimuli, approximately 15 Pioneer transcription Factors and lineage specific regulators (p300, STAT1,T-bet, GATA3, Foxp3) initiate cell-type specific Enhancers in order to determine and maintain a specific immune phenotype [77]. While the T cell phenotype was previously thought to be immutable, Th2 cells can be "re-programmed" to a Th1 phenotype through inhibition of the Polycomb Repressive Complex (PRC) EZH2 protein and subsequent removal of the suppressive epigenetic marks [66]. Similar to biomarkers for innate immunity, identification of DNA methylation, histone post-translational modifications and/or miRNA should be evaluated for their potential as biomarkers to identify and elucidate the *M.tuberculosis* immune correlates of protection.

Epigenetically mediated down-regulation of the immune response is an evolutionary failsafe to temper an exuberant immune response that would otherwise induce host collateral damage [78]. Seminal research elucidating a pathogen's alteration of host epigenetic status demonstrated that HIV infection decreases IFN-γ production by increasing DNMT activity, resulting in DNA hypermethylation of the *IFNG* CpG promoter region [79]. Subsequent studies showed that the genes expressed by HIV early in infection directly induce host DNMT1 expression via the AP1 pathway in both T cells and non-T cells [80]. In addition to epigenetic silencing of IFN-γ, HIV-induced DNMT1 changes result in decreased IL-2 production via hypermethylation of the *IL2* promoter regions. HIV further epigenetically represses T cells by de-methylating the PD-1 promoter and hypermethylates the IL-2 promoter [81, 82]. Similarly, *Mtb* induces epigenetic changes detrimental to host immune control. Specifically, HDAC activity at the *IL12B* loci decreases *Mtb*-infected macrophage IL-12 production and increasing *Mtb* intracellular survival [83]. Similarly, after *Mtb* infection, deacetylation of IFN-γ -inducible genes *MHC2TA* results in decreased MHCII via CIITA (class II transactivator) [84, 85]. In addition to HDAC-mediated changes, *Mtb* induces epigenetic changes in EZH2 and JMJD3 alterations in H3K27me3 suppressing CITTA with a net resultant decrease in classically activated macrophage phenotype [86, 87]. In addition, macrophages undergo global DNA hyper-methylation after *Mtb* infection with wide-spread alterations in gene expression, including perturbations in the NLRP inflammasome [88, 89]. On CD8+ Cytotoxic T Lymphocytes, *Mtb*-induces epigenetic changes in long noncoding RNA (ncRNA) and EZH2 recruitment to the *IFNG* and *TNF* promoters to suppress TNF and IFN-γ production [90]. To date, the majority of epigenetic studies have been implemented in in animal models and cell lines. With a growing body of evidence denoting the importance in epigenetic gene regulation in immune control of *Mtb* infection, cohort studies should be implemented to identify epigenetic differences between infection and disease and predicting incident disease [92].

Summary

Global TB elimination will require a global commitment to identify individuals at risk of TB infection and disease while expanding preventive efforts. Evidence and risk-based approaches to deliver preventive therapy can help to pave the path toward the end of TB.

More than one-hundred and twenty years after the identification of *M.tuberculosis* as the causative agent of TB, molecular techniques have provided "game changing" diagnostics, such as Gene Xpert's automated *M. tuberculosis* PCR-based platform. Gene Xpert has improved early microbiologic confirmation of TB. But much work remains. With 2 billion individuals harboring asymptomatic infection, we lack prognostic tests able to guide preventative therapy to those at highest need. Further, with treatment failure rates of 12% accompanied by a 3–9% case fatality rate that is dependent upon HIV-co-infection, prognostic tests will help clinicians identify high-risk individuals and guide personalized targeted therapeutics. Finally, recent paradigm shifting studies have shown that persistent *M.tuberculosis* mRNA after clinically successful TB therapy failed to correlate with relapse [91]. As an estimated 5% of TB patients suffer relapse, there is a need to identify a combination of host and microbe-specific prognostic tests that will help clinicians improve outcomes in TB affected patients. Scientific advancements in response to these important questions have the potential to fuel our journey to reach the global goal of TB elimination. Nevertheless, the impact of these knowledge gains will be critically dependent on our ability to successfully transform these sophisticated technologies into feasible, cost-effective point-of-care tests that may be used in TB high burden and resource constrained settings.

References

1. Uplekar M, Weil D, Lonnroth K, Jaramillo E, Lienhardt C, Dias HM, Falzon D, Floyd K, Gargioni G, Getahun H, et al. WHO's new end TB strategy. Lancet. 2015;385(9979):1799–801.
2. WHO. Global tuberculosis report, 2016. Geneva: WHO; 2016.
3. WHO. Recommendations for investigating contacts of persons with infectious tuberculosis in low- and middle-income countries. Geneva: WHO; 2012.
4. Comstock GW, Baum C, Snider DE Jr. Isoniazid prophylaxis among Alaskan Eskimos: a final report of the bethel isoniazid studies. Am Rev Respir Dis. 1979;119(5):827–30.
5. Efficacy of various durations of isoniazid preventive therapy for tuberculosis: five years of follow-up in the IUAT trial. International Union Against Tuberculosis Committee on Prophylaxis. Bull World Health Organ. 1982;60(4):555–64.
6. Sharma SK, Sharma A, Kadhiravan T, Tharyan P. Rifamycins (rifampicin, rifabutin and rifapentine) compared to isoniazid for preventing tuberculosis in HIV-negative people at risk of active TB. Cochrane Database Syst Rev. 2013;(7):CD007545.
7. Ayieko J, Abuogi L, Simchowitz B, Bukusi EA, Smith AH, Reingold A. Efficacy of isoniazid prophylactic therapy in prevention of tuberculosis in children: a meta-analysis. BMC Infect Dis. 2014;14:91.
8. Diel R, Loddenkemper R, Nienhaus A. Predictive value of interferon-gamma release assays and tuberculin skin testing for progression from latent TB infection to disease state: a meta-analysis. Chest. 2012;142(1):63–75.
9. Dodd PJ, Gardiner E, Coghlan R, Seddon JA. Burden of childhood tuberculosis in 22 high-burden countries: a mathematical modelling study. Lancet Glob Health. 2014;2(8):e453–9.
10. Smieja M, Marchetti C, Cook D, Smaill F. Isoniazid for preventing tuberculosis in non-HIV infected persons. Cochrane Database Syst Rev. 1999;(1):CD001363.
11. Woldehana S, Volmink J. Treatment of latent tuberculosis infection in HIV infected persons. Cochrane Database Syst Rev. 2004;(1):CD000171.
12. Hsu KH. Isoniazid in the prevention and treatment of tuberculosis. A 20-year study of the effectiveness in children. JAMA. 1974;229(5):528–33.
13. WHO. Global tuberculosis report 2016. World Health Organization; 2016.
14. Beyers N, Gie RP, Schaaf HS, Van Zyl S, Talent JM, Nel ED, Donald PR. A prospective evaluation of children under the age of 5 years living in the same household as adults with recently diagnosed pulmonary tuberculosis. Int J Tuberc Lung Dis. 1997;1(1):38–43.

15. Lienhardt C, Sillah J, Fielding K, Donkor S, Manneh K, Warndorff D, Bennett S, McAdam K. Risk factors for tuberculosis infection in children in contact with infectious tuberculosis cases in the Gambia, West Africa. Pediatrics. 2003;111(5 Pt 1):e608–14.
16. Morrison J, Pai M, Hopewell PC. Tuberculosis and latent tuberculosis infection in close contacts of people with pulmonary tuberculosis in low-income and middle-income countries: a systematic review and meta-analysis. Lancet Infect Dis. 2008;8(6):359–68.
17. Smith S, Jacobs RF, Wilson CB. Immunobiology of childhood tuberculosis: a window on the ontogeny of cellular immunity. J Pediatr. 1997;131(1 Pt 1):16–26.
18. Schluger NW, Rom WN. The host immune response to tuberculosis. Am J Respir Crit Care Med. 1998;157(3 Pt 1):679–91.
19. Barnes P. Immunology of tuberculosis. Semin Pediatr Infect Dis. 1993;4:232.
20. Barnes PF, Grisso CL, Abrams JS, Band H, Rea TH, Modlin RL. Gamma delta T lymphocytes in human tuberculosis. J Infect Dis. 1992;165(3):506–12.
21. Young DB, Gideon HP, Wilkinson RJ. Eliminating latent tuberculosis. Trends Microbiol. 2009;17(5):183–8.
22. Barber DL, Mayer-Barber KD, Feng CG, Sharpe AH, Sher A. CD4 T cells promote rather than control tuberculosis in the absence of PD-1-mediated inhibition. J Immunol. 2011;186(3):1598–607.
23. Gideon HP, Phuah J, Myers AJ, Bryson BD, Rodgers MA, Coleman MT, Maiello P, Rutledge T, Marino S, Fortune SM, et al. Variability in tuberculosis granuloma T cell responses exists, but a balance of pro- and anti-inflammatory cytokines is associated with sterilization. PLoS Pathog. 2015;11(1):e1004603.
24. Nunes-Alves C, Booty MG, Carpenter SM, Jayaraman P, Rothchild AC, Behar SM. In search of a new paradigm for protective immunity to TB. Nat Rev Microbiol. 2014;12(4):289–99.
25. Roca FJ, Ramakrishnan L. TNF dually mediates resistance and susceptibility to mycobacteria via mitochondrial reactive oxygen species. Cell. 2013;153(3):521–34.
26. Tobin DM, Vary JC Jr, Ray JP, Walsh GS, Dunstan SJ, Bang ND, Hagge DA, Khadge S, King MC, Hawn TR, et al. The lta4h locus modulates susceptibility to mycobacterial infection in zebrafish and humans. Cell. 2010;140(5):717–30.
27. Nardell EA, Wallis RS. Here today--gone tomorrow: the case for transient acute tuberculosis infection. Am J Respir Crit Care Med. 2006;174(7):734–5.
28. Comstock G. Epidemiology of tuberculosis. In: Reichman LB, Hershfield E, editors. Tuberculosis: a comprehensive international approach. 2nd ed. New York: Marcel Dekker; 2000. p. 129–48.
29. Yates TA, Khan PY, Knight GM, Taylor JG, McHugh TD, Lipman M, White RG, Cohen T, Cobelens FG, Wood R, et al. The transmission of *Mycobacterium tuberculosis* in high burden settings. Lancet Infect Dis. 2016;16(2):227–38.
30. Mandalakas A, Kirchner HL, Lombard C, Wazyl G, Gie R, Hesseling A. Well quantified tuberculosis exposure is a reliable surrogate measure of tuberculosis infection in children. Int J Tuberc Lung Dis. 2012;16:1033.
31. Wood R, Johnstone-Robertson S, Uys P, Hargrove J, Middelkoop K, Lawn SD, Bekker LG. Tuberculosis transmission to young children in a South African community: modeling household and community infection risks. Clin Infect Dis. 2010;51(4):401–8.
32. Sutter RW, Haefliger E. Tuberculosis morbidity and infection in Vietnamese in Southeast Asian refugee camps. Am Rev Respir Dis. 1990;141(6):1483–6.
33. Mandalakas AM, Kirchner HL, Iverson S, Chesney M, Spencer MJ, Sidler A, Johnson D. Predictors of *Mycobacterium tuberculosis* infection in international adoptees. Pediatrics. 2007;120(3):e610–6.
34. Saiman L, Aronson J, Zhou J, Gomez-Duarte C, Gabriel PS, Alonso M, Maloney S, Schulte J. Prevalence of infectious diseases among internationally adopted children. Pediatrics. 2001;108(3):608–12.
35. Marais BJ, Gie RP, Schaaf HS, Hesseling AC, Obihara CC, Starke JJ, Enarson DA, Donald PR, Beyers N. The natural history of childhood intra-thoracic tuberculosis: a critical review of literature from the pre-chemotherapy era. Int J Tuberc Lung Dis. 2004;8(4):392–402.

36. Horsburgh CR Jr. Priorities for the treatment of latent tuberculosis infection in the United States. N Engl J Med. 2004;350(20):2060–7.
37. den Boon S, van Lill SW, Borgdorff MW, Verver S, Bateman ED, Lombard CJ, Enarson DA, Beyers N. Association between smoking and tuberculosis infection: a population survey in a high tuberculosis incidence area. Thorax. 2005;60(7):555–7.
38. Bhat GJ, Diwan VK, Chintu C, Kabika M, Masona J. HIV, BCG and TB in children: a case control study in Lusaka, Zambia. J Trop Pediatr. 1993;39(4):219–23.
39. Hesseling AC, Cotton MF, Jennings T, Whitelaw A, Johnson LF, Eley B, Roux P, Godfrey-Faussett P, Schaaf HS. High incidence of tuberculosis among HIV-infected infants: evidence from a South African population-based study highlights the need for improved tuberculosis control strategies. Clin Infect Dis. 2009;48(1):108–14.
40. Schaaf HS, Marais BJ, Whitelaw A, Hesseling AC, Eley B, Hussey GD, Donald PR. Culture-confirmed childhood tuberculosis in Cape Town, South Africa: a review of 596 cases. BMC Infect Dis. 2007;7:140.
41. Marais BJ. On the definition of relevant disease. Arch Dis Child. 2004;89(5):497.
42. Mandalakas AM, Kirchner HL, Lombard C, Walzl G, Grewal HM, Gie RP, Hesseling AC. Well-quantified tuberculosis exposure is a reliable surrogate measure of tuberculosis infection. Int J Tuberc Lung Dis. 2012;16(8):1033–9.
43. Chan PC, Shinn-Forng Peng S, Chiou MY, Ling DL, Chang LY, Wang KF, Fang CT, Huang LM. Risk for tuberculosis in child contacts. Development and validation of a predictive score. Am J Respir Crit Care Med. 2014;189(2):203–13.
44. Jones-Lopez EC, Acuna-Villaorduna C, Ssebidandi M, Gaeddert M, Kubiak RW, Ayakaka I, White LF, Joloba M, Okwera A, Fennelly KP. Cough aerosols of *Mycobacterium tuberculosis* in the prediction of incident tuberculosis disease in household contacts. Clin Infect Dis. 2016;63(1):10–20.
45. Fennelly KP, Jones-Lopez EC. Quantity and quality of inhaled dose predicts immunopathology in tuberculosis. Front Immunol. 2015;6:313.
46. Fennelly KP. What is in a cough? Int J Mycobacteriol. 2016;5(Suppl 1):S51.
47. Weiss G, Schaible UE. Macrophage defense mechanisms against intracellular bacteria. Immunol Rev. 2015;264(1):182–203.
48. Herbst S, Schaible UE, Schneider BE. Interferon gamma activated macrophages kill mycobacteria by nitric oxide induced apoptosis. PLoS One. 2011;6(5):e19105.
49. Vandal OH, Nathan CF, Ehrt S. Acid resistance in *Mycobacterium tuberculosis*. J Bacteriol. 2009;191(15):4714–21.
50. Keiser TL, Purdy GE. Killing *Mycobacterium tuberculosis* in vitro: what model systems can teach us. Microbiol Spectr. 2017;5(3). https://doi.org/10.1128/microbiolspec.TBTB2-0028-2016.
51. Venketaraman V, Dayaram YK, Amin AG, Ngo R, Green RM, Talaue MT, Mann J, Connell ND. Role of glutathione in macrophage control of mycobacteria. Infect Immun. 2003;71(4):1864–71.
52. Sakai S, Kauffman KD, Sallin MA, Sharpe AH, Young HA, Ganusov VV, Barber DL. CD4 T cell-derived IFN-gamma plays a minimal role in control of pulmonary *Mycobacterium tuberculosis* infection and must be actively repressed by PD-1 to prevent lethal disease. PLoS Pathog. 2016;12(5):e1005667.
53. Andrews JR, Nemes E, Tameris M, Landry BS, Mahomed H, McClain JB, Fletcher HA, Hanekom WA, Wood R, McShane H, et al. Serial QuantiFERON testing and tuberculosis disease risk among young children: an observational cohort study. Lancet Respir Med. 2017;5(4):282–90.
54. Basu Roy R, Sotgiu G, Altet-Gomez N, Tsolia M, Ruga E, Velizarova S, Kampmann B. Identifying predictors of interferon-gamma release assay results in pediatric latent tuberculosis: a protective role of bacillus Calmette-Guerin?: a pTB-NET collaborative study. Am J Respir Crit Care Med. 2012;186(4):378–84.

55. Soysal A, Millington KA, Bakir M, Dosanjh D, Aslan Y, Deeks JJ, Efe S, Staveley I, Ewer K, Lalvani A. Effect of BCG vaccination on risk of *Mycobacterium tuberculosis* infection in children with household tuberculosis contact: a prospective community-based study. Lancet. 2005;366(9495):1443–51.
56. Harari A, Rozot V, Enders FB, Perreau M, Stalder JM, Nicod LP, Cavassini M, Calandra T, Blanchet CL, Jaton K, et al. Dominant TNF-alpha+ Mycobacterium tuberculosis-specific CD4+ T cell responses discriminate between latent infection and active disease. Nat Med. 2011;17(3):372–6.
57. Adekambi T, Ibegbu CC, Cagle S, Kalokhe AS, Wang YF, Hu Y, Day CL, Ray SM, Rengarajan J. Biomarkers on patient T cells diagnose active tuberculosis and monitor treatment response. J Clin Invest. 2015;125(5):1827–38.
58. Kling J. Cytometry: measure for measure. Nature. 2015;518(7539):439–43.
59. Shenai S, Ronacher K, Malherbe S, Stanley K, Kriel M, Winter J, Peppard T, Barry CE, Wang J, Dodd LE, et al. Bacterial loads measured by the Xpert MTB/RIF assay as markers of culture conversion and bacteriological cure in pulmonary TB. PLoS One. 2016;11(8):e0160062.
60. Anderson ST, Kaforou M, Brent AJ, Wright VJ, Banwell CM, Chagaluka G, Crampin AC, Dockrell HM, French N, Hamilton MS, et al. Diagnosis of childhood tuberculosis and host RNA expression in Africa. N Engl J Med. 2014;370(18):1712–23.
61. Zak DE, Penn-Nicholson A, Scriba TJ, Thompson E, Suliman S, Amon LM, Mahomed H, Erasmus M, Whatney W, Hussey GD, et al. A blood RNA signature for tuberculosis disease risk: a prospective cohort study. Lancet. 2016;387(10035):2312–22.
62. de Lannoy C, de Ridder D, Risse J. The long reads ahead: de novo genome assembly using the MinION. F1000Res. 2017;6:1083.
63. Gause WC, Wynn TA, Allen JE. Type 2 immunity and wound healing: evolutionary refinement of adaptive immunity by helminths. Nat Rev Immunol. 2013;13(8):607–14.
64. Barron L, Wynn TA. Macrophage activation governs schistosomiasis-induced inflammation and fibrosis. Eur J Immunol. 2011;41(9):2509–14.
65. Kleinnijenhuis J, Quintin J, Preijers F, Joosten LA, Ifrim DC, Saeed S, Jacobs C, van Loenhout J, de Jong D, Stunnenberg HG, et al. Bacille Calmette-Guerin induces NOD2-dependent non-specific protection from reinfection via epigenetic reprogramming of monocytes. Proc Natl Acad Sci U S A. 2012;109(43):17537–42.
66. Tumes DJ, Onodera A, Suzuki A, Shinoda K, Endo Y, Iwamura C, Hosokawa H, Koseki H, Tokoyoda K, Suzuki Y, et al. The polycomb protein Ezh2 regulates differentiation and plasticity of CD4(+) T helper type 1 and type 2 cells. Immunity. 2013;39(5):819–32.
67. DiNardo CD, Ravandi F, Agresta S, Konopleva M, Takahashi K, Kadia T, Routbort M, Patel KP, Mark B, Pierce S, et al. Characteristics, clinical outcome, and prognostic significance of IDH mutations in AML. Am J Hematol. 2015;90(8):732–6.
68. Zumla A, Rao M, Dodoo E, Maeurer M. Potential of immunomodulatory agents as adjunct host-directed therapies for multidrug-resistant tuberculosis. BMC Med. 2016;14:89.
69. Bhatt K, Verma S, Ellner JJ, Salgame P. Quest for correlates of protection against tuberculosis. Clin Vaccine Immunol. 2015;22(3):258–66.
70. Rodriguez RM, Suarez-Alvarez B, Mosen-Ansorena D, Garcia-Peydro M, Fuentes P, Garcia-Leon MJ, Gonzalez-Lahera A, Macias-Camara N, Toribio ML, Aransay AM, et al. Regulation of the transcriptional program by DNA methylation during human alphabeta T-cell development. Nucleic Acids Res. 2015;43(2):760–74.
71. Hirahara K, Vahedi G, Ghoreschi K, Yang XP, Nakayamada S, Kanno Y, O'Shea JJ, Laurence A. Helper T-cell differentiation and plasticity: insights from epigenetics. Immunology. 2011;134(3):235–45.
72. Kanhere A, Hertweck A, Bhatia U, Gokmen MR, Perucha E, Jackson I, Lord GM, Jenner RG. T-bet and GATA3 orchestrate Th1 and Th2 differentiation through lineage-specific targeting of distal regulatory elements. Nat Commun. 2012;3:1268.

73. Peine M, Rausch S, Helmstetter C, Frohlich A, Hegazy AN, Kuhl AA, Grevelding CG, Hofer T, Hartmann S, Lohning M. Stable T-bet(+)GATA-3(+) Th1/Th2 hybrid cells arise in vivo, can develop directly from naive precursors, and limit immunopathologic inflammation. PLoS Biol. 2013;11(8):e1001633.
74. Ishii M, Wen H, Corsa CA, Liu T, Coelho AL, Allen RM, Carson WF, Cavassani KA, Li X, Lukacs NW, et al. Epigenetic regulation of the alternatively activated macrophage phenotype. Blood. 2009;114(15):3244–54.
75. Deaton AM, Cook PC, De Sousa D, Phythian-Adams AT, Bird A, MacDonald AS. A unique DNA methylation signature defines a population of IFN-gamma/IL-4 double-positive T cells during helminth infection. Eur J Immunol. 2014;44(6):1835–41.
76. Tough DF, Tak PP, Tarakhovsky A, Prinjha RK. Epigenetic drug discovery: breaking through the immune barrier. Nat Rev Drug Discov. 2016;15(12):835–53.
77. Evans CM, Jenner RG. Transcription factor interplay in T helper cell differentiation. Brief Funct Genomics. 2013;12(6):499–511.
78. Zhang Q, Zhao K, Shen Q, Han Y, Gu Y, Li X, Zhao D, Liu Y, Wang C, Zhang X, et al. Tet2 is required to resolve inflammation by recruiting Hdac2 to specifically repress IL-6. Nature. 2015;525(7569):389–93.
79. Mikovits JA, Young HA, Vertino P, Issa JP, Pitha PM, Turcoski-Corrales S, Taub DD, Petrow CL, Baylin SB, Ruscetti FW. Infection with human immunodeficiency virus type 1 upregulates DNA methyltransferase, resulting in de novo methylation of the gamma interferon (IFN-gamma) promoter and subsequent downregulation of IFN-gamma production. Mol Cell Biol. 1998;18(9):5166–77.
80. Youngblood B, Reich NO. The early expressed HIV-1 genes regulate DNMT1 expression. Epigenetics. 2008;3(3):149–56.
81. Youngblood B, Noto A, Porichis F, Akondy RS, Ndhlovu ZM, Austin JW, Bordi R, Procopio FA, Miura T, Allen TM, et al. Cutting edge: prolonged exposure to HIV reinforces a poised epigenetic program for PD-1 expression in virus-specific CD8 T cells. J Immunol. 2013;191(2):540–4.
82. Nakayama-Hosoya K, Ishida T, Youngblood B, Nakamura H, Hosoya N, Koga M, Koibuchi T, Iwamoto A, Kawana-Tachikawa A. Epigenetic repression of interleukin 2 expression in senescent CD4+ T cells during chronic HIV type 1 infection. J Infect Dis. 2015;211(1):28–39.
83. Chandran A, Antony C, Jose L, Mundayoor S, Natarajan K, Kumar RA. *Mycobacterium tuberculosis* infection induces HDAC1-mediated suppression of IL-12B gene expression in macrophages. Front Cell Infect Microbiol. 2015;5:90.
84. Pennini ME, Pai RK, Schultz DC, Boom WH, Harding CV. *Mycobacterium tuberculosis* 19-kDa lipoprotein inhibits IFN-gamma-induced chromatin remodeling of MHC2TA by TLR2 and MAPK signaling. J Immunol. 2006;176(7):4323–30.
85. Kincaid EZ, Ernst JD. *Mycobacterium tuberculosis* exerts gene-selective inhibition of transcriptional responses to IFN-gamma without inhibiting STAT1 function. J Immunol. 2003;171(4):2042–9.
86. Holla S, Prakhar P, Singh V, Karnam A, Mukherjee T, Mahadik K, Parikh P, Singh A, Rajmani RS, Ramachandra SG, et al. MUSASHI-mediated expression of JMJD3, a H3K27me3 demethylase, is involved in foamy macrophage generation during mycobacterial infection. PLoS Pathog. 2016;12(8):e1005814.
87. Ghorpade DS, Holla S, Sinha AY, Alagesan SK, Balaji KN. Nitric oxide and KLF4 protein epigenetically modify class II transactivator to repress major histocompatibility complex II expression during *Mycobacterium bovis* bacillus Calmette-Guerin infection. J Biol Chem. 2013;288(28):20592–606.
88. Sharma G, Sowpati DT, Singh P, Khan MZ, Ganji R, Upadhyay S, Banerjee S, Nandicoori VK, Khosla S. Genome-wide non-CpG methylation of the host genome during M. tuberculosis infection. Sci Rep. 2016;6:25006.

89. Wei M, Wang L, Wu T, Xi J, Han Y, Yang X, Zhang D, Fang Q, Tang B. NLRP3 activation was regulated by DNA methylation modification during *Mycobacterium tuberculosis* infection. Biomed Res Int. 2016;2016:4323281.
90. Wang Y, Zhong H, Xie X, Chen CY, Huang D, Shen L, Zhang H, Chen ZW, Zeng G. Long noncoding RNA derived from CD244 signaling epigenetically controls CD8+ T-cell immune responses in tuberculosis infection. Proc Natl Acad Sci U S A. 2015;112(29):E3883–92
91. Malherbe ST, Shenai S, Ronacher K, Loxton AG, Dolganov G, Kriel M, Van T, Chen RY, Warwick J, Via LE, et al. Persisting positron emission tomography lesion activity and *Mycobacterium tuberculosis* mRNA after tuberculosis cure. Nat Med. 2016;22(10):1094–100.
92. Netea MG, Joosten LA, Latz E, Mills KH, Natoli G, Stunnenberg HG, O'Neill LA, Xavier RJ. Trained immunity: a program of innate immune memory in health and disease. Science. 2016;352(6284):aaf1098.

Index

J. D. Cirillo, Y. Kong (eds.), *Tuberculosis Host-Pathogen Interactions*,
https://doi.org/10.1007/978-3-030-25381-3

The manufacturer's authorised representative in the EU is Springer Nature Customer Service Centre GmbH, Europaplatz 3, 69115 Heidelberg, Germany. If you have any concerns regarding our products, please contact ProductSafety@springernature.com

Printed and bound by CPI Group (UK) Ltd, Croydon, CR0 4YY
30/09/2026
02225651-0007